Minimally Invasive Cardiac Surgery

Minimally Invasive Cardiac Surgery
A Practical Guide

Edited by
Theo Kofidis, MD, PD(Ger), FRCS, FAHA, FAMS
Department of Cardiac, Thoracic and Vascular Surgery
NUHCS, National University of Singapore
National University Health System
Singapore

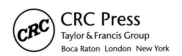

CRC Press is an imprint of the
Taylor & Francis Group, an **informa** business

First edition published 2021
by CRC Press
6000 Broken Sound Parkway NW, Suite 300, Boca Raton, FL 33487-2742

and by CRC Press
2 Park Square, Milton Park, Abingdon, Oxon, OX14 4RN

© 2021 Taylor & Francis Group, LLC

CRC Press is an imprint of Taylor & Francis Group, LLC

This book contains information obtained from authentic and highly regarded sources. While all reasonable efforts have been made to publish reliable data and information, neither the author[s] nor the publisher can accept any legal responsibility or liability for any errors or omissions that may be made. The publishers wish to make clear that any views or opinions expressed in this book by individual editors, authors or contributors are personal to them and do not necessarily reflect the views/opinions of the publishers. The information or guidance contained in this book is intended for use by medical, scientific or health-care professionals and is provided strictly as a supplement to the medical or other professional's own judgement, their knowledge of the patient's medical history, relevant manufacturer's instructions and the appropriate best practice guidelines. Because of the rapid advances in medical science, any information or advice on dosages, procedures or diagnoses should be independently verified. The reader is strongly urged to consult the relevant national drug formulary and the drug companies' and device or material manufacturers' printed instructions, and their websites, before administering or utilizing any of the drugs, devices or materials mentioned in this book. This book does not indicate whether a particular treatment is appropriate or suitable for a particular individual. Ultimately it is the sole responsibility of the medical professional to make his or her own professional judgements, so as to advise and treat patients appropriately. The authors and publishers have also attempted to trace the copyright holders of all material reproduced in this publication and apologize to copyright holders if permission to publish in this form has not been obtained. If any copyright material has not been acknowledged please write and let us know so we may rectify in any future reprint.

Except as permitted under U.S. Copyright Law, no part of this book may be reprinted, reproduced, transmitted, or utilized in any form by any electronic, mechanical, or other means, now known or hereafter invented, including photocopying, microfilming, and recording, or in any information storage or retrieval system, without written permission from the publishers.

For permission to photocopy or use material electronically from this work, access www.copyright.com or contact the Copyright Clearance Center, Inc. (CCC), 222 Rosewood Drive, Danvers, MA 01923, 978-750-8400. For works that are not available on CCC please contact mpkbookspermissions@tandf.co.uk

Trademark notice: Product or corporate names may be trademarks or registered trademarks and are used only for identification and explanation without intent to infringe.

Library of Congress Cataloging-in-Publication Data

Names: Kofidis, Theo, 1969- editor.
Title: Minimally invasive cardiac surgery : a practical guide / edited by Theo Kofidis.
Other titles: Minimally invasive cardiac surgery (Kofidis)
Description: First edition. | Boca Raton : CRC Press, [2021] | Includes bibliographical references and index.
Identifiers: LCCN 2020035597 (print) | LCCN 2020035598 (ebook) | ISBN 9781498736466 (hardback) | ISBN 9780367641740 (paperback) | ISBN 9780429188725 (ebook)
Subjects: MESH: Heart Diseases–surgery | Cardiac Surgical Procedures–methods | Minimally Invasive Surgical Procedures–methods
Classification: LCC RD598.35.C35 (print) | LCC RD598.35.C35 (ebook) | NLM WG 169 | DDC 617.4/12–dc23
LC record available at https://lccn.loc.gov/2020035597
LC ebook record available at https://lccn.loc.gov/2020035598

ISBN: 9781498736466 (hbk)
ISBN: 9780429188725 (ebk)

Typeset in Georgia
by Deanta Global Publishing Services, Chennai, India

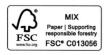

Printed and bound in Great Britain by
TJ Books Limited, Padstow, Cornwall

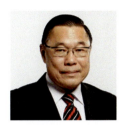

To

Professor Chuen Neng Lee

…for shaping my career and transforming my life.

CONTENTS

Prologue	xxv
Acknowledgments	xxix
Our Editorial Team	xxxi
Contributors	xxxv

1 Foreword/Introduction — 1
Theo Kofidis

How to Get the Most Out of the Present Book	4
Who Is the Primary and Secondary Readership of the Book?	5

2 History of Minimally Invasive Cardiac Surgery — 7
Chang Guohao and Theo Kofidis

History or Introduction	7
How It Has Been Done	7
Tools/Instruments and Devices	12
Perioperative Consideration	15
Alternative Approaches	17
Caveats and Controversies	17
Research, Trends and Innovation	18
Where and How to Learn	18
References	19

3 How to Set up a Minimally Invasive Program — 21
Theo Kofidis and Chang Guohao

History or Introduction	21
How to Do It/Step by Step	22
Tools/Instruments and Devices	23
Perioperative Consideration	26
Alternative Approaches	28
Caveats and Controversies	28
Where and How to Learn	29
References	30

4 Instrumentation and Operating Theater Set up in Minimally Invasive Cardiac Surgery — 31
Faizus Sazzad and Theo Kofidis

Introduction	31
How to Do It/Step by Step	32

Minimally Invasive Valve Surgery	32
Minimally Invasive Mitral Valve Surgery	32
Minimally Invasive Aortic Valve Surgery	33
Minimally Invasive CABG Surgery	33
Positioning Draping of Patient	33
Special Considerations	33
Special Instruments and Consumables	34
TAVI (Transfemoral and Transapical)	34
Femoral Cannulation Technique	34
Cannula Selection	35
Cannula Sizing	35
The Insertion Technique	36
Cannula Positioning	36
Cannula Securing	36
Open Cannulation for Endoballoon (Thruport)	36
Percutaneous Femoral Cannulation	37
Tools/Instruments and Devices	37
General Instrumentation	37
Special Retractor for Minimally Invasive Mitral Valve Surgery	38
Special Instruments for MICS CABG Surgery	39
ThoraTrak Retractor	39
Octopus Nuvo Stabilizer and Starfish NS Positioner	39
Femoral Cannula	42
Special Instruments	42
Perioperative Consideration	44
Alternatives	45
Alternative Stabilizers	45
Aesculap FLEXHeart	45
Valve XS Atrium Retractor	45
Alternative Cannulation Technique for CPB	45
Axillary Artery Cannulation	45
SVC Cannulation	45
Conventional Cannulation	46
Peripheral Cannulation Technique	46
Robotic Surgery	46
TAVI	47
Caveats and Controversies	47
Heart Valve Surgery	47
MIS AVR: Approach – Upper J Sternotomy vs RATS	47
TAVI vs SAVR	47
MiMVR: Mini MVR vs Robotic-Assisted	48
MICS CABG	48
References	49

5 Anesthesia for Minimally Invasive Cardiac Surgery — 51
Ti Lian Kah, Sophia Ang Bee Leng, Wei Zhang, Lalitha Manickam and Jai Ajitchandra Sule

History and Introduction — 51
How to Do It/Step by Step — 53
    Monitoring — 53
    Anesthetic Preparation — 53
    Transesophageal Echocardiography (TOE) — 55
    Ventilation Strategy — 59
    Principles Guiding Conduct of Anesthesia — 59
Tools/Instruments and Devices — 60
Perioperative Considerations — 61
    Pre-Anesthetic Evaluation — 61
    Positioning — 62
    Postoperative Management — 62
Alternative Approaches — 63
Caveats and Controversies — 63
    One-Lung Ventilation — 63
    Postoperative Pulmonary Edema — 64
    Surgical Techniques Impacting Anesthesia — 64
        Deairing of the Heart — 64
        Mitral Valve and Right Mini-Thoracotomy — 64
        Long-Acting Cardioplegia — 65
    MICS CABG — 65
        Proximal Anastomosis — 65
        Reinflating the Left Lung — 65
Research, Trends and Innovation — 65
Where and How to Learn — 66
References — 67

6 Surgical Approaches in Minimally Invasive Cardiac Surgery — 69
Faizus Sazzad and Theo Kofidis

History or Introduction — 69
How to Do It/Step by Step — 70
    Patient Selection, Preparation and Positioning — 70
    Perioperative Considerations — 72
Tools/Instruments and Devices — 83
Alternative Approaches — 83
    Alternative Caval Isolation for Right Heart — 84
    Trans-areolar Endoscopic approach — 84
Caveats and Controversies — 85
    Potential Complications and Troubleshooting — 85
References — 85

7.1 The Aortic Valve: Minimally Invasive Aortic Valve Replacement. The Right Anterior Minithoracotomy — 87
Igo B Ribeiro and Marc Ruel

Introduction — 87
How to Do It/Step by Step — 88
    Step 1: Patient Preparation and Exposure — 88
    Step 2: CPB Installation – Cannulation, Cardioplegia and LV Venting — 89
    Step 3: AVR – Aortotomy, Aortic Valve Exposure and Replacement — 90
Tools/Instruments and Devices — 92
    Medtronic ThoraTrak (MICS Retractor System) — 92
Perioperative Considerations — 92
Alternative Approaches — 94
Caveats and Controversies — 94
Research, Trends and Innovation — 96
Where and How to Learn — 97
References — 97

7.2 Minimally Invasive Aortic Valve Replacement: Upper "J" Sternotomy — 99
Faizus Sazzad and Theo Kofidis

Introduction — 99
How to Do It/Step by Step — 100
    Special Considerations — 102
Tools/Instruments and Devices — 104
    Saw: Oscillating Saw — 104
    Aortic Cannula: EOPA™ — 104
    Aortic Cross Clamp — 104
    Automated Knot Fastener — 104
Perioperative Consideration — 104
    Preoperative CT Scan of the Patient (CT Thorax, Abdomen and Pelvis) — 104
    Chest Wall Deformity — 104
    Severe Calcified Ascending Aorta — 104
    Reoperations/Redo Surgery — 105
    Status Post-Pneumonectomy — 105
    Obesity — 106
    Post-Radiation Therapy — 106
Alternative Approaches — 106
    Manubrium-Limited Sternotomy — 106
    Suprasternal AVR — 106
Caveats and Controversies — 106
Research, Trends and Innovation — 108
    Trans-Apical TAVI — 108
    Valve-in-Valve — 108

Where and How to Learn	108
Professional Education: LivaNova	108
EACTS Academy	108
National University Health System (NUHS), Singapore (ASTC)	108
Aortic Valve and Root Boot Camp	108
References	109

7.3 The Aortic Valve: Sutureless Valves in the Setting of MICS AVR — 111
Theodor Fischlein and Giuseppe Santarpino

History and Introduction	111
How to Do It/Step by Step	113
Patient Selection	113
Perceval	113
Intuity Elite Valve	114
Tools/Instruments and Devices	115
Perceval S (LivaNova Group, Milan, Italy)	115
Intuity (Edwards Lifesciences, Irvine, CA)	116
Perioperative Consideration	117
Alternative Approaches	117
Caveats and Controversies	118
Research, Trends and Innovation	119
Perceval	119
Intuity	119
Perceval versus Intuity	119
Current Evidence and Future Prospects	121
Where and How to Learn	122
International Valvular Surgery Study Group (IVSSG)	122
References	122

7.4 The Aortic Valve: Endoscopic Aortic Valve Surgery — 125
Giovanni Domenico Cresce and Loris Salvador

History and Introduction	125
OT Setup and Instrumentation	126
How to Do It/Step by Step	126
Cardiopulmonary Bypass (CPB)	126
Aortic Cross Clamping, Cardioplegia and Ventricular Venting	127
Surgical Technique	127
Prosthetic Choice	128
Summarized Experience	128
Caveats and Controversies	128
Where and How to Learn	129
Conclusions	130
References	130

8.1 Transcatheter Aortic Valve Implantation (TAVI): Transapical Transcatheter Aortic Valve Replacement — 133

Amalia Winters, Jessica Forcillo and Vinod H Thourani

History and Introduction	133
How to Do It/Step by Step	134
The Transapical Approach	134
Operative Technique	135
Tools/Instruments and Devices	137
Perioperative Consideration	137
Preoperative Assessment and Planning	137
Alternative Approaches	138
Caveats and Controversies	138
Research, Trends and Innovation	140
Where and How to Learn	140
References	141

8.2 Transfemoral Transcatheter Aortic Valve Implantation — 143

Ivandito Kuntjoro and Edgar Tay

History and Introduction	143
How to Do It/Step by Step	144
Patient Selection	144
Setup and Equipment	144
Vascular Access	145
Temporary Pacemaker Placement	146
Aortic Root Angiogram	146
Delivery Sheath Insertion	146
Aortic Valve Crossing	146
Balloon Aortic Valvuloplasty (BAV)	147
Valve Implantation	147
Post-Valve Implantation Assessment	148
Tools/Instruments and Devices	148
Sapien 3 (Edwards Lifesciences, Irvine, CA, USA)	148
Evolut R (Medtronic, Fridley, MN, USA)	148
Lotus Edge (Boston Scientific, Marlborough, MA, USA)	148
Portico (Abbott, Chicago, IL, USA)	150
Perioperative Considerations	151
Preoperative Assessment and Screening	151
Echocardiogram	151
Cardiac Catheterization	151
Computed Tomography (CT) Angiography	155
Associated Co-Morbidities	156
Alternative Approaches	157

Caveats and Controversies	158
Paravalvular Regurgitation (PVR)	158
Cardiac atrioventricular conduction abnormalities	160
Stroke	160
Vascular Complications	161
Specific Caveats	162
Research, Trends and Innovation	162
Current Status of TAVI	162
Balloon Valvuloplasty Catheter	164
Delivery Sheath Design	164
Future of Transfemoral TAVI	165
Where and How to Learn	166
Medtronic TAVI course	166
PCR Online TAVI Atlas	166
ESC Courses	166
References	167

8.3 Transcatheter Aortic Valve Implantation (TAVI): Alternative Approaches for Transcatheter Aortic Valve Implantation — 171

Faizus Sazzad and Theo Kofidis

Introduction	171
Alternative Approaches	172
How to Do It/Step by Step	172
Subclavian Transcatheter Aortic Valve Replacement (SC-TAVI)	172
Technique	172
Pros and Cons	173
Transaxillary Transcatheter Aortic Valve Replacement (TAX-TAVI)	173
Technique	173
Pros and Cons	174
Direct Aortic Transcatheter Aortic Valve Replacement (DA-TAVI)	174
Technique	174
Pros and Cons	175
Transcarotid Transcatheter Aortic Valve Replacement (TC-TAVI)	175
Technique	175
Pros and Cons	175
Transcaval Transcatheter Aortic Valve Replacement (TCA-TAVI)	176
Technique	176
Pros and Cons	177
Devices	177
Peri-Procedural Considerations	179
Where and How to Learn	179
TAVI Fellowship	180
References	181

9.1 The Mitral Valve: Minimally Invasive Mitral Valve Surgery — 183
Hugo Vanermen

History and Introduction — 183
How to do it/Step by Step — 184
    Position the Patient — 184
    Installing Extracorporeal Circulation — 184
    Myocardial Preservation — 187
    Exposure — 188
    Mitral Valve Repair Technique — 193
Tools/Instruments and Devices — 195
    Medtronic Extracorporeal Cannula — 195
    ThruPort IntraClude from Edwards Lifesciences — 195
Perioperative Considerations — 196
Caveats and Controversies — 196
Research, Trends and Innovation — 197
Where and How to Learn — 197
    FOCUS Valve Workshops — 197
    NUHCS Singapore Minimally Invasive Mitral Valve Programme — 197
    Cleveland Clinic Minimally Invasive Mitral Repair — 197
References — 199

9.2 The Mitral Valve: Alternative Approaches to Minimally Invasive Mitral Valve Surgery — 201
Chang Guohao and Theo Kofidis

History or Introduction — 201
How to Do It/Step by Step — 202
    Right Paramedian Approach — 202
    Upper Sternotomy Approach — 203
    Right Thoracotomy Approach — 203
Tools/Instruments and Devices — 203
    MitraClip™ — 203
    Tiara Valve — 204
    AccuFit Valve — 204
    Tendyne™ Valve — 205
    Cardiaq Valve — 206
    Coronary Sinus-Based Percutaneous Mitral Annuloplasty — 206
    Valtech Cardioband — 207
    Mitralign — 207
    GDS Accucinch — 208
    Transapical Off-Pump NeoChord Implantation — 208
    Valtech V-Chordal — 209
    Mitra-Spacer — 209
Perioperative Consideration — 209
Alternative Approaches — 210

Transcatheter Mitral Valve Replacement	210
Percutaneous Mitral Valve Repair	211
Where and How to Learn	213
References	214

9.3 The Mitral Valve: Robotic Mitral Valve Surgery — 215

Nirav C Patel, Meghan K Torres and Jonathan M Hemli

History and Introduction	215
How to Do It/Step by Step	216
Patient Selection	216
Preparation	218
Surgical Exposure and Access	219
Cardiopulmonary Bypass and Myocardial Protection	220
Operating on the Mitral Valve	222
Concluding the Operation	223
Tools/Instruments and Devices	225
Da Vinci Xi System	225
Alexis Wound Protector	225
Endo Close™ Trocar Site Closure Device	225
LivaNova Venous Return Cannulas	225
Optisite Arterial Cannulas	225
MiaR™ Cardioplegia Cannula	226
Chitwood Debakey Aortic Cross-Clamp	226
StrykeFlow II Suction Irrigation Pump	226
Perioperative Consideration	226
Preoperative Assessment	226
Previous Cardiac Surgery	227
Clinical Outcomes	227
Alternative Approaches	230
LEAR Technique	230
Cardioplegia	230
Cross-Clamp	230
Reoperative Surgery	230
Caveats and Controversies	230
Research, Trends and Innovation	231
Where and How to Learn	232
Annals of Cardiothoracic Surgery (ACS) Video Atlas	232
STS workshop on Robotic Cardiac Surgery	232
References	232

9.4 The Mitral Valve: Percutaneous Mitral Valve Repair: MitraClip® — 235

Mohammad Abdulrahman Al Otaiby

History and Introduction	235
Percutaneous Mitral Valve Repair Using the MitraClip® System	235
How to Do It/Step by Step	236

Steps	236
Surgical Approach	236
Transseptal Puncture	236
Anatomy of the septum	238
Tools/Instruments and Devices	240
Perioperative Consideration	241
Indications for MICS Procedure	241
Patient Selection	243
Contraindications	243
Alternative Approaches	244
A look to current and soon-to-come transcatheter mitral valve repair options	244
Caveats and Controversies	245
From the Cardiologist's point of view	245
Transcatheter Mitral Valve Repair Today and Tomorrow	245
Experiences so far	245
Real-World Experience	245
Butterfly in the Heart	245
Beyond EVEREST	247
Research, Trends and Innovation	247
ACCESS-EU PHASE I	250
ACCESS-EU PHASE II	250
Where and How to Learn	252

10 Minimally Invasive Tricuspid Valve Surgery — 253

Christos Alexiou and Theo Kofidis

History and Introduction	253
Tricuspid Regurgitation	253
TR at the Time of Left-Sided Heart Surgery	254
Tricuspid Stenosis	254
How to Do It/Step by Step	254
Exposure of the Heart and Right Atrium	256
Cannulation and Cardiopulmonary Bypass	257
Aortic Clamping and Cardioplegia Delivery	258
Main Operation (TV Repair or Replacement)	258
Completion of the Procedure	259
Redo Right Mini Thoracotomy TV Surgery (after Previous Pericardiotomy)	259
Tools/Instruments and Devices	259
Perioperative Consideration	260
Alternative Approaches	260
Caveats and Controversies	260
Research, Trends and Innovation	261
Where and How to Learn	263
References	263

11	**Minimally Invasive Combined Heart Valve Surgery**	**267**
	Faizus Sazzad and Theo Kofidis	

Introduction	267
How to Do It/Step by Step	268
Upper J sternotomy Approach for Double Valve Repair/Replacement (AVR+MVR)	268
Upper T Sternotomy Approach	269
Right Mini-Thoracotomy Approach	269
Caval Isolation	269
Caval Occlusion	270
Concomitant Procedures	271
Tools/Instruments and Devices	272
External Defibrillator Pads	272
Soft Tissue Retractor	272
Atrial Lift System and Visor	272
Alternatives	272
Conventional Full Sternotomy Approach	272
Caval Isolation	273
Caveats and Controversies	273
Combined Procedures in Minimally Invasive versus Conventional Approaches	273
Research, Trends and Innovation	273
Soft Robotics in Minimally Invasive Surgery	273
Where and How to Learn	275
Minimally Invasive Techniques in Adult Cardiac Surgery (MITACS)	275
International Society for Minimally Invasive Cardiothoracic Surgery (ISMICS) Courses	275
References	275

12.1	**The Coronaries: Minimally Invasive Coronary Artery Bypass Grafting Surgery**	**277**
	Janet M. C. Ngu, Ming Hao Guo and Marc Ruel	

History or Introduction	277
How to Do It/Step by Step	277
Patient Positioning	277
Chest Marking and Incision	278
Harvesting the Left Internal Thoracic Artery (LITA)	278
Proximal Anastomosis	279
Distal Anastomosis	280
Chest Closure	281
Post-Operative Care	281
Tools/Instruments and Devices	282
Perioperative Consideration	282
Anesthesia	282

Alternative Approaches	283
Caveats and Controversies	284
Research, Trends and Innovation	284
Where and How to Learn	284
References	284

12.2 The Coronaries: Robot Facilitated Coronary Artery Bypass Grafting — 285
László Göbölös and Johannes Bonatti

History and Introduction	285
How to Do It/Step by Step	288
Patient Selection	288
Preparation	288
Operative Guide	288
Step 1: Patient Placement and Operative Start-Up	288
Step 2: Port Insertion and Robot Docking	288
Step 3: Internal Mammary Artery Takedown	289
Step 4: Utility Port Placement	290
Step 5: Precordial Fat Pad Resection and Pericardial Exposure	290
Step 6: Vascular Cannulation and Application of Endoclamp (Endoballoon Occlusion)	291
Step 7: Cardiopulmonary Bypass	291
Step 8: Identification and Exposure of the Target Vessels	291
Step 9: Robot-Facilitated Endoscopic Coronary Anastomosis	293
Step 10: Final Actions	294
Tools/Instruments and Devices	294
Perioperative Consideration	294
Preoperative Assessment and Work-Up	294
Anesthetic Considerations	295
Postoperative Care	295
Time Demand	295
Alternative Approaches	297
Cannulation	297
Cardioplegia	297
TECAB Approaches	297
Coronary Grafting Options	298
TECAB as Hybrid Coronary Procedure	298
Caveats and Controversies	298
Contraindications to TECAB	298
Endoballoon	299
Extracorporeal Circulation	300
Coronary Anastomosis	300
Other Caveats	301
Research, Trends and Innovation	302
Reduced Surgical Trauma Advantages	302
Intermediate- and Long-Term Outcomes	302

Predictors of Success and Safety, Further Patient Aspects	303
Summary and Future Aspects	304
Where and How to Learn	306
References	306

12.3 Anaortic, Off-Pump, Total-Arterial Coronary Artery Bypass Grafting Surgery: The Coronaries — 309

Michael Seco, J James B Edelman, Fabio Ramponi, Michael K Wilson, and Michael P Vallely

History and Introduction	309
Introduction	309
History of OPCAB and Technical Innovation	310
Research, Trends and Innovation	310
Stroke and Other Peri-Operative Complications	310
High-risk Patients	311
Caveats and Controversies	313
Complete Revascularization and Long-Term Outcomes	313
How to Do It/Step by Step	314
Anaortic OPCAB Surgical Technique	314
Tools/Instruments and Devices	317
Alternative Approaches	319
Where and How to Learn	319
EACTS OPCAB Fellowship	319
EBM Beat + YOUCAN Simulator	319
Summary	320
References	320

12.4 The Coronaries: Hybrid Coronary Artery Bypass Grafting Surgery — 323

Claudio Muneretto, Chang Guohao and Theo Kofidis

History and Introduction	323
How to Do It/Step by Step	324
Tools/Instruments and Devices	326
Perioperative Consideration	326
Alternative Approaches	327
Caveats and Controversies	327
Research, Trends and Innovation	328
ISMICS 2014 Annual Meeting presentation	328
References	329

13 Minimally Invasive Atrial Ablation Surgery — 331

Anil K Gehi and Andy C Kiser

History and Introduction	331
How to Do It/Step by Step	333
Minimally Invasive Cox Maze Procedure	333
Pulmonary Vein Isolation	333

Pruitt Box Lesion		334
Wolf Mini Maze		334
PVI via Right Minithoracotomy		334
Pulmonary Vein Isolation and Autonomic Denervation		335
Dallas Lesion Set		335
Five Box Ablation		335
Tools/Instruments and Devices		336
Perioperative Considerations		337
Paroxysmal versus Persistent AF		337
Minimally Invasive Surgical versus Catheter Ablation		338
Comorbidities		339
Alternative Approaches		340
Hybrid Ablation		340
Thoracoscopic Approach		341
Subxiphoid Pericardioscopic Approach		344
Transdiaphragmatic Combined Subxiphoid and Laparoscopic Approach		345
Concomitant Minimally Invasive AF Ablation and Mitral Valve Surgery		345
Left Atrial Appendage Exclusion		345
Caveats and Controversies		345
Epicardial Ablation for AF		345
Hybrid Ablation for AF		348
Research, Trends and Innovation		349
Minimally Invasive Cox Maze		349
Minimally Invasive Pulmonary Vein Isolation		349
Pruitt Box Lesion		349
Wolf Mini Maze		349
Pulmonary Vein Isolation via Right Minithoracotomy		350
Pulmonary Vein Isolation and Autonomic Denervation		351
Dallas Lesion Set		351
Five-Box Ablation		352
Hybrid Surgery for AF		352
Thoracoscopic Approach		353
Subxiphoid Pericardioscopic Approach		355
Transdiaphragmatic Combined Subxiphoid and Laparoscopic Approach		355
Concomitant Atrial Ablation with Minimally Invasive Mitral Surgery		355
Conclusion		356
Where and How to Learn		356
International Society of Minimally Invasive Cardiac Surgery (ISMICS) Workshop		356
AtriCure Education and Training		356
The Journal of Innovations in Cardiac Rhythm Management		356
References		356

14.1 Aortic Surgery: Minimally Invasive Ascending Aortic Surgery — 359
Ourania Preventza
History or Introduction — 359

Minimally Invasive Aortic Surgery for Cardiovascular Surgeons	359
History	359
How to Do It/Step by Step	360
Surgical Approach	360
Aortic Root, Ascending Aorta with or without Proximal Arch, Total Arch	360
Endovascular Repair of the Ascending Aorta	362
Endovascular Repair of Aortic Arch	363
Descending Thoracic Aorta	365
Thoracoabdominal Aorta	365
Tools/Instruments and Devices	366
FDA-Approved Stent Grafts	366
Perioperative Consideration	367
Indications for Minimally Invasive Aortic Surgery	367
Ascending Aorta and Aortic Arch	367
Descending Thoracic Aorta	367
Alternative Approaches	368
Caveats and Controversies	368
Research, Trends and Innovation	369
Current Results	369
Ascending Aorta: Endovascular Repair	369
Arch and Descending Thoracic Aorta	369
Hybrid Results	369
Endovascular Repair	369
Descending Thoracic Aorta	369
Where and How to Learn	370
References	370

14.2 Aortic Surgery: Endovascular and Hybrid Approaches for Distal Arch and Descending Thoracic Aorta — 373

Cem Alhan, Sahin Senay, Julian Wong and Andrew MTL Choong

History or Introduction	373
Distal Arch Aneurysms	374
Descending Aortic Aneurysms	374
Traumatic Aortic Injury	374
Penetrating Aortic Ulcers	376
Intramural Hematoma	376
Coarctation of Aorta	376
Type B Aortic Dissections	377
Other Pathologies	377
How to Do It/Step by Step	377
Arch Debranching	377
Evolution of the "Visceral Hybrid" Repair for Thoracoabdominal Aortic Pathology	377
General Principles	379
Treatment Techniques	380
Zone 1 Pathologies	380

Zone 2 Pathologies	382
Zone 3 Pathologies	382
St Mary's Visceral Hybrid Repair Technique	382
Alternative Approaches	384
Standard Approach (Transfemoral)	384
Conduits	384
Iliac/Infra-Renal Abdominal Aortic Approach	384
Thoracic Aortic Approach	384
Tools/Instruments and Devices	385
Tools/Instruments	385
Devices	385
Standard TEVAR Devices	385
Custom-Made TEVAR Devices	385
Hybrid Open TEVAR Devices	386
Perioperative Considerations	386
Device and Stock Considerations	386
Radiation Protection	386
Lumbar Spinal Drainage	386
Caveats and Controversies	386
Subclavian Artery Coverage	386
Chimney Techniques	386
References	387

15 Minimally Invasive Heart Failure Surgery   389

Faizus Sazzad and Theo Kofidis

Introduction	389
Operations for Heart Failure	389
How to Do It/Step by Step	390
Minimally Invasive LVAD Implantation	390
Technique	391
Surgical Access	391
Circulatory Support	391
Operation	391
Special Concerns	392
Tools/Instruments and Devices	392
Acorn CoreCap	392
HeartWare VAD (HVAD)	392
HeartMate III	392
Alternatives	392
Conventional Full Sternotomy Approach	392
Caveats and Controversies	393
Abandoned Surgical Options	393
Managing Arrhythmias in LVAD Patients	395
Park's Plication Stitch for AI at the Time of LVAD	395
Bilateral Mini-Thoracotomy vs Separate Incisions	395

	Sternal-Sparing Approach	395
	Off-Pump vs On-Pump LVAD Implantation	395
	Minimally Invasive vs Conventional LVAD Implantation	396
Research, Trends and Innovation		396
	Heart Failure Therapy Update	396
Where and How to Learn		396
	ISHLT	396
	Postgraduate Courses on Heart Failure in London	397
References		397

16 EPILOGUE — 399
Theo Kofidis

Annex — 401

Index — 417

PROLOGUE

"True ignorance is not the absence of knowledge, but the refusal to acquire it" wrote Karl Popper.

José L. Pomar, MD, PhD
Professor of Surgery
The Cardiovascular Institute
Hospital Clinic & University of Barcelona
Spain
jlpomar@clinic.cat
Past President of EACTS
Past Councillor AATS

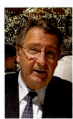

According to Wikipedia, the word *education* derives from Latin and means breeding, or bringing up or rearing. Education has the objective to improve knowledge, skills and habits through teaching, training or research, and research includes, by definition, creativity and innovation.

In many areas and professions, reasonable training is linked to a good outcome. But in our specialty, this assumption, similar to musicians or painters, architects or even soccer players, may be far from actual practice, when it comes to the inculcation of excellence.

Becoming a good cardiovascular or thoracic surgeon takes time, a lot of time, and devotion but also a rather peculiar behavior, something you have or you do not have, something we could also call *talent*.

Talent is aptitude, or a group of aptitudes, useful but also essential for a given activity.

In ancient times, talent was a measure of weight, approximately the mass of the water required to fill an amphora. It established itself as a unit of weight and value in Greece, Rome and the Middle East. A talent was a unit of measurement for weighing several metals, usually gold and silver. In the New Testament, a talent also referred to the value of money or coins.

A talent, therefore, represents value. In today's terms, one talent would be worth about € 1,735,000. That's a lot of value!

Training refers to the acquisition of knowledge, skills and competencies towards accomplishing specific goals in improving one's capability, productivity and performance. Training requires repetition, and repetition again. In Tirone David's words "training is the mother of skills", crucial indeed in our specialty.

Indeed, nowadays not everybody may choose to enter our specialty. Among the many medical students, already more than 60% claim they are not "made" for surgery. About 20% think it is a too demanding and stressing, and only 5–10% feel, a priori, surgery of the heart and lungs is what they would like to be able to learn once they graduate, provided they have a good teacher. Despite that, some still recognize that their hand tremor is prohibitive or their sight is not sufficient, that the learning time is too long and the possibilities of getting a good and well-remunerated position minute. And they choose something else. Fair enough.

In the last 30 years, the landscape has also changed dramatically. The dinosaurs of the field, the early pioneering heart surgeons, are not any more the reflective mirrors for our medical students or residents. Today's leading surgeons are not considered stars anymore. They are involved in a more horizontal scheme. The likes of DeBakey, Cooley, Shumway, Kirklin, Lillehei, McGoon or Fontan, Borst, Barnard, Ross, Yacoub, Carpentier, Miller, David, Duran, Stark, Schaff, Senning, Mohr and so many others were – and are for many of us – the fathers of our still young medical specialty. They were able to develop a completely new world in medicine. Not easily, that is, and with a lot of work, sacrifice and, and for sure, with exceptional talent.

A famous British thoracic surgeon once told me: "teach a monkey how to do a CABG and after some time it will become an expert".

However, cardiac surgery is not just a set of manual skills. Learning our specialty requires a lot of basic knowledge, quite as much as that of any colleague in cardiology; one needs to visualize the procedures many times, performing them step by step from the easiest to the most complex interventions and, indeed, with frequent replication. The more you exercise, the quicker you master the operation but this is also the way to troubleshoot complications. In addition, understanding the indications and selection of the most appropriate therapy, having the capacity to teach, manual dexterity, managing the operating team, offering help to partners or other specialists in difficult situations, handling all postoperative situations, the implementation of ideas into innovation through scientifically based research and the ability to write about your experience to disseminate the knowledge are some of those values. Now, lacking one of them is not a demerit, yet it will require training and grind. In fact, as many things in life, the lack of some may enhance and accelerate those already existing. Some are *gifted* in certain skills…

Cardiac surgery has evolved in the last decades at its own pace and pattern. Some other disciplines subspecialized sooner, such as cardiology. However, the "*Superman*-surgeon" who is able to cover the entire spectrum, neonates to aged patients, is a rare specimen nowadays.

The advent of new imaging technologies for diagnosis and therapy, the development of percutaneous approaches and the constant need for updates in our daily activity, but also evolving patient needs have prompted surgeons to search for less traumatic interventions ensuring a quicker recovery and therefore a sooner return to patients' professional and personal activities.

The so-called "minimally invasive" approach to the aortic valve was most likely, together with some attempts at the CABG, the first to be standardized through a smaller access. Lateral thoracotomies or partial sternotomies were proposed in many diverse configurations. Europe, the USA, Asia, Latin America and Australia slowly added new modalities to enter the chest and heart in a less traumatic but safe manner, using central or peripheral cannulation for extracorporeal circulation.

Port access, for instance, was designed by a group of surgeons from Palo Alto in the late 1990s; they utilized the femoral artery and vein for cannulation to attain an empty and quiet heart and perform, through a limited left thoracotomy, a complete myocardial revascularization. But Benetti, a surgeon from Argentina, was rather simultaneously reporting that he could do the same coronary surgery on a beating heart and, therefore, avoid the burden of extracorporeal circulation and the levels of anticoagulation required. The off-pump surgery was born.

The port access for CABG was initially not convincing, due to extended operation times, amongst other reasons, such as neurological complications, induced by the reverse flow from the periphery and the lack of visual control. In fact it was largely abandoned.

However, elements of this approach were found useful by a number of surgeons for mitral valve repair and replacement and some congenital defects, such as ASD and left atrial myxomas. A few iconic surgeons, such as Carpentier and Mohr, pioneered this field, but it was the perseverance of colleagues such as Vanermen who, convinced of the approach, had the dexterity and the vision, in the adequate environment, to develop what is today a technique well accepted and performed by many surgeons. An operation nearly impossible to follow, even by the first assistant, could now be shown on several screens, visible to all of the operating room crew and even extramurally, for educational purposes. A new outstanding educational tool emerged.

Yet, it has taken more than 25 years to consolidate this specific approach to minimally invasive mitral surgery. Why is that?

We were talking about talent and training. And this approach had two main problems. A prominent one is that of talent, skills or dexterity. Not every surgeon has the same ability, technically speaking. Any surgeon knows that. Some may have brilliant ideas and tons of knowledge, the capability of deliver fantastic speeches or write outstanding papers, but may only be bestowed with average skills.

This talent seems obvious with regard to minimally invasive excellence. Patrick Perier, a great contributor to the evolution in the field, said in many of his lectures that "Geoff Colvin was right in saying that *Talent is overrated*". No doubt.

Perier was also stated: "in doing MICS, you have to leave your comfort zone to step into a less familiar territory".

Off-pump CABG is a good example. It is true that not a single properly randomized paper has been able to demonstrate significant advantages of the standard myocardial revascularization, not to speak about the percutaneous use of stents. Trial after trial, a lot of money from industry has been devoted to show ... non-inferiority. Still, 20 years later, we are faced with multiple times more PCIs than surgeries. The recent controversy around the EXCEL trial is a glaring example.

It seems clear to me that individualization is crucial. Some patients will certainly benefit from a given technique more than others; its only very rarely that "one size fits all".

Concurrently, materials and instruments are evolving; visualization is outstanding, allowing for an incredible 3D image with thinner endoscopes. Still, the number of units performing this type of surgery at high standards is still relatively small. The young generation of surgeons may still find it difficult to obtain condensed and specialized knowledge and practical guidance beyond lectures, or identify the go-to places to train.

And there is not an easy solution in the equally diverse field of MICS. Not many centers can provide have the volume and the credentials for foreign fellows to get real hands-on experience. Some large public institutions are not open to teaching this set of skills. Some scientific societies may provide funds for fellowships. Oftentimes, it is not easy to leave a busy practice to go an acquire a full set of skills.

To the relief of both teacher and pupil, a novel, perfectly designed book, not only exquisitely well-written by the most acclaimed experts in the field, but cleverly utilizing the audio-visual power of QR-code scans, has been edited. The reader will find in every chapter Quick Response (QR) boxes, linking the text to the relevant images and videos required to better understand a procedure. Something unique.

The book's concept proposer and editor, Theodoros Kofidis, has prolific academic experience: Hannover, Stanford, Zürich and Singapore. He has written many papers and books, but most importantly he has huge surgical experience, which very few surgeons around the world may have under their belt. This fact, along with the wishes of many surgeons he has been able to teach, was the trigger for engaging him in such an extraordinary endeavor.

The classic aim of minimally invasive surgery to achieve less trauma, better safety and less risk, together with shorter operating times and length of stay, faster recovery and better cosmesis has to be redefined. For some colleagues, the minimally invasive practice may be a vehicle to survive, by differentiating themselves from others. Furthermore, however, patients are nowadays well informed and ask for this new modality. Clinical cardiologists, involved in the heart-team decision-making, are inclined to provide their patients with novel and minimally invasive procedures. Today all cardiovascular professionals have many diverse therapeutic tools to offer, searching for the best for the particular patient. The operating rooms, the staff and the technological ecosystem are nowadays ready to adapt to novel MICS or percutaneous techniques and deal with complications.

Minimally invasive cardiac surgery is here to stay as part of our surgical armamentarium. The chapters which follow this preface will certainly aid the newcomers but also those colleagues already immersed in minimally invasive surgery in their approach to their patients. All professionals, passionately involved in modern surgical care, will find this book a passion by itself.

Jose L Pomar

ACKNOWLEDGMENTS

Special thanks…

To **Professor Yeoh Khay Guan**, Chief Executive, NUHS, for having faith in me through thick and thin.

To **Professor Chong Yap Seng**, Dean, Yong Loo Lin School of Medicine, for his continued support in academia and enterprise.

To **Professor Tan Huay Cheem**, Director of the National University Heart Center, for fervently supporting the Minimally Invasive and Hybrid Program, since its inception.

To **Professor Aymeric Lim**, Group Chief of Medical Board, NUHS, for the inspirational guidance.

To **Professor Quek Swee Chye**, our Chief of Medical Boards for promoting the inclusive platform, the "Peak of Excellence" in Minimally Invasive Cardiothoracic Surgery.

To **Professor Eugene Liu**, our CEO, for teaching us to bid, to frame and to structure our program.

To **Professor Ho Teck Hua**, Senior Deputy President and Provost, NUS, for his encouragement and genuine interest in the MICS program and support for its related research.

This book would not have materialized without the effort of my partners in establishing our minimally invasive program: our anesthesiologist, Professor Ti Lian Kah in particular, our perfusionists, nurses, but also surgeons and researchers. My gratitude also goes to the cardiologists for entrusting their patients to our team's care. I would like to acknowledge our industry partners for supporting numerous events, as well as our Center of Excellence in MICS. I am fortunate to be bestowed with the tolerance, understanding and incessant support by my wife and love, Persephone, who even took to the "pen" to push and cut the finish line, along with the rest of my editorial team. To her and our ten-year-old daughter, Danae, I owe not only thanks, but also sincere apologies, for countless missed weekends, evenings and squandered opportunities for family bonding. Last, we would have never reached this far without our patients, their relatives, as well as donors' generosity and enthusiastic cooperation.

OUR EDITORIAL TEAM

My profound and foremost thanks go to Dr. Faizus Sazzad, the multitasker, whom I proudly call my "pupil", now a solid minimally invasive heart surgeon himself, an innovator, a researcher and a great prospect in the field in Asia. He contributed as co-author, and dedicated endless hours on my side to accomplish the present daunting task. My special thanks and appreciation to our young surgeons, Doctors Chang Guohao, Jai Sule and Qian Qi, for harmonizing several of the individual chapters to their final shine. Our students Ashlynn and Shaye also helped with sketch and text edit. Moreover, the present piece of work would not have been possible without the diligent assistance of our secretarial team, Mrs. Peggy Hu, Joanna Goh and Cheryl Chong.

EDITOR IN CHIEF

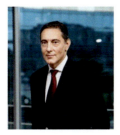

Theo Kofidis, MD, PD(Ger), FRCS, FAHA and FAMS
Assoc. Professor and Head
Department of Cardiac, Thoracic and Vascular Surgery
NUHCS, National University of Singapore
National University Health System
Singapore, Singapore

Professor Theo Kofidis is Head of the Department of Cardiac, Thoracic and Vascular Surgery, at the National University Hospital of Singapore, Senior Consultant Cardiothoracic Surgeon, an expert minimally invasive heart surgeon and avid researcher. He is a renowned cardiac surgeon and strongly sought-after proctor and surgical teacher around the world. He is one of only two AATS members in SE Asia. He is founder and owner of the company Kardia Pte Ltd., aiming at the development of disruptive heart valve and minimally invasive heart surgery technology. He is chairman of the Initiative for Research and Innovation in Surgery (IRIS), has introduced various new technologies and launched new types of less invasive surgery. Over the last ten years in Singapore, he has established the most complete, pioneering and advanced minimally invasive heart surgery program in the region, and set up the most advanced hemodynamic research laboratory and cardiovascular surgical research group in Singapore, after winning numerous grants. His enthusiastic involvement in the field of minimally invasive cardiac surgery now encompasses a prototype simulation center in minimally invasive cardiac, thoracic and vascular surgery, featuring manual and digital surgical simulators, virtual reality and more, in a high-tech environment at NUS.

Professor Kofidis has trained in some of the world's leading institutions (Rochester, NY/Texas Heart, Houston, TX/Hannover, Germany/Stanford, CA). He has been decorated with various international awards and carries various offices and commitments internationally. He has lectured for the American Medical Association, the FDA, the Bill Gates Research Institute and more. As an academic teacher, proctor and consultant for a number of companies in the field-related industry, he holds events and workshops in various countries around the world. He is a trailblazer for the bringing of minimally invasive knowhow to doctors in South East Asia.

Professor Theo Kofidis lives in Singapore with his wife Persephone and daughter Danae, and loves to fly airplanes, photograph, work out and read.

MEMBERS

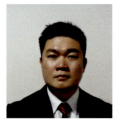

Chang Guohao, MBBS (Singapore), MRCSEd (Surgery), MMed (Surgery), FRCSEd (CTh)
National University Heart Centre
Singapore

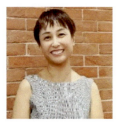

Hu Xinpei, Peggy
Department of Cardiac, Thoracic and Vascular Surgery
National University Heart Centre
Singapore

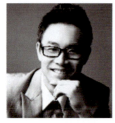

Qian Qi
Department of Cardiac, Thoracic and Vascular Surgery
National University Heart Centre
Singapore

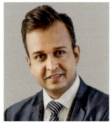

Faizus Sazzad
Research Fellow/Cardiac Surgeon, Department of Surgery (CTVS)
Yong Loo Lin School of Medicine, National University of Singapore
MD-6 Building, Level 08 #South, 14-Medical Drive
Singapore 117599, Singapore

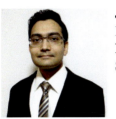

Jai Ajitchandra Sule
Department of Cardiac, Thoracic and Vascular Surgery
National University Heart Centre
Singapore

CONTRIBUTORS

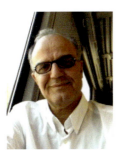

Christos Alexiou
Department of Cardiac Surgery
Interbalkan European Medical Centre
Thessaloniki, Greece

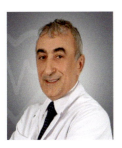

Cem H Alhan
Acibadem University
Acibadem Maslak Hospital
Department of Cardiovascular Surgery
Istanbul, Turkey

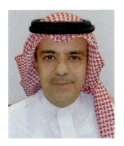

Mohammad Abdulrahman Alotaiby
Prince Sultan Cardiac Center – Riyadh
Kingdom of Saudi Arabia

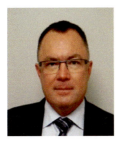

Johannes Bonatti
Vienna North Hospital
Vienna, Austria

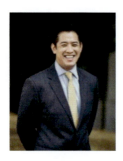

Andrew MTL Choong
National University Heart Centre

and

Department of Surgery
National University of Singapore
Singapore

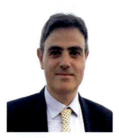

Giovanni Domenico Cresce
Division of Cardiac Surgery
San Bortolo Hospital
Vicenza, Italy

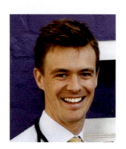

J James Edelman
Department of Cardiothoracic Surgery
Fiona Stanley Hospital
Murdoch, Australia

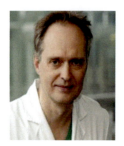

Theodor Fischlein
Department of Cardiac Surgery
Klinikum Nürnberg, Cardiovascular Center
Paracelsus Medical University
Nuremberg, Germany

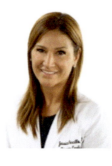

Jessica Forcillo
University of Montreal Hospital Center (CHUM)

and

University of Montreal
Montreal, Canada

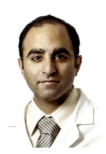

Anil K Gehi
Division of Cardiology
University of North Carolina (UNC) School of Medicine
Chapel Hill, North Carolina

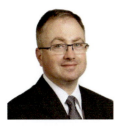

László Göbölös
Cleveland Clinic Lerner College of Medicine
Case Western Reserve University
Heart and Vascular Institute Cleveland Clinic Abu Dhabi
Sowwah Square-Al Maryah Island, Abu Dhabi, UAE

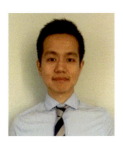

Ming Hao Guo
Division of Cardiac Surgery
University of Ottawa Heart Institute
University of Ottawa
Ottawa, Canada

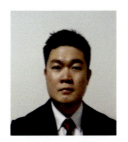

Chang Guohao
Department of Cardiac, Thoracic and Vascular Surgery
National University Heart Centre
Singapore

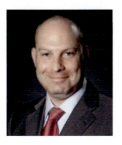

Jonathan M Hemli
Zucker School of Medicine at Hofstra/Northwell

and

Department of Cardiovascular and Thoracic Surgery
Lenox Hill Hospital
New York, New York

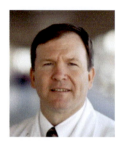

Andy C Kiser
St. Clair Cardiovascular Surgery Associates
Pittsburgh, Pennsylvania

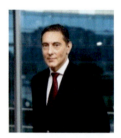

Theo Kofidis
Department of Cardiac, Thoracic and Vascular Surgery
NUHCS, National University of Singapore
National University Health System
Singapore

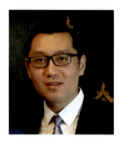

Ivandito Kuntjoro
Department of Cardiology
National University Heart Centre
Singapore

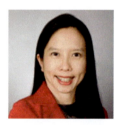

Sophia Ang Bee Leng
Department of Anesthesia
Yong Loo Lin School of Medicine
National University of Singapore
Singapore

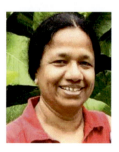

Lalitha Manickam
Department of Anesthesia
National University Hospital Singapore
National University Health System
Singapore

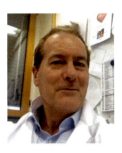

Claudio Muneretto
Italian College of Cardiac Surgeons
School of Cardiac Surgery
University of Brescia
Brescia, Italy

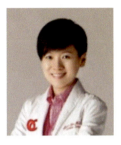

Janet MC Ngu
Division of Cardiac Surgery
University of Ottawa Heart Institute
Ottawa, Canada

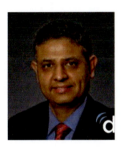

Nirav C Patel
Robotic Cardiac Surgery
Northwell Health

and

Cardiovascular and Thoracic Surgery
Zucker School of Medicine at Hofstra/Northwell

and

Department of Cardiovascular and Thoracic Surgery
Lenox Hill Hospital
New York, New York

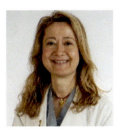

Ourania Preventza
Division of Cardiothoracic Surgery
Baylor College of Medicine

and

Adult Cardiac Surgery
Department of Cardiovascular Surgery
Texas Heart Institute
Houston, Texas

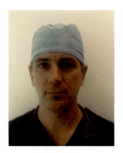

Fabio Ramponi
Department of Cardiothoracic Surgery
The Royal Adelaide Hospital
Adelaide, Australia

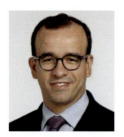

Igo B Ribeiro
Department of Surgery
Queen's University

and

Kingston Health Science Centre
Kingston General Hospital
Kingston, Canada

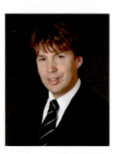

Marc Ruel
Division of Cardiac Surgery
University of Ottawa Heart Institute

and

Departments of Surgery and Cellular and Molecular Medicine
University of Ottawa
Ottawa, Canada

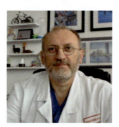

Loris Salvador
Cardiac Surgery Division
San Bortolo Hospital
Vicenza, Italy

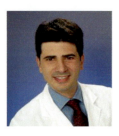

Giuseppe Santarpino
Klinikum Nürnberg
Cardiovascular Center
Paracelsus Medical University
Nuremberg, Germany

and

Magna Graecia University of Catanzaro
Department of Experimental and Clinical Medicine
Catanzaro, Italy

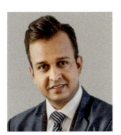

Faizus Sazzad
Department of Surgery (CTVS)
Yong Loo Lin School of Medicine
National University of Singapore
Singapore

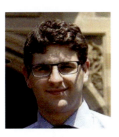

Michael Seco
Sydney Medical School
The University of Sydney
Sydney, Australia

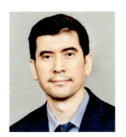

Şahin Şenay
Cardiovascular Surgery
Acibadem Mehmet Ali Aydınlar University School of Medicine
Acibadem Maslak Hospital
Department of Cardiovascular Surgery
Istanbul, Turkey

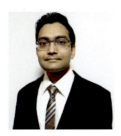

Jai Ajitchandra Sule
Department of Cardiac, Thoracic and Vascular Surgery
National University Heart Centre
Singapore

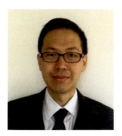

Edgar Tay
Department of Cardiology
National University Heart Centre
Singapore

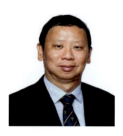

Lian Kah Ti
Department of Anesthesia
National University Hospital, Singapore

and

Department of Anesthesia
Yong Loo Lin School of Medicine
National University of Singapore
Singapore

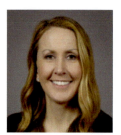

Meghan K Torres
Department of Cardiovascular and Thoracic Surgery
Lenox Hill Hospital
New York, New York

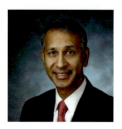

Vinod H Thourani
Department of Cardiovascular Surgery
Marcus Heart and Vascular Center
Piedmont Heart Institute
Atlanta, Georgia

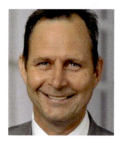

Michael P Vallely
The Ohio State University
Wexner Medical Center
Division of Cardiac Surgery
Columbus, Ohio

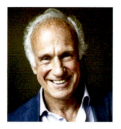

Hugo K Vanermen
OLV-Clinic
Aalst, Belgium

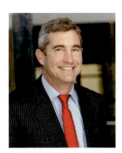

Michael K Wilson
Department of Cardiothoracic Surgery
Macquarie University Hospital
New South Wales, Australia

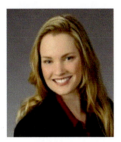

Amalia Winters
Division of Cardiothoracic Surgery
Emory University School of Medicine
Atlanta, Georgia

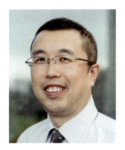

Julian Wong
Division of Vascular and Endovascular Surgery
Department of Cardiac, Thoracic and Vascular Surgery
National University Heart Centre
Singapore

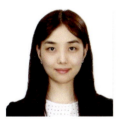

Wei Zhang, MBBS, MRCS
Department of Anesthesia
National University Hospital Singapore
National University Health System
Singapore

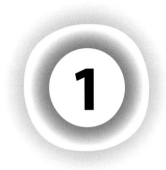

FOREWORD/INTRODUCTION

THEO KOFIDIS

Mantra: "We went bankrupt slowly… slowly…slowly…, then suddenly."

Ernest Hemingway

"We can't reach somewhere we haven't been before, without doing things we haven't done before."

Unknown

Cardiac surgeons don't read anymore. At least not as they used to do a generation ago, when Kirklin and Cohn's book was devoured by all of us as the "Cardiac Surgery Bible". The multimedia pluralism in 2021 offers much better, and certainly more impregnable educational material to train the cardiac surgeon of the modern era. Heart surgeons are presently spoiled by choice: CTSNet offers a domain-specific content, reasonably and sensibly structured, and constitutes a go-to page for surgical content, industry ads, colleague search, the latest news and event calendar. VuMedi and webinars have revolutionized surgical education, and hence virtualized lectures, so that the surgeon can watch their subject of choice, by their speakers of choice, without moving an inch. The majority of our annual cardiothoracic surgery conferences offer off-line digital material for purchase. An impressive example: the AATS, EACTS, or Mitral Conclave, which I wouldn't miss, no matter the cost. The content is THAT substantial. Furthermore, journals offer online submission, and PubMed is a universal link to all available literature, particularly for the corporate or university audience. Next, many surgeons post their own material on their own webpages; see for instance an amazing and rich page created and regularly refreshed by

Prof. Joe Lamelas on minimally invasive heart valve techniques.

Last but not least: where do we all turn for advice ... the day before a demanding or controversial procedure for reference? We ask "Professor GOOGLE"; we watch how it's done on YouTube! The content there in the meantime is very rich and spans from basic procedural steps (EVH, minimally invasive mammary harvest, robotic setup, and more) all the way to full, complex procedures, which feature both minimally invasive tool setup techniques, as well as core procedures, such as mitral valve repair techniques, or MICS CABG anastomoses. Having shared the above, nothing can replace the hands-on training and regular exposure, and also, increasingly, surgical simulation. There is a visible trend away from in-patient hands-on training for the young surgeon, more towards in-silico training, hence simulations and workshops, aiming at reducing the learning curve on the actual patient and teaching both surgical skill as well as – recently – troubleshooting.

- ∞ As a matter of fact, why would you need another hardcopy book in the modern era?

Let me start by referring to the needs of the "market", that is to say, the patients' and surgeons' needs in this relatively new, yet rapidly expanding, field of surgery, minimally invasive cardiac surgery.

Minimally invasive cardiac surgery is not just another feat of surgical bravado nor is it a fashion trend to abate soon. Is it here to stay? While started by a number of surgeons, on a number of occasions around the globe, we don't profess to claim who was the "first" in each case, as this would spark controversy, and certain first-time achievements often cannot be attributed to one single surgeon; it has now reached the main stage, as a well-accepted methodology that can provide the same efficacy and safety as the so-called "Gold Standard" – allow me a neologism, or a small teaser here: sometimes indeed the "Comfort Standard" – particularly for the older-generation surgeon who, by force of habit, and for lack of competition, sticks to the old habits. This is not to denigrate median sternotomy, which is still the traditional and well-proven approach for the majority of cardiac cases.

Hence, MICS surgery is not only a sub-specialty niche, but started co-defining the cardiac surgeon's training, as more cardiac surgeons incorporate MICS techniques in their specialty training. Furthermore, at times of aggressive cardiology pursuit and evolving patient demands, MICS surgery is not only in compliance with those needs and the most primary Hippocratic principles; it is a breadwinner, and a crucial remaining platform for the continuation and expansion of the cardiac surgery métier. Cardiac surgeons recognize this, and there is now a huge wave towards MICS, with developing countries showing greatest interest. A growing number of cardiac surgeons train in MICS surgery. It is a mode of survival, and it's also in compliance with evolving patient demands. There is a huge and pressing trajectory around the globe towards less invasive techniques. The cardiologist and cardiac surgeon nowadays form "heart teams" to provide patients with novel, minimally invasive procedures. Those aim at less trauma, better safety, less risk, faster recovery and better cosmesis.

There is a great demand to learn and apply less invasive techniques. These are often complex and require special know-how and skills. There is no dedicated and comprehensive book to teach this know-how with an up-to-date methodology and modern materials. The last systematic work was edited by Dr. Mehmet Oz in 2001, and is now totally outdated. The demand is high. The training colleagues around the world are well-saturated with the basic knowledge "Bibles", such as Kirklin, Edmunds, Sabiston, etc. But, beyond that, they do care about acquiring knowledge that will help them earn a living, and find a niche in our fields' competitive environment. MICS is a MUST-do and -learn issue for another reason. In modern heart teams and with the advent of the hybrid era, a surgeon will only be able to survive if he has state-of-the-art skills in less invasive technologies, which can be incorporated in the hybrid theatre and/or trans-catheter arena. The hybrid portfolio has not been exploited fully yet. There is a long way to go, including anecdotal combinations of procedures which will soon be undergoing systematic study, such as mitral valve repair and stenting, aortic valve TAVI plus minimally invasive bypass procedure, etc., in all kinds of combinations. The field of cardiac surgery as we know it will change for ever. We need a book to accompany the surgeon along this path, and provide true hints and solutions, beyond the necessary basic knowledge. Which courses to visit, which videos to watch, which centers to join for serious training? How to exploit public and multimedia best? How to consent a patient into a MICS procedure? How to set up a MICS program/practice?

Finally, the patient demand is huge, particularly in developing countries, which pursue development and innovation at great speed and with great investment. SE Asia, India, and China expand their health services aggressively, with a clear domination of less invasive procedures.

As a MICS surgeon and tutor/proctor, I have been setting up a few MICS courses and programs around Asia and Europe; I

FIGURE 1.1 Scan the QR code to go to the ISMICS webpage.

am astounded by the volume and intensity of the demand. I often wish for an accompanying book to use as teaching foundation, reference and handout at those courses. In conclusion, it is time for a dedicated MICS book, written by embedded surgeons, who routinely do it and teach it. A practical guide.

So, what makes the present book special? It's the newly adopted concept of using Quick Response (QR) codes to link the text with multimedia material on the Internet. The QR code has infiltrated both the market as well as the educational community, as a gateway to richer large-volume or audiovisual material on the Internet. Medical journals have long adopted it to link to such material, lectures or how-to-do-it videos. Societies employ QR codes for various functions, mainly for the purpose of one-action step transfer to relevant pages. The utilization of QR codes has in fact just started, and their potential will only expand as an educational tool, to append material on a secured Internet space. There is a plethora of apps out there, which anyone can download onto his smartphone, and exploit the full potential of QR codes. Last, any amateur can now easily generate QR codes from any http//: link, hence any Internet address, and refer to that respective link (Figure 1.1).

Cardiac surgeons nowadays learn from CTSNet, Heart Surgery Forum, online

TABLE 1.1 There is a need for an updated educational tool in minimally invasive cardiac surgery

- By doing MICS you are all applying the most primary Hippocratic principles
- MICS is the way to go
- MICS will be our breadwinner in the 21st century
- MICS covers evolving patient expectations
- There is high demand for a practical guide in today's CS profession, not just an exam review
- It is knowledge that will earn the surgeon a living
- Technologies outpace books
- A book that never ages
- A "smartbook" that employs the latest technology and media

PubMed access, YouTube videos, webinars, conferences, etc. Today's cardiac surgeons (and today's young generation altogether) are more visual, and more practically oriented. They appreciate live media, they want pictures, sounds and links. Here, we offer them a novel concept, namely all the above elements in an unprecedented book, which "comes alive" with meaningful tips, videos, checklists, instrument lists, YouTube videos and app references, and automatic updates, a fully loaded educational script, which brings it to the point, using audiovisual content.

The book has a new, practice-oriented layout of the chapters, updated content (since a dedicated book on MICS is missing in the market), and new modalities (QR codes for Internet referrals and visualization), dispersed within the paragraphs of the text. It is book compatible with iPhones, iPads, YouTube, learning libraries, industry-, and product- webpages. It makes use of special tools, educational videos, online- and recorded video material, related courses and other educational means (Table 1.1).

Hence, it should not only be viewed as a textbook (rather succinct and practical); it will be a gateway and directory to whatever makes sense in the field of MICS. This way it will not lose its relevance so easily. It will close the gap between reading about something, and actually seeing how something is done, by a click (or QR code scan).

In summary: we want to introduce a new paradigm of cardiac surgery education.

HOW TO GET THE MOST OUT OF THE PRESENT BOOK

This book is based on both relevant text for a series of mainstream MICS procedures, but also on QR codes – links to visual material from the Web. Armed with a QR code reading application on our smartphone, this book comes alive, as a tutor and a reference to what really matters, and to learn how to perform the technique or achieve further learning. Every chapter of the book is harmonized to the same structure, featuring:

1. General thoughts/history/introduction
2. How to do it/surgical approach/step by step
3. Tools/instruments and devices
4. Operative and perioperative considerations/troubleshooting

TABLE 1.2 A new educational concept, aimed at the established, or potential, MICS surgeon and trainee

- A book that guides you in how to become an MICS and hybrid surgeon
- A book that tells you which courses to visit – anywhere in the world, and in your backyard
- A book that tells you which videos to watch on YouTube, VuMedi or various fora
- A book that tells you which centers to join for observations or serious hands-on training
- A book that shows you how to use the multimedia space (the cardiac surgeon's social media bible)
- A book that tells you how to set up your MICS program
- A book that tells you how and where to purchase which equipment for your practice
- An "honest" book, that discloses caveats, pitfalls and both pros and cons from experts' mouths
- A book that links you (via itself or an app) to all relevant pages on CTS.net, Heart Surgery Forum, further reading (PubMed), YouTube videos, VuMedi, webinars, conferences, symposia, live transmissions, industry and representatives and, of course, surgeons' blogs!

5. Alternative approaches
6. Caveats and controversies
7. Research, trends and innovations
8. Where and how to learn
9. References/further reading

QR codes will be dispersed throughout the above paragraphs, linking to rich Internet material. We don't claim completeness for the latter, as it would be a futile task, considering the vast ocean of content, which breaks the boundaries of the present work (Table 1.2).

The paragraphs are marked by icons, for easy identification. Being a practical and unbiased guide, the content does not take sides, or show any kind of partiality to one technique, albeit demonstrating those perceived to be most popular. Chapters were appointed/assigned according to surgical target (aortic valve, mitral valve, coronaries, etc.): all chapters will function as gateways to webinars and continuing medical education (CME) reading. All chapters will involve a critical view and "caveats" section.

WHO IS THE PRIMARY AND SECONDARY READERSHIP OF THE BOOK?

Primary: Cardiac surgeons in training and subspecializing cardiac surgeons. Some hybrid cardiologists. Secondary: All companies involved in MICS surgery or any cardiac surgical implant and imaging technology involved; they could distribute the book to the workshop, booth and event delegates; MICS programs within hospitals; cardiac surgery programs. Geographically: Globally. The demand for MICS surgery is strong in Asia, where patients don't want large incisions and surgery altogether.

We – the authors – feel privileged that the renowned publishing house CRC Press (Taylor & Francis) accommodated our idea of using QR codes in a niche subject with enthusiasm and appropriate urgency. The present book started with a proposal which, by the rules of conduct of our publisher, was reviewed and approved unanimously by a selected group of key opinion leaders (KOL) and deemed essential in the field. We thank them, for inspiring motivation and vigor in our effort (Table 1.3).

Let me close on a light-hearted note: A few years ago, at the inauguration of the Indian Society of Minimally Invasive Surgery, I was given the privilege of the podium for

TABLE 1.3 A practical guide in MICS, using QR codes: Scan and watch!
A book that is "alive"
A book that never ages
A book that gets you connected
A book that gets you started
A book that continuously educates you
A book that speaks through image and video
A book that closes the gap between "reading" – "seeing" – and actually … "doing" something

a holistic presentation on the needs and current spectrum of minimally invasive cardiac surgery. As a known proponent of the minimally invasive agenda, I declared myself – at various stages of my lecture – a "minimally invasive cardiac surgeon". Little did I know that an inspired heart surgeon from the audience was about to raise his hand – and by license of his skill with trans-apical mitral cords – pronounce "And … I am a micro-invasive heart surgeon", dully justified! The audience could hardly hold back loud laughter, when a cardiologist rushed to the microphone and proclaimed: "And … I am a nano-invasive heart surgeon!", to a massively entertained audience, and a stunned speaker on the podium.

Let's face it, professional Darwinism is a fact in our domain, and the lion–zebra partnership we all eulogize as the heart team (eventually the better term would be a "multidisciplinary team"), is heavily leaning towards the cardiology side. So I fail to see why the modern or training heart surgeon would not insist on acquainting him-/herself with the minimally invasive quiver, in our time. I hope that the present effort, as imperfect as it may be, will provide valuable and practical assistance.

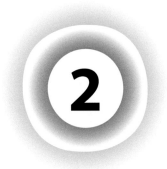

HISTORY OF MINIMALLY INVASIVE CARDIAC SURGERY

CHANG GUOHAO AND THEO KOFIDIS

HISTORY OR INTRODUCTION

The first cardiopulmonary bypass (CPB) machine was used successfully on a human patient by John Gibbon in 1953. Cardiac surgery has since made countless brilliant advancements. In 1960, it was considered safe to use the CPB machine, devised by Gibbons, in combination with hypothermia to perform cardiac surgery. This led to the birth of coronary artery bypass graft (CABG) surgery. Subsequently, other aspects of cardiac surgery, involving the opening of cardiac chambers to tackle valvular lesions and aortic pathology, were made possible (Figure 2.1).

HOW IT HAS BEEN DONE

Even before the birth of CPB, Alexis Carrel first described operating on the coronary circulation in 1910. He was the first surgeon to fully understand the relationship between angina and stenotic coronary artery disease and to carry out canine experiments to perform "complementary circulation" for the diseased native coronary arteries.

Over the past decade, CABG has undergone three distinct eras in its evolution. The first (also known as the "experimental") period was dominated by surgeons with vision who pioneered and established direct coronary artery surgery. The second (era of vein grafts) period was the time when the use of saphenous vein grafts as conduits

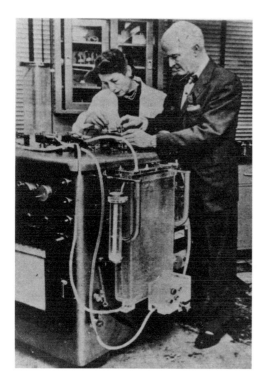

FIGURE 2.1 Dr Gibbon and his wife Mary ("Maly") Gibbon with the newer version of the heart-lung machine (IBM II). This was the second and more refined model that Dr Gibbon used on his first patients. (Reprinted from *Thorac Cardiovasc Surg*, 147(3), Theruvath TP, Ikonomidis JS. Historical perspectives of The American Association for Thoracic Surgery: John H. Gibbon, Jr (1903-1973), 833-836, © 2014, The American Association for Thoracic Surgery, with permission from Elsevier.)

FIGURE 2.2 QR code for "On the Experimental Surgery of the Thoracic Aorta and Heart".

FIGURE 2.3 This video shows an interview with Brian Buxton on the evolution of CABG.

dominated, and routine CABG became the mainstay in the management of coronary artery disease. The third and current era is that of "mixed arterial and venous grafting". It can be said that we're currently moving into the fourth era where the new generation of cardiac surgeons are entering the field of minimally invasive surgery (Figure 2.2 and Figure 2.3).

Options for conduit harvest include the long saphenous vein, radial artery, left internal thoracic artery (LITA) and the less commonly used right gastroepiploic artery. The long saphenous vein and radial artery are conventionally harvested via an open technique. It was not until 1995 that Al Chin from Aalst, Belgium, performed the first endoscopic vein harvesting. Jordan WD et al. was the first surgeon who reported the technique of subcutaneous video-assisted saphenous vein harvest in a series of 30 cases in 1996. He then described this technique in 1997 after performing the largest series in the world, numbering 68 cases. The LITA was first used in 1945 by Arthur Vinberg. He described the "Vinberg Procedure" which involved implanting the LITA directly into the myocardium of the left ventricle. This had variable success but did lead to symptomatic improvement in some patients. Demikhov first described using the LITA to directly graft the LAD in dogs in 1952 and reported graft patency of up to 2 years. At the same time other surgeons, Gordon Murray and Sabiston, reported success with the use of LITA as well. The group led by Floyd Loop in the Cleveland Clinic was the first to report improved clinical outcomes with the usage of the LITA when compared to using saphenous vein grafts

FIGURE 2.4 Technique of subcutaneous video-assisted saphenous vein harvest.

FIGURE 2.5 History of cardiac surgery. An interview with Professor Alain Carpentier.

alone. This led to the third era of "mixed arterial and venous grafting" (Figure 2.4).

Alain Carpentier was the first surgeon to report the use of the radial artery in 1971. Due to early inferior patency rates as compared to the saphenous vein, the radial artery was not widely used until Christopher Acar reported his experience in 1992 where he managed to demonstrate 100% radial artery patency on post-operative coronary angiography. Terada Y reported the first endoscopic harvesting of the radial artery as a conduit for CABG in Ibaraki-ken, Japan, in 1998, with good short-term results. Subsequently, in 2002, Mark Connolly published the largest study of 300 patients who underwent endoscopic radial artery harvesting, reporting satisfactory results (Figure 2.5).

The advent of MICS may be so variable, concurrent and plethoric, that a clear identification of one single surgeon as the birth father of a procedure may be difficult, negotiable or, at times, even a matter of dispute. Table 2.1 gives a summary of the procedures in cardiac surgery with their pioneers and the years that they were first performed (Figure 2.6 and Figure 2.7).

Mitral valve surgery is an area in cardiac surgery extensively influenced by the art of minimal access. Its humble beginnings date back to the mid-1990s when Cosgrove and Cohn independently described techniques of the first minimally invasive mitral valve surgery (MIMVS) [1, 2]. These were done via the parasternal and hemisternotomy accesses. The next major milestone in 1996 saw the first video-assisted mitral valve repair through a mini-thoracotomy, done by Carpentier [3]. Chitwood subsequently described the use of his trans-thoracic aortic clamp in MIMVS, now widely known as the "Chitwood Clamp" (Scanlan International, MN, USA) [4]. In 1998, surgeons in Leipzig, Germany, employed a port-access approach and voice-activated robotic assistance. In the same year, Carpentier and Mohr successfully completed the world's first robotic mitral valve repair using the da Vinci Robotic System [5, 6] (Figure 2.8).

Minimally invasive aortic valve surgery was first reported in 1996 by Cosgrove and Sabik [7]. Since then, various means for exposing the aortic valve have been explored. The first minimally invasive aortic valve replacement (MIAVR) was done via a right parasternal incision with rib cartilage resection. Since then, other surgeons have developed variations of hemi- or mini J-shaped sternotomy and right anterior thoracotomy [8]. The current access of choice is the J-shaped mini-sternotomy as it has many advantages over other incisions. Whilst minimizing post-operative pain and maintaining thoracic wall integrity, this incision does provide adequate exposure [9]. Furthermore, when the need arises, it can be extended for additional exposure. Compared to the parasternal approach, the internal mammary artery can be preserved. In patients who require isolated aortic valve surgery, MIAVR is a safe and feasible alternative to

TABLE 2.1 First reported MICS procedures

Procedure	First Reported by	Year
Coronary revascularization	Alexis Carrel	1910
Left internal mammary artery as CABG conduit	Arthur Vinberg	1945
Cardiopulmonary bypass	John Gibbon	1953
Off-pump coronary artery bypass (OPCAB)	Kolesov	1960
Radial artery as CABG conduit	Alain Carpentier	1971
Minimally invasive direct coronary artery bypass (MIDCAB)	Frederico Benetti	1994
Complete coronary revascularization via MIDCAB	Joseph T McGinn	1994
Video-assisted mitral valve repair via mini-thoracotomy	Carpentier	1996
Minimally invasive aortic valve replacement (AVR)	Cosgrove	1996
Minimally invasive mitral valve repair (MVR)	Cosgrove	1996
Endoscopic harvest of long saphenous vein	Jordan WD	1997
Ambulatory coronary artery bypass graft	Frederico Benetti	1997
Endoscopic harvest of radial artery	Terada Y	1998
Robotic mitral valve repair	Carpentier	1998
Hybrid coronary revascularization (HCR)	Lloyd CT	1999
Awake CABG	Karagoz	2000
Minimally invasive implantation of left ventricular assist device (LVAD)	Hill JD	2000
Awake CABG with aortic valve replacement (AVR)	Vivek Jawali	2002
Transcatheter aortic valve implantation (TAVI)	Alain Cribier	2002
Hybrid atrial ablation for atrial fibrillation	Andy Kiser	2013

Footnote: List of MICS procedures first performed in the world. (Disclaimer: We do not claim strict accuracy and cannot prevent or predict that any surgeon around the world may provide evidence of being the "first". Our table is based on "first published" following our personal search of Internet resources.)

conventional sternotomy. Besides surgical aortic valve replacement, AVR can now be performed via the transcatheter route. The first transcatheter aortic valve implantation (TAVI) was described by Alain Cribier in Rouen, France, on 16 April 2002 in an inoperable patient using a trans-septal antegrade approach and a balloon-expandable aortic valve prosthesis. The study demonstrated the feasibility of percutaneous valve implantation. TAVI has since been developed for patients who require aortic valve replacement, but who are poor candidates for surgery [10]. These patients with multiple comorbidities can now consider the option of TAVI for the treatment of symptomatic aortic stenosis (Figure 2.9).

Atrial fibrillation (AF) is a common cardiac arrhythmia. Conventionally, surgical treatment of AF takes the form of Cox Maze III procedures that involve median sternotomy, cardiopulmonary bypass and complex biatrial incisions. This is associated with a high risk of bleeding and longer surgical time [11]. Currently, Cox Maze IV has been developed and involves the use of different energy modalities to bring about myocardial scarring, resulting in a conduction block to thereby terminate re-entrant circuits, which are the culprits of AF (Figure 2.10).

Cox Maze first performed the procedure on 25 September 1987. Many approaches for Cox Maze IV have been described. They include bilateral or unilateral mini-thoracotomies, a total endoscopic approach, a video-assisted thoracoscopic approach and the robotic maze. This video (Figure 2.11)

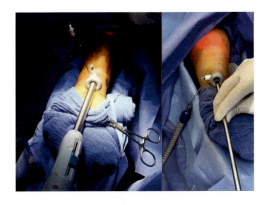

FIGURE 2.7 Interview with Professor Friedrich Mohr.

FIGURE 2.6 Endoscopic radial artery harvesting technique. A. The endoscopic port with the conical tip inserted in the forearm. B. The VasoView cannula inserted through the forearm. (With kind permission from Springer Science+Business Media: Springer Nature, *Cardiothorac Surg*, Endoscopic versus open harvesting of radial artery for CABG, 28(2), Fouly, M.A.H. © 2020.)

demonstrates Cox Maze IV via a right anterior thoracotomy.

Energy modalities used for Cox Maze IV include radiofrequency, cryoablation, high-intensity focused ultrasound, microwave (pioneered by Pruitt JC) and laser. The last two have fallen out of favor as studies have demonstrated that they are not as efficacious and are unable to reliably produce transmural scarring on a beating heart [12–14]. Radiofrequency uses alternating currents to emit electromagnetic energy and heat deeper layers of tissues by conduction

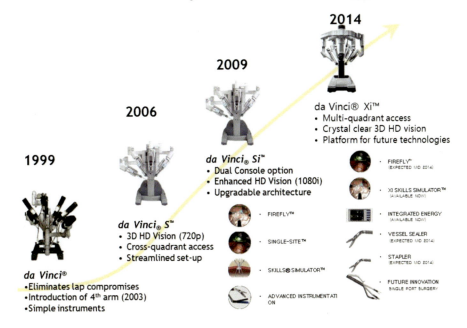

FIGURE 2.8 The da Vinci Robotic System evolution. (After Lee W et al, Ten-year Experience of the da Vinci Robotic Surgery At Severance Yonsei University Hospital in Korea. *Hanyang Medical Reviews*, 36, 215-224, © 2016 Hanyang University College of Medicine.)

FIGURE 2.9 Alain Cribier and the history and development of TAVI.

FIGURE 2.10 First Cox Maze procedure.

FIGURE 2.11 Demonstration of Cox Maze IV.

FIGURE 2.12 Bipolar RF Maze, Wolf mini-Maze.

FIGURE 2.13 The Epicor Cardiac Ablation System.

to cause transmural myocardial scarring. Randall Wolf developed the bipolar RF clamp and performed the Maze procedure via small non-rib spreading incisions, which was named the Wolf mini-Maze procedure. Cryoablation uses rapid cooling of the probe to cause cell death by freezing and results in a full-thickness scar. Charles Mack was one of the first surgeons who reported his results of argon-based cryoablation using a novel argon-based clamp [15] for atrial fibrillation. High-intensity focused ultrasound (Epicor – first used by Michael Harostock) generates thermal energy by using ultrasound waves to harmonically oscillate water molecules (Figure 2.12 and Figure 2.13).

TOOLS/INSTRUMENTS AND DEVICES

Initial attempts at MICS were hindered by the paucity of appropriate technology, such as visualization systems, anastomotic devices, stabilizers and alternative methods of vascular cannulation for cardiopulmonary bypass, as well as the durability of stent patency. This increased technical difficulty in MIDCAB spurred the development of advanced surgical instruments to facilitate the procedure. In collaboration with industrial partners, namely Medtronic Inc, a novel retractor – ThoraTrak® – was developed to improve visualization of the operative target and is currently in use in every MIDCAB procedure (Figure 2.14, Figure 2.15, Figure 2.16 and Figure 2.17).

Even now, new equipment is being developed. Surgical technology is an important factor for MICS to be successful. Robotic surgical systems have been developed to

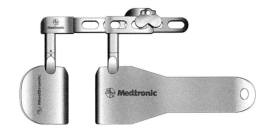

FIGURE 2.14　ThoraTrak Mics Retractor: A reusable, stainless steel retractor for minimally invasive heart surgery. Reproduced with permission of Medtronic, Inc.

FIGURE 2.15　Thoracoscopic LITA harvesting.

FIGURE 2.16　Totally endoscopic coronary artery bypass (TECAB).

FIGURE 2.17　Robotic CABG (Francis P Sutter).

permit the manipulation of surgical instruments through limited thoracic incisions. Early success at endoscopic LIMA harvest has fueled the development of totally endoscopic coronary artery bypass (TECAB), and this has been made possible with the development of high-resolution visualization systems as well as shafted robotic equipment to enable CABG through chest wall ports (Figure 2.18).

The da Vinci Surgical System (Intuitive Surgica, Inc, Mountain View, CA) was one of the most successful robotic systems with highly articulating mechanical joints which maintain the dexterity of the surgeon's forearm and wrist at the operative sites via sub-centimeter entry ports. As cardiac surgeons begin exploring MICS, improvements were made with the intention of minimizing or circumventing the systemic inflammatory response as a result of circulating blood through a perfusion circuit. Cannulae have decreased in size over the years, are now specially coated to be less thrombogenic and are made with non-kinking materials so as to maximize the operative space. Improvements in transesophageal echocardiography techniques aid in the visualization of intraoperative conditions for the confirmation of cannulae placement and ensuring adequate deairing in a limited operative space in MICS. The new challenge of surgery in limited operative space has driven developments in the area of CPB access. Alternative arterial access sites are established – peripheral cannulation via the femoral or axillary artery. Venous cannulation with traditional vacuum-assisted drainage via a two-stage cannula in the right atrium or via bicaval cannulation has been made impossible through a MICS access. Instead, MICS requires venous cannulation percutaneously from the femoral or internal jugular veins. MICS has fostered the development of newer technologies and specialized instruments to facilitate antegrade cardioplegia and aortic cross-clamp through the MICS access. The port-access method is an example – a combination of endovascular balloon aortic occlusion with antegrade cardioplegia administration. It

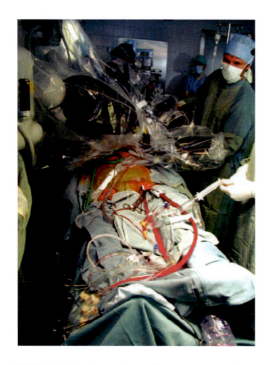

FIGURE 2.18 Operation theater setup for a totally endoscopic coronary artery bypass (TECAB) surgery. (With kind permission from Springer Science+Business Media, Springer Nature, *Eur Surg*, Robotically assisted minimal invasive andendoscopic coronary bypass surgery, 43, 195–197, Schachner, T., Bonaros, N., Wiedemann, D. et al. © 2011.)

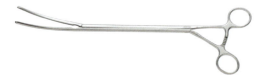

FIGURE 2.19 Chitwood aortic cross-clamp. Reproduced with permission of Scanlan International, Inc. © 2020.

has been useful in MIDCAB as well as minimally invasive mitral valve surgery. Another innovation is the Chitwood aortic cross-clamp that enables aortic cross-clamping to be done with a right thoracotomy in MIMVS (Figure 2.19).

This video (Figure 2.20) describes the concept of hybrid atrial ablation for atrial fibrillation by Dr Andy Kiser and the various

FIGURE 2.20 Hybrid atrial ablation by Andy Kiser.

FIGURE 2.21 COBRA Fusion by Dr Mark Groh.

accesses. This hybrid procedure consists of a surgical ablation procedure and incorporates intra-operative electrophysiological testing by the electrophysiologist to confirm that the erratic electric signals have been blocked. September 2012 witnessed the market launch of the COBRA Fusion® ablation system by Estech. This system overcomes the most significant challenge faced in minimally invasive epicardial ablation – the cooling effect of the circulating blood within the heart – and reproducibly creates transmural box lesions on a beating heart. Cardiothoracic surgeon Andy Kiser was one of the first to use this system in humans. COBRA Fusion system is employed to bring about epicardial ablation. Subxiphoidal endoscopic atrial ablation was first reported by Guillermo E Sosa [16], a cardiac electrophysiologist, who developed a novel access for epicardial mapping in patients with Chagas disease and recurrent ventricular tachycardia (Figure 2.21).

Besides Cox Maze IV bringing about myocardial scarring, left atrial appendage exclusion is commonly employed in the same surgery as this is the most significant

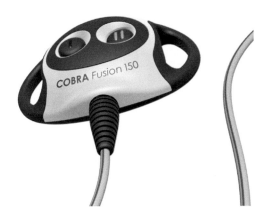

FIGURE 2.24 Different surgical strategies for implantation of continuous-flow VADs.

FIGURE 2.22 The COBRA Fusion 150 Ablation System. The COBRA Fusion 150 Surgical Ablation System facilitates intuitive, real-time temperature-controlled radiofrequency (TCRF). Reproduced with permission of AtriCure, Inc. © 2020.

FIGURE 2.23 Minimally invasive LAA exclusion with LARIAT.

thromboembolic source in AF. This, too, has been described as possible using the minimally invasive approach using the LARIAT device via the percutaneous route (Figure 2.22 and Figure 2.23).

The implantation of ventricular assist devices (VADs) has always been performed via a median sternotomy. Hill JD introduced the concept of minimally invasive implantation in the year 2000. He used a combination of a right mini-thoracotomy and small left subcostal incision to implant the Thoratec® left ventricular assist device (LVAD). This video (Figure 2.24) shows the strategies for the implantation of VADs. Besides the incision, the implantation of VADs evolved from on-pump implantation to off-pump strategies. This avoids the harmful inflammatory response associated with CPB. Sun BC was the first surgeon to report his series of 25 patients who underwent off-pump implanted LVAD in 2008 and concluded that these techniques have acceptable outcomes (Figure 2.25).

PERIOPERATIVE CONSIDERATION

Minimally invasive cardiac surgery (MICS) is like a "chameleon". It is an ever-evolving entity of surgical practice and even amongst groups of surgeons and laymen alike, its definition changes. It has undergone numerous transformations in techniques and philosophy (Figure 2.26).

MICS has not only transformed over time, but has also transcended international boundaries – first beginning largely in the USA, it rapidly influenced surgical practice in parts of Europe (Germany, France, Belgium). Most recently, this innovative technique has been taken up by surgeons in Japan, China and Southeast Asia. Evidently, the fourth era of cardiac surgery is making steady progress (Figure 2.27).

Minimally invasive direct coronary artery bypass (MIDCAB) grafting via an anterolateral thoracotomy was pioneered by Kolesov in 1967. However, this novel approach was not well received at that time due to the

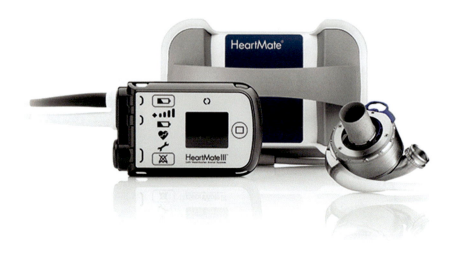

FIGURE 2.25 HeartMate 3™ left ventricular assist device (LVAD). Reproduced with permission of Abbott, © 2020.

FIGURE 2.26 First worldwide MIDCAB by Federico Benetti.

FIGURE 2.27 Dr. Joseph McGinn discusses his revolutionary minimally invasive bypass surgery method.

FIGURE 2.28 Minimally invasive CABG – "The McGinn Technique".

technical complexity and poor quality of the anastomoses performed as a consequence of the inadequacy of the technological armamentarium. A better understanding of cardiac surgical anatomy, physiology and more confidence in the safety and efficacy of minimally invasive procedures led to the inception of minimally invasive cardiac surgery. This video shows the first MIDCAB done by Federico Benetti in the US in April 1994. In addition, Dr Benetti performed the first ambulatory surgery in October 1997 and the patient was discharged 22 hours after the operation.

Joseph T McGinn, the pioneer of minimally invasive direct coronary artery full revascularization, once said, "I clearly saw there was a need for a change in the way we did heart surgery". The first MIDCAB to achieve complete coronary revascularization was performed on 21 January 2005, at what was then the Heart Institute of Staten Island, by a highly trained team led by Joseph T McGinn. This technique involves anastomosis of proximal grafts to the aorta or the mammary artery (as a T graft) and was performed over the next 2 years with favorable outcomes (Figure 2.28).

ALTERNATIVE APPROACHES

With thoracotomy being proven to be a reliable means of access to the heart, MICS has taken flight. It is now used as an alternative, if not standard of care, to traditional surgery for operations involving hybrid revascularization, mitral valve, aortic valve, atrial septal defects and for atrial fibrillation.

The accomplishment of CABG without the CPB has been explored and the first off-pump coronary artery bypass (OPCAB) surgery was reported by Kolesov in the 1960s. Now it constitutes up to 30% of CABG performed worldwide.

Hybrid coronary revascularization (HCR) is a new development as part of the evolution of minimally invasive access treatment for multivessel coronary artery disease (CAD). It was first performed by Lloyd CT in 1999 as an integrated small left anterior thoracotomy and angioplasty as a staged procedure. During its early developmental stages, PCI and single-graft CABG (LIMA to LAD) were done on two separate occasions. John Puskas conducted the first multicenter study of HCR and presented at the American College of Cardiology, demonstrating that the technique of HCR has a similar rate of major adverse events in the first year, compared with percutaneous intervention, namely stenting. Currently, HCR can be performed in one setting, with LIMA to LAD graft commonly being done off-pump followed by PCI.

CAVEATS AND CONTROVERSIES

The term minimally invasive cardiac surgery does not have a standard definition, nor does it refer to a single approach. It is an amalgamation of innovations in techniques and strategies with the aid of surgical technologies to achieve the primary aims of reducing the impact of the surgical procedure and achieving a satisfactory if not excellent therapeutic result but at the same time to allow faster recovery and quicker rehabilitation. MICS achieves basic Hippocratic principles and covers evolving patient expectations. According to one, elimination of CPB in CABG is considered minimally invasive as it reduces the morbidity associated with CPB. Other authors view the median sternotomy as a significant source of morbidity, in particular postoperative respiratory impairment, sternal wound infections, chest instability and chronic pain. As a result, alternative means of access to the heart and great vessels have been sought. This has fueled the development of alternative routes and methods of CPB for cardiac surgeries (Figure 2.29).

Over the past 5 decades, cardiac surgery for coronary artery disease and valvular lesions has been perfected to a high success rate with years of proven reliability. However, the access – the median sternotomy – continues to make cardiac surgery an "invasive and perceived-traumatic experience". To date, a flurry of progressive advancements into less invasive forms of

FIGURE 2.29 Discussion – getting comfortable with MICS.

heart surgery has taken place. They all aim to achieve similar if not better effects of surgery without the pain and trauma associated with this major operation. Over the past decade, minimally invasive cardiac surgery has increased in popularity and has gained wide acceptance in the cardiac surgeon fraternity. There is the desire to translate the myriad of observed benefits of minimal access surgery – e.g. reduced surgical trauma, decreased pain, reduced hospital length of stay – to the cardiac surgical arena. This video is an interview with cardiac surgeons on embarking on a journey of MICS for the benefit of the patients.

RESEARCH, TRENDS AND INNOVATION

Kofidis et al. [17] demonstrated that there are no significant differences between a conventional single-vessel CABG and a MIDCAB in terms of myocardial infarction rates, re-operations for bleeding and cerebrovascular accidents. In addition, there are multiple advantages of MIDCAB as it avoids sternotomy, thereby reducing the time to ambulation and rates of sternal wound infections. It avoids CPB and its attendant complications brought about by the systemic inflammatory response syndrome.

Cardiac surgeons then went on to explore "more minimal" techniques in the area of "awareness". The first awake CABG in the world was reported by Karagoz in 2000 where high thoracic epidural anesthesia was employed without the need for general anesthesia. Later on in 2002, this technique was further popularized by Vivek Jawali who performed the first awake aortic valve replacement with CABG (Figure 2.30).

WHERE AND HOW TO LEARN

Cardiac surgery has developed in leaps and bounds over the past 50 years. The benefits of minimally invasive cardiac surgery have been well-documented, and for suitable candidates, the minimal access is starting to become the access of choice. In conclusion, as we embark on the journey into the fourth era of cardiac surgery, this video serves to remind us of the pros and cons of the traditional open heart surgery and those of the innovative MICS (Figure 2.31).

In addition, there are various organizations, e.g. the European Association for Cardio-Thoracic Surgery (EACTS): EACTS provides high-quality training courses that are attended by delegates from all over the

FIGURE 2.30 Awake cardiac bypass and valve surgery.

FIGURE 2.31 Open heart versus MICS – pros and cons.

FIGURE 2.32 EACTS course calendar.

FIGURE 2.34 Multimedia platform of MICS.

FIGURE 2.33 STS course 2019.

FIGURE 2.35 Establishment of MICS program.

world. As an educational institution, their goal is to promote a non-dogmatic learning environment that brings together people, cultures and ideas from around the world, changing lives, and helping to transform through education (Figure 2.32).

The Society of Thoracic Surgeons (STS): Founded in 1964, the mission of the STS is to enhance the ability of cardiothoracic surgeons to provide the highest quality patient care through education, research and advocacy. STS provides online training programs, panel discussions and Online video resources (Figure 2.33).

There are other institutions around the world that provide courses in the field of minimally invasive cardiac surgery via online platform, e.g. Multimedia Manual of Cardiothoracic Surgery (Figure 2.34). Some institutions even discuss how the minimally invasive cardiac surgery program was established [18] (Figure 2.35).

REFERENCES

1. Navia JL, Cosgrove DM. Minimally invasive mitral valve operations. *Ann Thorac Surg.* 1996; 62:1542–1544.
2. Cohn LH, Adams DH, Couper GS, et al. Minimally invasive cardiac valve surgery improves patient satisfaction while reducing costs of cardiac valve replacement and repair. *Ann Surg.* 1997; 226(4):421–428.
3. Carpentier A, Loulmet D, Carpentier A, et al. Open heart operation under videosurgery and minithoracotomy first case (mitral valvuloplasty) operated with success. *C R Acad Sci.* 1996; 319(3):219–223.
4. Chitwood WR Jr, Elbeery JR, Chapman WH, et al. Video-assisted minimally invasive mitral valve surgery: the 'micromitral' operation. *J Thorac Cardiovasc Surg.* 1997; 113(2):413–414.
5. Carpentier A, Loulmet D, Aupècle B, et al. Computer assisted open heart surgery: First case operated on with success. *C R Acad Sci III.* 1998; 321:437–42.
6. Modi P, Hassan A, Chitwood WR. Minimally invasive mitral valve surgery: a systematic review and meta-analysis. *Eur J Cardio-thorac Surg.* 2008; 34:943–952.

7. Cohn LH, Adams DH, Couper GS, et al. Minimally invasive cardiac valve surgery improves patient satisfaction while reducing costs of cardiac valve replacement and repair. *Ann Surg.* 1997; 226(4):421–428.
8. Estrera AL, Reardon MJ. Current approaches to minimally invasive aortic valve surgery. *Curr Opin Cardiol.* 2000; 15(2):91–95.
9. Walther T, Falk V, Metz S, et al. Pain and quality of life after minimally invasive versus conventional cardiac surgery. *Ann Thorac Surg.* 1999; 67:1643–1647.
10. Wolf PA, Mitchel JB, Baker CS, Kannel WB, D'Agostino RB. Impact of atrial fibrillation on mortality, stroke, and medical costs. *Arch Intern Med.* 1998; 158:229–234.
11. Gaynor SL, Diodato MD, Prasad SM, et al. A prospective, single-center clinical trial of a modified Cox maze procedure with bipolar radiofrequency ablation. *J Thorac Cardiovasc Surg.* 2004; 128:535–542.
12. Gaynor SL, Byrd GD, Diodato MD, et al. Microwave ablation for atrial fibrillation: dose–response curves in the cardioplegia-arrested and beating heart. *Ann Thorac Surg.* 2006; 81:72.
13. Gaynor SL, Byrd GD, Diodato MD, et al. Dose response curves for microwave ablation in the cardioplegia-arrested porcine heart. *Heart Surg Forum.* 2005; 23:331–336.
14. Van Brakel TJ, Bolotin G, Salleng KJ, et al. Evaluation of epicardial microwave ablation lesions: histology versus electrophysiology. *Ann Thorac Surg.* 2004; 78:1397–1402.
15. Federico M, Nikolaos S, William MB, et al. Epicardial beating heart cryoablation using a novel argon-based cryoclamp and linear probe. *J Thorac Cardiovasc Surg.* 2006; 131:403–411. doi: 10.1016/j.jtcvs.2005.10.048
16. Sosa E, Scanavacca M, d'Avila A, et al. A new technique to perform epicardial mapping in the electrophysiology laboratory. *J Cardiovasc Electrophysiol.* 1996; 7(6):531–6. doi: 10.1111/j.1540-8167.1996.tb00559.x
17. Kofidis T, Emmert MY, Paeschke HG, et al. Long-term follow-up after minimal invasive direct coronary artery bypass grafting procedure: a multi-factorial retrospective analysis at 1000 patient-years. *Interact Cardiovasc Thorac Surg.* 2009; 9(6):990–994.
18. Kofidis T, Chang GH, Lee CN. Establishment of a minimally invasive cardiac surgery programme in Singapore. *Singapore Med J.* 2017; 58(10):576–579.

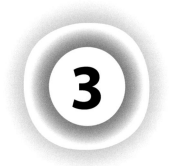

HOW TO SET UP A MINIMALLY INVASIVE PROGRAM

THEO KOFIDIS AND CHANG GUOHAO

HISTORY OR INTRODUCTION

Mantra: "Analysis Paralysis".

"Shoot first, aim later".

For any new venture to thrive in the medical world you need resources and skill. Resources may be money and space, or even access to the right people. Skill is all about yourself: looking for change in our portfolio, change in our patient clientele, change in our sphere of influence or even change of income … then we need to change, and leave the comfort zone of median sternotomy, as much as we still use and appreciate this access. Hence, change starts within.

In brief, first comes the conviction that you wish to learn and focus. In our excruciating daily 36/7 routines, there is little time left for extracurricular things, and let's face it, there is no "Extra Time". When the day is over, that's about it. Hence, something has to give, that is, you need to commit the time and discipline to learn. You may be lucky to "grow up" as a surgeon in a high-volume, high-efficiency MICS program, such as in Leipzig, Germany, or Aalst, Belgium, where MICS had started at a large scale. That's the best-case scenario, whereby you have to learn as part of your everyday exposure to the high standards of those exemplary programs. But these are exceptions. Most likely, the rest of us have grown up in rather otherwise-focused programs, like myself (aortic surgery, transplantation: the latter could not fill my plate nor provide for my family, as much as it used to be *en vogue* and glorious for three decades), Others "matured" in private environments, where training is not high on the agenda, or just off-shot, where innovation is not the primary focus. From my experience of tutoring around the world, this is what I have mostly encountered: hungry, talented young surgeons with good skill and reasonable exposure to the full circle of heart surgeries, however oppressed under an omnipotent guru-boss, who doesn't have any interest in changing the status quo, may not be in your favor or is too insecure to allow progress and the inevitable ascent and freedom of his subjects. In a few words: militaristic organizations with top-down vertical leadership. The two programs mentioned above are examples of the opposite: two megastar-pioneers of MICS who have basically trained the rest of the world, and their own people. It boils down to the same old principles of leadership: either you have a leader who leads from the trenches, or one who leads from the safety of the hill, above the battleground, who minds himself first (Figure 3.1).

FIGURE 3.1   How should I set up a minimally invasive program? By Paul Modi.

HOW TO DO IT/STEP BY STEP

Let's start with what you should not do when contemplating changing course in your surgical career and considering MICS.

- ∞ Don't hesitate
- ∞ Don't procrastinate
- ∞ Don't listen to nay-sayers
- ∞ Don't fear competition
- ∞ Don't isolate
- ∞ Don't keep it for yourself

Instead:

While our program is neither the largest in the world nor the first to have pioneered most of the herein-described methodologies, it is a very complete one, and has thrived amidst difficult conditions of competition and scrutiny, due to the very nature of the profession in the region. Hence, we do not claim that we have invented the wheel, but we do speak of our own experience over the past 10 years (Figure 3.2).

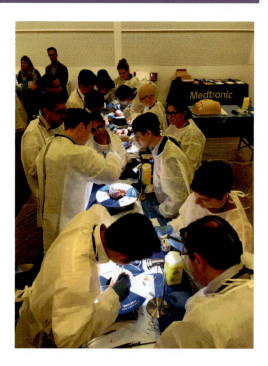

FIGURE 3.2   Simulation/hands-on training on explanted hearts and mannequins; organized by our NUHS team during an overseas conference.

22   Minimally Invasive Cardiac Surgery

Human nature is, at its core, the desire to preserve, protect and delineate one's territory, a strategy that is detrimental to innovation and progress. The other negative force that stands in your way of becoming an excellent MICS surgeon is habit. Entropy can be a massive disruption in your progress. Why trouble yourself to spend 45 extra minutes to set up properly for an MICS mitral valve procedure? Why bother your anesthetist to insert a double lumen tube? Why stress your nurses and perfusionists to learn something totally new? Why force the surgeon following you in the same theater to risk postponing their case? These are important logistic considerations that you will face in the beginning. Therefore, as long as you live and work within a group of people, you must win their buy-in and their enthusiasm. How? Be inclusive. Even with those who are not born to be pioneers and will watch you fall and stand up again, strike through the bush and get bruised, produce a few complications and struggle through the consequences, until your program "stands" and they can harvest the benefits.

TOOLS/INSTRUMENTS AND DEVICES

All of the above are valid considerations, but they are not deterrents in your quest for progress and self-improvement. It all starts with focus and conviction. Once you have made up your mind, you start educating yourself. Get a flavor of what's out there, which courses to visit, which programs to spend time with, and ask, ask, ask! Ask questions humbly and incessantly. Read this book or parts of it. It's supposed to guide you with realism and focus. Subscribe to the Innovations journal (instrument of the International Society for Minimally Invasive Cardiothoracic Surgery); go to CTSNet and find out how to best contact the relevant people (the present work will guide you to this end).

Secondly, time for the diplomatic part: you are not alone in your department, and most likely you are not the boss. Hence, you must win over your peers, reporting officers, nursing and perfusionists, allied health, your boss, your CEO and last but not least, the gatekeepers: the cardiologists around you. This will involve long and onerous work, but there is now a way around it. They all need to know, and better yet, co-own the program, thus becoming part of your success in setting up the program. That's fine. Fifty percent of zero is … zero. Better start somewhere, and things will fall your way if you insist and get good at it. In business terms, you must achieve incentive alignment. Younger doctors in your team will see a new perspective for their careers and their training in your efforts. Your reporting officer or boss will see benefit for his program or get a larger picture of things. Your nurses and perfusionists will eventually see … stress (not all of them). Your CEO and administrator will look at the financial side of things. Your patient will see an opportunity to have less trauma and go back to full functionality faster. Basically you start by promoting the patient's interest first, which is inherently what we are doing all this for. Secondly, you must achieve incentive alignment with your boss and CEO/admin, and display sufficient data on how minimally invasive heart surgery can promote value-driven outcomes (VDOs), hence better outcomes by various metrics (better quality) over the same or even less cost AND bill to the patient (these are two different things). Further down (Figure 3.6), you will find preliminary data

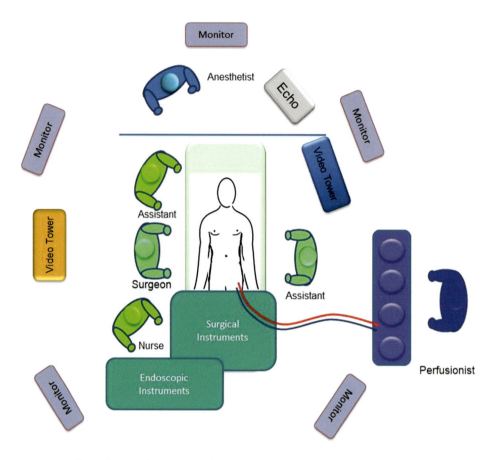

FIGURE 3.3 Outline of general operation theater set up for the minimally invasive cardiac surgery.

from our own learning curve, showing a clear VDO advantage of MICS MVR, as compared to "open" MVR through median sternotomy. The shorter hospital stay in the MICS group renders smaller costs and a smaller bill to the patient himself. With more experience, you will see this effect enhancing, and the split between classical sternotomy and MICS widening further. Therefore, in no time, with some reasonable outcomes, you will see benefits to the advantage of MICS from an economical and value standpoint Figure 3.3.

Here are situations whereby the institutional governance and structure or hospital administration is paralyzed by stringent rules and slow-turning mills. There are other situations whereby the local government policy changes and the purchase programs are frozen. The authors' team has experienced all these situations in developing countries, so they find brief mention here, and we would like to share what our fellow colleagues exposed to such conditions have figured out. When there are limited resources … be resourceful: often times, surgeons will save to buy their own instruments, particularly in the private domain. We have seen surgeons making beneficial deals with companies who are willing to sell their tools at heavily discounted prices to get the program started (kudos to them), for the sake of progress and benefit to the patient. Or, in other cases, donations or endowments can help to get a program off the ground (as with our simulation center on MICS) (Table 3.1).

TABLE 3.1	Important considerations before the start

- Focus, don't waste time: shape it in your mind: vision and unflinching purpose
- Persuade by incentive alignment
- Self-reflect and self-assess
- Go for your training (in stages, if you cannot go for all at once)
- Start cases and don't get discouraged
- Stand your ground/get your HOD's support
- Perform cases with proctor or spend some time at an MICS center (depending on your training and skill level). Take courses
- After experience: define differentiator, and go for it
- Be inclusive
- Educate and share it

TABLE 3.2	Basic instruments to get started with the first level of MICS (usually MVR, AVR)

- Specialized instruments to start with:
  - Shafted tools (Geister, Delacroix-Chevalier, Fehling, etc.)
  - Femoral cannulas (Edwards, Medtronic, etc.) and long cardioplegia cannula
  - LA retractor
  - LA retractor holder
  - Aortic cross-clamp (Chitwood, Cygnet, etc.)
  - Adequately sized Finocietto retractor with blades of different sizes or specialized wound retractors
- Key enablers for optimization of the learning curve
  - Knot-tying instruments, e.g. knot pusher, Cor-Knot
  - With experience, expand your armamentarium (camera, tower, others)

The investment required to start a minimally invasive program does not have to exceed 50,000 euros or 75,000 USD initially: you don't need the full quiver, with camera and video-tower, and the Ferraris of equipment. Below is the minimal set that is required in general, to start doing your first MVRs and AVRs, while MICS CABG may be a bit more costly. These expenses are aimed at getting you started and will cater for the most basic instruments. A differentiation needs to be made upfront, with regard to the various levels of minimally invasive cardiac surgery:

- ∞ Manual, direct vision
- ∞ Manual, camera-enhanced
- ∞ Endoscopic/robotic
- ∞ Hybrid, or trans-catheter

We usually start with level one, and I bet you, if executed correctly and diligently, it will not make too much difference for the patient, pertaining to his overall experience, complications and length of hospital stay. Most probably, it will save any inexperienced surgeon a substantial amount of money. I have witnessed countless novices visiting very advanced third- and fourth-level centers, who are then discouraged upon going back to their countries of origin and finding themselves in front of an unachievable task. So, they never get started in the first place. Our recommendation is: start simple, use simple equipment and begin with the low-hanging fruit (Table 3.2).

The rest of the instruments can be as per usual. Good-quality instruments, such as good-quality cannulas, will of course make a difference, but are not essential if the initial budget does not permit. Often times we scrap and collect whatever we have from various other programs or mixed brands. Other times we borrow from our VATS thoracic surgeons, laparoscopic surgeons, etc. As we go around proctoring in developing countries, we often find ourselves making do with whatever is on the instrumentation table, including longer 9- and 11-inch forceps, Castroviejo needle holders, any needle holders, one-time, hand-held cardioplegia, all sorts of rib retractors, including gynecological equipment! Thus, having a new set of specialized tools for MICS is already a luxury for many a program, and you will be

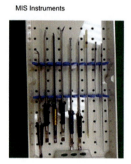
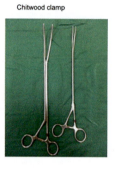
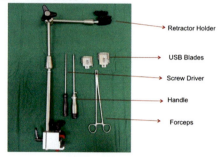

FIGURE 3.4 Sample armamentarium for the start of MICS MVR and AVR, the mainstay of MICS. MIS instruments and the most popular cross-clamp: the Chitwood clamp.

FIGURE 3.5 Commonly used left atrial retractor: the HV retractor, introduced by Hugo Vanermen, with its table fixator.

privileged to have them for a start. In conclusion, you don't have to replicate whatever you see in the preceptorships you visit, in some of the world's most advanced programs (Figure 3.4 and Figure 3.5).

PERIOPERATIVE CONSIDERATION

It goes without saying that the best ingredients for success in any human venture, surgery in particular, are people and their skills, by far. The above paragraphs were dedicated to strategy, be it diplomatic, instrumental or financial. The skill and culture of people involved in the emerging program is, I would say, the most crucial component for success. "Culture eats strategy for breakfast, anytime", is very accurately postulated. You will need pursuant, ambitious, dedicated people around you, i.e. a strong team (Table 3.3).

It is essential to build rapport, and inculcate co-ownership and motivation along the same vector, with all team members. The surgeon is the main driver of such an endeavor, and he cannot be an individualist. Optimally, the surgeon, who is usually the one to be invited by sponsors for both proctorships and preceptorships elsewhere, invites his anesthetist for a start. Next, if a proctorship on site is arranged, make sure the syllabus encompasses the perfusionists and nurses, and adapts to their level of training. There are indeed aspects (to be handled in the respective chapters), which are of particular interest for the anesthetist (intraoperative transesophageal echocardiography skills, double-lumen intubation and single-lung ventilation, etc.), for the nurse (handling a variety of new tools, even robots) and perfusionist (special cardioplegia solutions, dealing with femoral

TABLE 3.3 A harmonious and dedicated team is key
• A dedicated and well-trained team
• Surgeons
• Anesthetists
• Perfusionists
• Scrub nurses
• Train together, progress together
• Lecture them
• Simulate
• Take them for training elsewhere

cannulas and potentially special ones, such as endoballoons, suction techniques, etc.), so make it a team effort. With the advancement of simulation (in-silico) training, opportunities exist to get the whole team trained all at once. The author and team have developed a lengthy syllabus to train teams in an interactive fashion, which we deploy in our preceptorship programs in Singapore, and equivalent programs exist in some of the world's leading programs, consisting of theory lectures, hands-on wet-labs and case observations in the operating theater.

The ultimate key to your success as a budding MICS surgeon is a happy patient: patients with little or no complications, as few as possible mishaps and conversions, happy allies and quiet challengers of the MICS agenda (you will always face those when you start a new program). Our advice there is:

- Be self-aware, self-reflective and play smart!

Don't start with difficult, high-risk and challenging or controversial cases. Don't try and surprise anyone. Get all, friends and foes, to buy into the first few cases, in frequent weekly M&Ms and case discussions; ask humbly and seek support. Make the first successes – and failures – co-owned ones. Even as experience grows, one should not enter the field with fanaticism and rigidity. Clear, well-documented and transparent consent is of equal importance. Don't overpromise, and do not leave any information (particularly that of conversion to median sternotomy) concealed during the preoperative consent-taking. You will often find yourself confronted with the question: "Doc, how many of those have you done?". There is no point concealing your lack of expertise. That's where a proctor is key in the first few cases, or even better, a preceding fellowship in a large-volume center.

Next, patient selection is key. Let's take the mitral valve as an example: it would be of no use to start with a Barlow's, or even a rheumatic heart disease when MV repair is planned, for that matter. How about a straightforward mitral valve replacement in a non-obese, non-frail, patient with mitral valve stenosis, neither too old nor too young? Or a male patient, not too obese, non-Marfan, with a singular mitral valve pathology (no aortic or tricuspid valve affected) with a P2-prolapse? These are optimal patients to start with (Table 3.4).

TABLE 3.4 Practical tips for a good and safe start

Off to a good start
1. Avoid very flat-chested patients with verticalized hearts
2. Avoid very pyknic habitus with severe obesity and high-standing diaphragms
3. Avoid extremely low EF
4. Avoid severely impaired RV function
5. Avoid very severe PHT (>90 mmHg)
6. Avoid inaccessible, combined pathology
7. Avoid severely calcified aorta
8. Avoid severe adhesions
9. Don't be fanatical about it
10. Don't drive a Ferrari the day you get your driver's license; start simple: easy cases first (M. Mack)
11. MICS heart surgery is … heart surgery first
12. Consider cost
13. Train your team
14. Individualize approach and access
15. Don't compromise the quality of repair for the fancy of MICS
16. Avoid extreme anatomy, very flat-chested tiny patients
17. Not every case needs to be done with an MICS technique (particularly in SE Asia)
18. Don't compromise the quality of revascularization for the fancy of MICS
19. Don't turn minimal into maximal
20. Take good informed consent

ALTERNATIVE APPROACHES

In spite of all Darwinistic professional pressure, evolution of technology and encouragement or competition, there will be hopeless naysayers, whenever a new approach arises. Some 30 years ago, the same controversy was in full bloom in the field of abdominal surgery. Next on the line was thoracic surgery, which faced rigid sceptics and skepticism before galloping into the VATS arena. Can you imagine any abdominal or thoracic surgeon nowadays having any sense of reputation or putting bread on the table if he is oblivious to laparoscopy, or VATS, not to speak of uniport VATS? MICS will eventually go through a similar phase, with growing rates of adoption around the world, and similar scrutiny from conservative circles. With evolving technology, improving techniques on both ends of the cardiology-cardiac surgery spectrum and novel, hybrid procedures entering the market, it is only a matter of time for MICS to be established as the staple of heart treatments.

CAVEATS AND CONTROVERSIES

The final question that arises is: when in the experience journey of a surgeon should one start converting to MICS approaches? How many cases of off-pump CABG, or open mitral valves must one have done, before transiting safely to MICS? Well, there is no definite answer to that, as it depends upon an array of confounding variables:

- ∞ The surgeon's prior experience
- ∞ The tradition and culture of the existing program
- ∞ The environmental, political and logistic pressures
- ∞ The collegial (or lack thereof) environment
- ∞ The nature of your practice (high-volume public hospital vs. low-volume private practice)
- ∞ The surgeon's personal gift of talent and brain-manual axis (Table 3.5)

Let's face it, there are some gifted surgeons out there, who go by the principle "See one – do one – teach one" and very successfully so! There are programs that have been teaching their surgeons in an optimal, very structured way, such as the ones in Aalst, spearheaded by Hugo Vanermen for decades now. And there are others that enjoy such referral inflows and the luxury of high volumes, that allow juniors to start their mitral valve exposure right through a lateral mini-thoracotomy, without prior median sternotomy experience. The authors would refrain from propagating or condemning any of those approaches, as they have all demonstrated reasonable success. That's where a circumspect, sensible and reflective entry by the novice is required, if he does not want to experience fall after fall, right at the start. In our experience,

TABLE 3.5 Frequently faced questions about MICS

To the conservative opponent of MICS
- You don't want to start due to age? Fear of failure? Scrutiny by the colleagues?
- Technical struggle? Cost? Weak team?
- Too small exposure and volume to sustain program? Entropy?
- Have you ever tried MICS and reverted to classical cardiac surgery and why?
- Too many headaches? Effort? Bad outcomes?

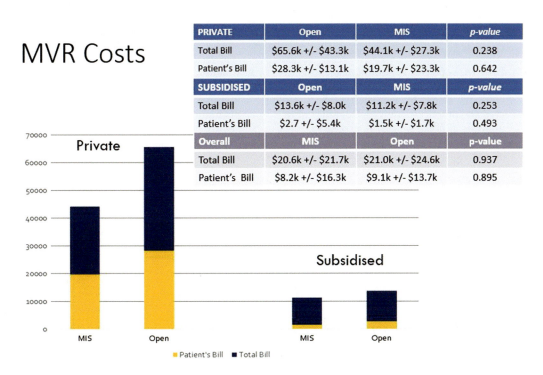

FIGURE 3.6   In spite of more technicalities and tools, MICS MVR renders shorter hospital stays and therefore less cost, as well as a smaller bill burden for the patient. Prices are in Singapore dollars. The graph reflects our starting experience with 50 MICS MVR vs. 50 open MVR cases. With growing experience, the economic benefit of MICS becomes even more obvious. Hence, you may very well find yourself making a good financial case to your hospital or department leadership right at the start of your program, making the initial investment worthwhile.

junior surgeons gather reasonable experience, of – I would say – roughly 100 MVRs before they venture into MICS. What would be the equivalent in MICS CABG? Similar rules apply here. Ruel et al. have delineated such learning curves in their paper in the Innovations journal, indicating a surprisingly short learning curve, provided embedment in a safe, well-standardized environment [1] (Figure 3.6).

WHERE AND HOW TO LEARN

Our team will be at the readers' disposal, via every means of communication, direct or audiovisual, to help you set up your programs successfully, seek and find support routes or point you to the right people and places to do so [2].

Godspeed.

Chapter 3 – How to Set up a Minimally Invasive Program   29

REFERENCES

1. Une, D., Lapierre, H., Sohmer, B., Rai, V., & Ruel, M. (2013). Can minimally invasive coronary artery bypass grafting be initiated and practiced safely? A learning curve analysis. *Innovations, 8*(6), 403–409.

2. Kofidis, T., Chang, G. H., & Lee, C. N. (2017). Establishment of a minimally invasive cardiac surgery programme in Singapore. *Singapore Medical Journal, 58*(10), 576.

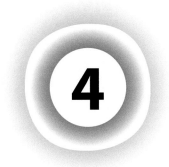

INSTRUMENTATION AND OPERATING THEATER SET UP IN MINIMALLY INVASIVE CARDIAC SURGERY

FAIZUS SAZZAD AND THEO KOFIDIS

INTRODUCTION

Minimally invasive cardiac surgery is a complex operative procedure with its most common concerns over surgical exposure and the potential need for prolonged operative time. All of it translates to overall patient safety. Assiduous instrumentation, appropriate operation theater set up, innovations in perfusion techniques, the use of cerebral oximetry and the development of specialized surgical instruments and robotic technology have changed the outcome of the minimally invasive cardiac surgery.

In this video (Figure 4.1) Dr Glenn Branhart talks about minimally invasive cardiac surgery, which requires expertise on many different levels. Good communication between the surgeon, anesthesiologist and the perfusionist is very important for a successful outcome, which will reflect the level of cohesiveness of the team. Apart from good team work, which is a fundamental component of success, a good start up always needs a good set up.

The operation theater demands specific infrastructure, resources and

FIGURE 4.1 Team work for minimally invasive heart surgery by Glenn Barnhart

instrumentation. It is not completely different from standard cardiac operative rooms, but substantial changes are more in its armamentarium i.e. MICS instruments. It largely varies by the type of proposed surgical procedure. In general a minimally invasive operation theater looks like that shown in Figure 4.2.

HOW TO DO IT/STEP BY STEP

Cardiac surgery has to be provided with the necessary tools to progress to less invasive approaches. The gross subdivision for an initial start up will be as follows:

- ∞ Operating room set up, special instruments and equipment for minimally invasive valve surgery
- ∞ Operating room set up, special instruments and equipment for minimally invasive CABG surgery
- ∞ Operating room set up, special instruments and equipment for transapical or transfemoral aortic valve implantation (Figure 4.3)

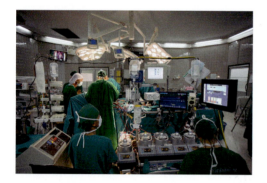

FIGURE 4.2 MICS operating room consists of surgeon, anesthesiologist, surgical assistant, nurses, perfusionist. Additional TEE, shafted and MICS instruments, endoscopic instruments are now a mandatory part of MICS operations.

A. MINIMALLY INVASIVE VALVE SURGERY

The anesthesiologist plays a role by guiding the placement of cannula (i.e. femoral venous cannula) with a transesophageal echocardiography (TEE). It is a mainstay of the procedure which requires excellent echocardiographic skills, usually from cardiac anesthesiologist personnel trained with the technology (Figure 4.4).

I. MINIMALLY INVASIVE MITRAL VALVE SURGERY

Positioning and draping of the patient:

- ∞ Supine position with right side up on gel roll (15° elevation).
- ∞ Drape the patient, exposing the axilla on right side and sternum.
- ∞ Keep both groins exposed.
- ∞ External defibrillator pads to be attached and secured in correct position.

FIGURE 4.3 Introduction to MICS instruments

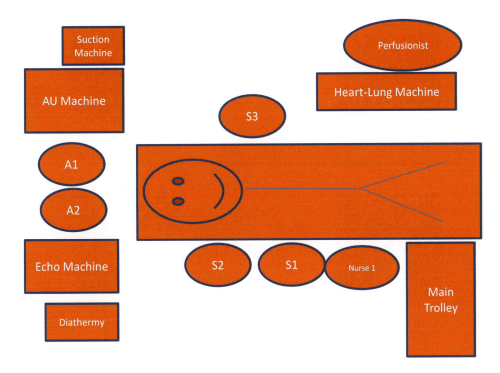

FIGURE 4.4 Operation theater lay out for MICS heart valve surgery.

(Keep the pads away from the surgical field)

Special considerations for operation theater set up:

- ∞ Special instruments and equipment required for the surgery (LA retractor).
- ∞ Always prepare the theater as for the open case.
- ∞ CO_2 insufflation arrangements.
- ∞ Prepare for femoral artery cannulation (Figure 4.5 and Figure 4.6).

II. MINIMALLY INVASIVE AORTIC VALVE SURGERY

Positioning and draping of the patient: always supine.

Draping: expose chest slightly more towards right side (below the right mid axillary line).

Incision: mid sternotomy or right anterior thoracotomy – second intercostal space (Figure 4.7).

B. MINIMALLY INVASIVE CABG SURGERY

Coronary artery bypass grafting is done, gaining access to thoracic cavity and heart itself through left mini thoracotomy incisions, usually a sub-mammary anterolateral incision.

POSITIONING DRAPING OF PATIENT

- ∞ Supine with left side elevated
- ∞ Make sure that operating theater table can be flexed intra-operatively
- ∞ Drape patient, exposing the left side and sternum (Figure 4.8)

SPECIAL CONSIDERATIONS

- ∞ Gather all the special equipment and instruments needed for the surgery
- ∞ Make sure that OR table can be flexed
- ∞ Perfusionist and heart lung machine stand by inside theater
- ∞ Always prepare the theater as for open cases

Chapter 4 – Instrumentation and Operating Theater Set up in MICS

FIGURE 4.5 Minimally invasive mitral valve surgery: tips, tricks and technique.

FIGURE 4.7 Pros and cons of keyhole aortic surgery.

FIGURE 4.6 Step-by-step mini mitral MICS.

FIGURE 4.8 MICS CABG preoperation to incision.

SPECIAL INSTRUMENTS AND CONSUMABLES

- ∞ Rultract Skyhook surgical retractor systems
- ∞ Thoratract retractor
- ∞ Octopus Nuvo Stabilizer
- ∞ Starfish NS Positioner
- ∞ Blower mister
- ∞ Soft tissue retractor
- ∞ US Army retractor
- ∞ Surg-I-Loop Plus Vascular Loop

C. TAVI (TRANSFEMORAL AND TRANSAPICAL)

Transcatheter aortic valve implantation (TAVI), a percutaneous treatment for severe aortic valve stenosis, is increasingly performed worldwide (read more in Chapter 8) (Figure 4.9).

D. FEMORAL CANNULATION TECHNIQUE

Diligent femoral cannulation is a compulsory part of peripheral cannulation technique for establishing cardiopulmonary bypass. "Open" groin cut down was a preferred technique for many years [1]. A mini incision is required in the groin, preferably on the right side due to a relatively straight course towards the right atrium. This technique is a direct cut down to expose the vessel. Some surgeons prefer a distal small incision in the thigh and complete the cannulation by percutaneous tunneling, which is believed to have a lower angle of entry to the femoral vessels and to reduce the risk of infection and bleeding [2]. The main advantage of the open surgical cut down technique is the direct visualization of the femoral vessels and confirmation of the cannulation directly into the femoral vessels and vessel security by a purse-string suture around the cannula [3] (Figure 4.10).

Lately, wire-reinforced and thin-walled, small-diameter peripheral cannulas were introduced into the market, which ensured an improved femoral cannulation outcome. The ultrasound-guided insertion has enhanced the more percutaneous insertion of femoral vessels [4].

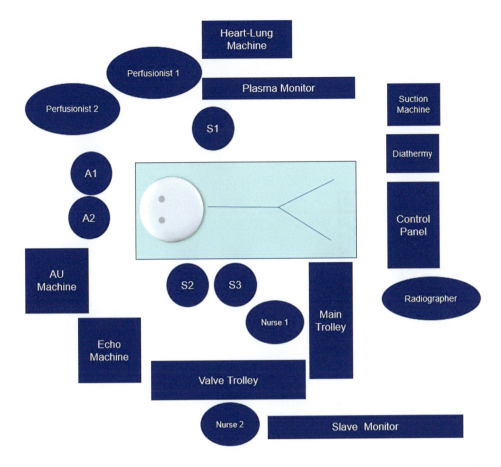

FIGURE 4.9 Operation theater lay out for TAVI.

I. CANNULA SELECTION

Fem-fem bypass requires both arterial and venous cannula to be placed in the proper position. Femoral arterial access may be warranted with or without a distal perfusion of the limb. There are usually single-stage venous cannulas, but a multistage cannula can also be used to drain the blood from SVC and IVC (Figure 4.11).

II. CANNULA SIZING

The diameter of the cannula is proportionate to the amount of blood drainage, but a bigger sized cannula possibly may result in vessel and tissue damage. Similarly the small size may result in poor venous drainage. Hence, the idea is to place a larger and safe cannula based on the size of the peripheral vessel. There are different methods of cannula size estimation. One common method is based on preoperative vascular duplex and use the femoral vessel diameter as given below [5]:

The diameter of the femoral vessel at the insertion point is measured and the circumference of the vessel calculated using the formula πD. The result in millimeters will give the largest French size cannula capable of being passed. For example:

- Measured vessel diameter = 10 mm
- Calculated circumference: $\pi D = 3.1 \times 10$ mm = 31 mm
- Max size of cannula = 31 F

FIGURE 4.10 Percutaneous femoral access.

FIGURE 4.11 Femoral cannulation by Joseph Lamelas.

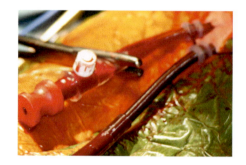

FIGURE 4.12 Open femoral cannulation without distal perfusion.

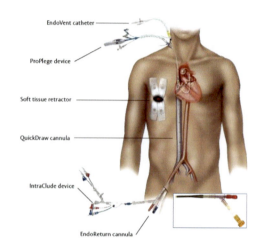

FIGURE 4.13 EndoReturn arterial cannula, integrated to Thruport™ system. Reproduced with permission of Edwards Lifesciences LLC, Irvine, CA.

III. THE INSERTION TECHNIQUE

A small incision open cut down insertion technique is the commonest technique, followed by a serial dilatation using the Seldinger technique [6] using various forms of purse-strings.

IV. CANNULA POSITIONING

During and after cannula insertion the position of wire and cannula should be confirmed by using a transesophageal echocardiography. The site of cannula insertion should also assessed for bleeding or hematoma formation during and at the end of the surgery.

V. CANNULA SECURING

Once the cannulas are correctly positioned they are secured to the skin by using silk sutures. Most of the time the arterial cannula can be secured by needle and suture technique, and the venous cannula with sharp clips. In particular multistage venous cannulas need to be adjusted preoperatively (Figure 4.12).

VI. OPEN CANNULATION FOR ENDOBALLOON (THRUPORT)

a. Thruport

The IntraClude intra-aortic occlusion device is indicated for use in patients undergoing cardiopulmonary bypass. The IntraClude intra-aortic occlusion device occludes and vents the ascending aorta when the balloon is inflated. It has proven itself in redo cases in particular, but also in larger-volume MICS centers (Figure 4.13).

b. Endoballoon

To facilitate transcatheter port access cardioplegia delivery, aortic root venting and

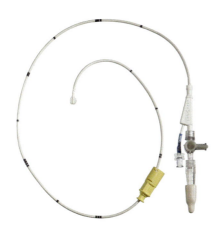

FIGURE 4.14 IntraClude™ is a composite endo-aortic balloon occlusion device. Reproduced with permission of Edwards Lifesciences LLC, Irvine, CA.

pressure monitoring for ascending aorta, the endoballoon has been introduced (Figure 4.14).

VII. PERCUTANEOUS FEMORAL CANNULATION

Device closure is a suitable alternative to femoral cutdown during the establishment of peripheral cardiopulmonary bypass

FIGURE 4.15 Percutaneous and open cannulation.

FIGURE 4.16 ProGlide Perclose Vascular Closure Device.

access by using femoral vessels. The placement of suture-mediated closure devices before cannulation allows surgeons to close the vascular access point percutaneously after removal of the cannula (Figure 4.15, Figure 4.16 and Figure 4.17).

TOOLS/INSTRUMENTS AND DEVICES

GENERAL INSTRUMENTATION

- Cardio basic set
  - Needle holder (Crilewood, microvascular, Mayo Hegar, Debakey), Rampley sponge holding forceps, atraumatic towel clips and Ligaclip applicator
  - Hemostatic forceps (Roberts, Schmidt, Criles, Halstead Mosquito), wire needle holder (Philin)
  - Scissors (Metzembaum, Nelson, Mayo, tubing scissors)
  - Others: Semb clamp, O'Shaughnessy, right-angled, tissue forceps Duval and Stille
- MIS instrument set: common MIS instruments consist of a shafted needle holder, forceps, scissors and knot pusher.
  - Potts scissor
  - ValveGate mini TC needle holder
  - ValveGate mini Potts scissors
  - ValveGate PRO clip applying forceps
    - ValveGate mini IMA holding forceps
  - ValveGate Debakey grasper
  - Chitwood aortic clamp
  - Diethrich atraumatic forceps
  - Felhing aortic punch
  - Ceramo HCR knot punch

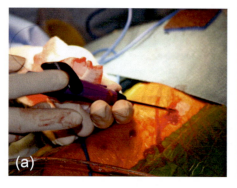
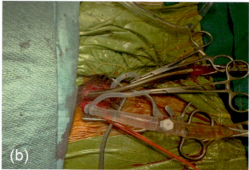

FIGURE 4.17 Operative image showing: A. preoperative placement of the percutaneous closure device and B. femoral cannulation for CPB.

- ∞ Cremao HCR valve scissor
- ∞ MICS suture hook
- ∞ Gester knot pusher
- ∞ Creamo TC HCR needle holder
- ∞ Aescualp long BP handle
- ∞ Estech straight needle holder
- ∞ Retractor US army, double ended
- ∞ Extra-long Debakey forceps
- ∞ Castroviejo needle holder
- ∞ The special instruments are usually divided into the following groups:
  - ∞ MICS shafted instruments: a number of established manufacturers produce long shafted instruments. Figure 4.18 shows a list of Felhing cardiovascular instruments.
  - ∞ MICS retractor system: The most commonly used retractor is the MICS rib retractor. Other retractors are different for MICS mitral valve, aortic valve and MICS CABG surgery. Figure 4.19 demonstrates the way to use different MICS retractors. Figure 4.20 displays a Basic set of instruments.

[Disclaimer: the list of instruments is an example of required MICS instrument; it may vary widely in institutional practice.]

FIGURE 4.18 Felhing cardiovascular Instruments.

FIGURE 4.19 MICS retractor system.

SPECIAL RETRACTORS FOR MINIMALLY INVASIVE MITRAL VALVE SURGERY

USB HV retractor: this left atrial retractor increases the visibility of the mitral valve during minimally invasive surgery. It is designed mechanically to evenly distribute pull force, reduce tissue damage and accommodate the patient's physiology. It also features a high-strength hinge at the distal end actuated by a control arm and knob at the proximal end, as well as an open-walled hinge blade, enabling tissue

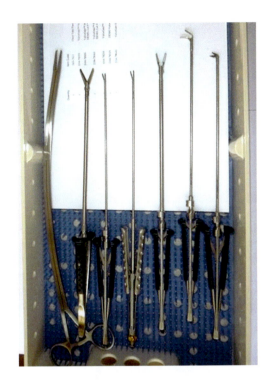

FIGURE 4.20 A set of commonly used MICS long shafted instruments.

FIGURE 4.21 HV USB retractor by Dr Smith.

FIGURE 4.22 HV USB retractor system.

FIGURE 4.23 Rultract Skyhook surgical retractor system.

manipulation while fully exposing the left atrium (Figure 4.21, Figure 4.22, Figure 4.23 and Figure 4.24).

SPECIAL INSTRUMENTS FOR MICS CABG SURGERY

There are different retractor systems available for IMA harvesting that at the same time can be used for MICS CABG. The Rultract Skyhook surgical retractor systems are commonly used: this retractor system is designed for a single operator and can easily be applied to the chest wall. It provides adequate exposure for dissection of the IMA from its origin to the distal bifurcation. Attach to table on the right side of the table, place at right shoulder level of patient and adjust the attachment while harvesting the distal part of IMA (Figure 4.25).

THORATRAK RETRACTOR

The ThoraTrak® MICS Retractor System has multiple interchangeable blades – including various lift blades and thoracotomy blades. This modular retractor system can accommodate various procedures and patient anatomies. It is a reusable, stainless-steel retractor, designed specifically for minimally invasive procedures. It has got different parts: rail clamp, long and short mounting rail, retractor tack and blades (Figure 4.25 and Figure 4.26).

OCTOPUS NUVO STABILIZER AND STARFISH NS POSITIONER

The Octopus Nuvo Tissue Stabilizer is a minimally invasive stabilizer that offers the

FIGURE 4.24 MICS CABG – basics of McGinn set up.

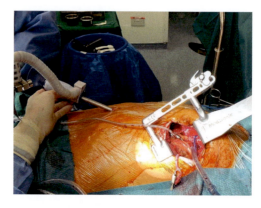

FIGURE 4.26 The ThoraTrak® MICS Retractor is in use for MICS CABG surgery. Long mounting rail placed on right side of patient at mid-thigh level, for Starfish NS. A short mounting rail also placed on left side of patient (not seen in photo) at mid-thigh for Octopus Nuvo.

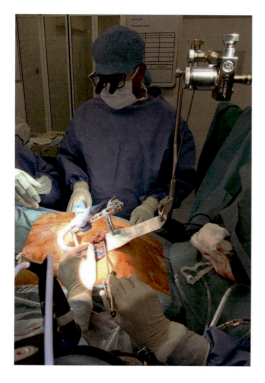

FIGURE 4.25 MICS IMA retractor in use.

FIGURE 4.27 Octopus® Nuvo Tissue Stabilizer by Medtronic.

flexibility, stability and ease-of-use of your OPCAB stabilizer (Figure 4.27). The Starfish NS Heart Positioner provides immediate tissue capture to the apex of the heart for effective positioning (Figure 4.28 and Figure 4.29).

Aortic Clamps for Minimally Invasive Cardiac Surgery:

- ∞ External clamps
- ∞ Rigid clamps
- ∞ Chitwood clamp
- ∞ Glauber clamp
- ∞ Flexible
- ∞ Cosgrove clamp
- ∞ Cygnet clamp
- ∞ Portaclamp
- ∞ Internal clamps
- ∞ Transfemoral clamps
- ∞ Endoclamp
- ∞ Intraclude
- ∞ Transaortic clamps
- ∞ Direct endoaortic clamp
- ∞ Endoclamp with endo direct flow cannula

Chitwood clamp: the clamp is typically used in minimally invasive cardiac procedures including mitral valve replacement or repair. It comes in a range of sizes that can accommodate a variety of patients with

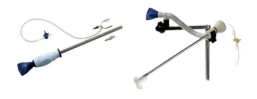

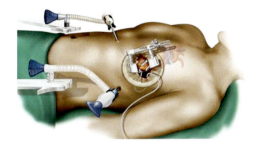

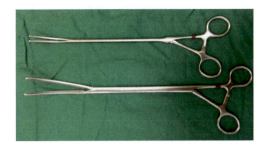

FIGURE 4.30 Chitwood transthoracic aortic cross clamp.

FIGURE 4.31 How to use Glauber clamp.

FIGURE 4.28 Stabilizer for MICS CABG. A. Octopus® Nuvo Tissue Stabilizer B. Octopus® Evolution Tissue Stabilizer C. Schematic for positioning of tissue stabilizer with mounting rails. Reproduced with permission of Medtronic, Inc

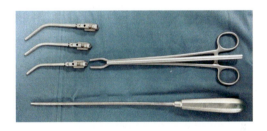

FIGURE 4.32 Glauber aortic cross clamp.

FIGURE 4.29 SCANLAN Chitwood Debakey clamp.

differing sizes and anatomy. The wider jaws of the clamp are more suitable for providing a more secure grip on the aorta without incurring damage to its walls (Figure 4.29 and Figure 4.30).

Glauber clamp: the Glauber Clamp is designed for use in minimally invasive heart surgery to clamp off major vessels such as the aorta and pulmonary artery. The clamp is designed with a mechanism for release and retrieval of the clamp portion, removing the handle and driver portion during the procedure to allow for more room to work (Figure 4.31 and Figure 4.32).

Cosgrove clamp: Cosgrove flex clamp features: strong, flexible, reliable shaft constructed of beaded stainless steel. Enough clamping force for total aorta occlusion without excessive pressure. Wide jaw opening for a secure grasp of all vessels. Gap between shaft beads to allow for thorough cleaning. Familiar ratchet design handle. Slim design, excellent for use in minimally invasive procedures (Figure 4.33 and Figure 4.34).

Cygnet flexible aortic clamp: the flexible neck makes it easier for maneuvering the clamp beyond the surgeon's working field. Additionally, the rigid shaft allows for greater ease in tunneling and

Chapter 4 – Instrumentation and Operating Theater Set up in MICS

FIGURE 4.33 Cosgrove™ flexclamp.

FIGURE 4.35 Cygnet® flexible aortic clamp.

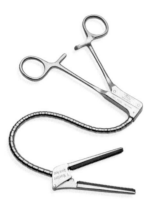

FIGURE 4.34 Cosgrove™ flexible aortic clamp. Reproduced with permission of Edwards Lifesciences LLC, Irvine, CA

placing the clamp in the appropriate position (Figure 4.35 and Figure 4.36).

FEMORAL CANNULA

The venous cannula serves to drain blood from the vena cava and/or right atrium during cardiopulmonary bypass. Commonly used MICS venous cannulas are Edwards Femflex cannulas and Medtronic arterial and venous (multistage) cannulas. Edwards venous cannula, known as the QuickDraw venous cannula, has a thin wall and wire-reinforced design (Figure 4.37 and Figure 4.38).

Medtronic arterial and venous (multistage) cannulas: Medtronic offers the EOPA™ and EOPA 3D arterial cannulas. In 3D model the arterial cannula has additional side holes at the distal end; hence the cannula tip has to be inserted beyond these side ports to a minimum depth. The Bio-Medicus™ NextGen femoral venous cannula has an elongated taper edge introducer. In addition, there is also the DLP™ arterial and venous cannula series for percutaneous and open femoral access (Figure 4.39 and Figure 4.40).

SPECIAL INSTRUMENTS

Rultract Skyhook surgical retractor system: it provides a range of cardio thoracic procedures to get adequate exposure by controlled retraction. Common use: IMA harvesting, re-sternotomy assist, redo cardiac surgery (xiphoid entry), subxiphoid pericardial procedures, pediatric/ASD, minimally invasive procedures, VATS sternal elevation, sternal elevation for NUSS procedure and panniculectomy assist (Figure 4.41 and Figure 4.42).

Blower mister: there are some accessories required for most open heart surgery as well as MICS. One of these is a blower mister. It's a fluid and gas (commonly CO_2) used to produce a blood-cleaning mist to clear the operative field during CABG surgery. The AccuMist® device has a malleable shaft and control on the handpiece (Figure 4.43 and Figure 4.44).

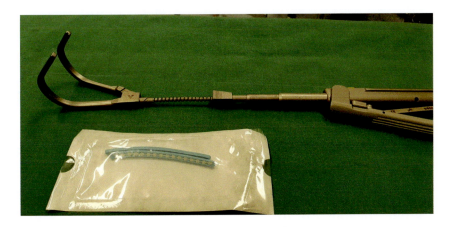

FIGURE 4.36   Cygnet® flexible aortic clamp – Novare Surgical Systems, Inc., Cupertino, CA.

FIGURE 4.37   Edwards peripheral cannula for CPB.

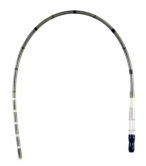

FIGURE 4.38   QuickDraw™ cannula. Reproduced with permission of Edwards Lifesciences LLC, Irvine, CA

FIGURE 4.39   Medtronic arterial and venous cannula.

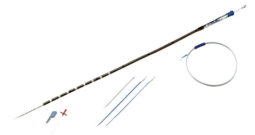

FIGURE 4.40   The Bio-Medicus™ NextGen femoral venous cannula with insertion set. Reproduced with permission of Medtronic, Inc.

FIGURE 4.41   Rultract Skyhook surgical retractor.

Chapter 4 – Instrumentation and Operating Theater Set up in MICS   43

PERIOPERATIVE CONSIDERATION

- ∞ **Appropriate instrumentation for the type of surgery**: the instrumentation largely depends on the type of surgery and surgical approach. The new armamentarium of minimally invasive heart surgery has widened the scope of different new approaches. The selection of appropriate instruments is a mandatory pre-requisite.
- ∞ **Operation theater set up and team training**: the set up for the minimally invasive operation theater differs from the conventional open heart surgery setup. A proper team orientation and team training should be carried out before a start up of minimally invasive surgery program.
- ∞ **Patient preparation and positioning and draping**: positioning of the patient also varies from procedure to procedure. Importantly, the operation table needs to be breakable. For draping it's important to keep the operative field clear and keep adequate exposure for conversion and emergency sternotomy.
- ∞ **Anesthetic preparation and consideration**: the use of transesophageal echocardiography for proper positioning of cannula and establishment of CPB is essential (Figure 4.45, Figure 4.46, Figure 4.47 and Figure 4.48).

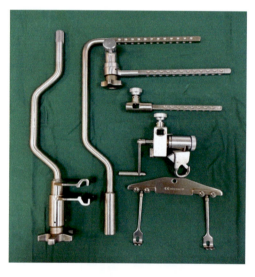

FIGURE 4.42 Rultract Skyhook surgical retractor.

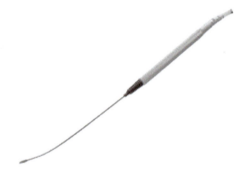

FIGURE 4.44 AccuMist® blower/mister device. Reproduced with permission of Medtronic, Inc.

FIGURE 4.43 AccuMist® device.

FIGURE 4.45 Consideration for MiAVR.

44   Minimally Invasive Cardiac Surgery

FIGURE 4.46 Which valve to choose? By Mayo Clinic.

FIGURE 4.48 MICS CABG set up by Mahesh Ramchandani.

FIGURE 4.47 Cannulation for MiAVR by Michael Mack.

FIGURE 4.49 FLEXHeart Tissue Stabilizer.

ALTERNATIVES

ALTERNATIVE STABILIZERS

AESCULAP FLEXHEART

The FLEXHeart® Tissue Stabilizer is based on one fundamental idea: it unifies stability AND flexibility. The innovative and completely new FLEXHeart® remains stable throughout the entire operation. Thanks to the single-hand control, the surgeon is able to react flexibly to every situation (Figure 4.49).

VALVE XS ATRIUM RETRACTOR

The Valve XS Atrium Retractor provides improved visibility and access for minimally invasive mitral valve procedures. It has a flexible blade joint connection, a blade angle, and position can be achieved to provide optimal valve visibility and access. Additional features: V-shaped blades for easier insertion and better conformance to the atrium, and optional lateral blade – malleable design increases lateral exposure (Figure 4.50).

ALTERNATIVE CANNULATION TECHNIQUE FOR CPB

AXILLARY ARTERY CANNULATION

Arterial perfusion through the axillary artery provides sufficient antegrade aortic flow, is a suitable alternative to femoral access in patients with peripheral vascular disease and is associated with fewer atheroembolic complications (Figure 4.51 and Figure 4.52).

SVC CANNULATION

The cannula for the superior vena cava (SVC) may be placed percutaneously from the neck or directly through the incision.[7-9] The presence of an IVC filter or occlusion of the IVC is a contraindication for femoral venous cannulation and thus for MICS mitral valve cases or MICS CABG cases that require CPB. However, MICS AVR cases can still be performed by placing a low-profile cannula into the right atrium directly through the chest incision [7,8].

FIGURE 4.50 Valve XS Atrium Retractor by B. Braun.

FIGURE 4.52 Cannulation of the superior vena cava for minimally invasive cardiac surgery.

FIGURE 4.51 Axillary cannulation in minimally invasive cardiac surgery.

FIGURE 4.53 CPB cannulation, cardioplegia, vent techniques by Ross Ruel.

CONVENTIONAL CANNULATION

Blood from the vena cava is usually drained via a venous cannula into a reservoir. A two-stage single venous cannula is commonly used, but the use of a selective venous cannula is not rare. A roller pump is used to send the venous blood to a heat exchanger and then into a membrane oxygenator. The oxygenated blood then splits into two separate stream – a left-sided flow passes through a bubble filter and is then delivered to the systemic circulation via ascending aorta (after aortic cross clamp), and a right-sided flow passes through a cardioplegia pump, a cardioplegia heat exchanger and is then delivered into the ascending aorta in the pre-cross clamp area. The operative site blood is returned to the CPB by cardiotomy suction, which then filters and defoams the blood before sending it back to the oxygenator (Figure 4.53).

PERIPHERAL CANNULATION TECHNIQUE

Peripheral cannulation, using the femoral veins and arteries, is occasionally used electively for cardiac surgery when central

FIGURE 4.54 Peripheral cannulation techniques in MICS.

cannulation is not technically possible, for initiating bypass before opening the chest in redo cases, for emergent situations, for aortic surgery and for extracorporeal membrane oxygenation [9] (Figure 4.54).

ROBOTIC SURGERY

Robotic cardiac surgery is done through various incisions in the chest. With the use of minimally invasive robotic instruments and robot-controlled tools, surgeons are able to execute more precise movements within smaller operating fields, and ultimately perform heart surgery in a way that is much less invasive than open heart surgery. The da Vinci surgical system,

FIGURE 4.55 Minimally invasive robotic mitral valve repair.

FIGURE 4.57 Mini-AVR – "Looking Down the Barrel".

FIGURE 4.56 Transcatheter aortic valve implantation by Robert Frankel.

TAVI

Transcatheter aortic valve implantation (TAVI) is a procedure that allows an aortic valve to be implanted by using a guidewire according to the Seldinger technique. The TAVI bioprosthetic valve is guided to and expanded at the site of implantation. Though the technique was initially reserved for use in patients at high risk of surgical valve implantation, it has since been extended to low- and intermediate-risk patients as well [12]. with postoperative patient outcomes comparable to those of conventional surgery [12]. Currently, TAVI is the "standard of care" for the treatment of high-risk and surgically inoperable patients with symptomatic AS [13], and more trials are needed for its role in low- and intermediate-risk patients to be accurately evaluated (detailed description in Chapter 8) (Figure 4.56).

created by Intuitive Surgical, is one such robotic surgical system that is designed for performing complex surgeries through a minimally invasive approach. It has been successfully used in robotically assisted mitral valve repair, demonstrating excellent mid-term outcomes [10]. The technique has also been determined to be safe and effective for use in a multitude of other cardiac surgery procedures, including minimally invasive CABG, cardiac myxoma treatment and atrial septal defects [11] (detailed description in Chapter 9.3) (Figure 4.55).

CAVEATS AND CONTROVERSIES

A. HEART VALVE SURGERY

MIS AVR: APPROACH – UPPER J STERNOTOMY VS RATS

Since 1993, minimally invasive AVR has been shown to have improved outcome like less bleeding, shorter mechanical ventilation time and reduced intensive care and hospital stay. Despite a better outcome there is no general conclusion regarding the surgical approach of minimally invasive AVR via upper J sternotomy and right anterior mini thoracotomy (Figure 4.57).

TAVI VS SAVR

For patients with severe calcific native aortic valve stenosis (AS) with an indication

FIGURE 4.58 TAVR vs SAVR – Dr Reardon on the SURTAVI trial.

FIGURE 4.59 Robotic approach to mitral valve repair: Mayo Clinic Experience.

for valve replacement, intervention options include surgical aortic valve replacement (SAVR) or transcatheter aortic valve implantation (TAVI, also known as transcatheter aortic valve replacement [TAVR]). A multidisciplinary team approach is recommended in approaching patients with severe AS, as the decisions involved here are complex (Figure 4.58).

MIMVR: MINI MVR VS ROBOTIC-ASSISTED

Mitral valve surgery has traditionally been performed through a conventional sternotomy approach. However, comparable repair techniques can be performed in selected patients through a minimally invasive right mini-thoracotomy approach with potentially superior perioperative outcomes. Despite technological improvements in miniature instrumentation and the development of operative techniques through increased experience, the extent of benefits derived from robotic surgery in patients with mitral valve disease remains uncertain [14] (Figure 4.59).

MICS CABG

MIDCAB/Hybrid vs Multivessel CABG in MICS

Minimally invasive multivessel coronary surgery–coronary artery bypass grafting (MICS-CABG) through a small thoracotomy has a well-known advantage over minimally invasive direct coronary artery bypass (MIDCAB), which is, MIDCAB is limited to a single anastomosis of the left internal mammary artery to the left anterior descending artery (LIMA-LAD). On the other hand, hybrid coronary revascularization (HCR) is an approach that aims to combine the best of both cardiology and cardiac surgery by attempting to achieve successful revascularization through the least invasive way possible. HCR was defined as a planned combination of LIMA-LAD with PCI to non-LAD coronary arteries (Figure 4.60 and Figure 4.61).

Robotic CABG

Robotic CABG is a relatively new minimally invasive surgical technique. It is a less invasive alternative to conventional open heart surgery where the breastbone, or sternum, is divided. It uses surgical instruments and a camera attached to the arms of a robotic manipulator device, which are controlled by the heart surgeon via a computer console [15] (Figure 4.62).

Endoballoon vs Transthoracic Clamp

To perform a minimally invasive mitral valve procedure, surgeons either use a transthoracic clamp, which can be applied across the ascending aorta from the right chest, or perform endoaortic balloon occlusion with the endoaortic balloon clamp (Johnson & Johnson Corp, New Brunswick, NJ, USA), which is introduced from the groin into the ascending aorta just above the sinotubular junction (Figure 4.63).

FIGURE 4.60 MICS CABG by Marc Ruel at Re-Evolution Summit (2017).

FIGURE 4.62 Robotic CABG by Francis P. Sutter.

FIGURE 4.61 Why MICS? By Sathyaki Nambala.

FIGURE 4.63 Debate – endoballoon vs transthoracic clamp.

REFERENCES

1. Migliari M, Marcolin R, Avalli L, et al. *Percutaneous Cannulation: Indication, Technique, and Complications. ECMO Extracorporeal Life Support in Adults.* Switzerland AG: Springer-Verlag Italia; 2014.
2. Reeb J, Olland A, Renaud S, et al. Vascular access for extracorporeal life support: tips and tricks. *J Thorac Dis* 2016;8:S353–63. doi:10.21037/jtd.2016.04.42
3. Stulak JM, Dearani JA, Burkhart HM, et al. ECMO cannulation controversies and complications. *Semin Cardiothorac Vasc Anesth* 2009;13:176–82. doi:10.1177/1089253209347943
4. Burrell AJ, Pellegrino VA, Sheldrake J, et al. Percutaneous cannulation in predominantly venoarterial extracorporeal membrane oxygenation by intensivists. *Crit Care Med* 2015;43:e595. doi:10.1097/CCM.0000000000001288
5. Burrell AJC, Ihle JF, Pellegrino VA, Sheldrake J, Nixon PT. Cannulation technique: femoro-femoral. *J Thorac Dis* 2018;10(Suppl 5):S616–S623. doi:10.21037/jtd.2018.03.83
6. Pellegrino V. Alfred ECMO guideline. 2012:1–64. Available online: http://www.alfredicu.org.au/assets/Documents/ICU-Guidelines/ECMO/ECMOGuideline.pdf
7. Franco KL, Vinod HT. *Cardiothoracic Surgery Review.* Philadelphia: Lippincott Williams & Wilkins; 2012, p. 1770.
8. Gravlee GP, editor. *Cardiopulmonary Bypass: Principles and Practice.* Philadelphia: Wolters Kluwer Health/Lippincott Williams & Wilkins; 2008, p. 783.
9. Mongero LB, Beck JR, editors. *On Bypass: Advanced Perfusion Techniques.* New York: Springer Science+Business Media; 2008, p. 576.
10. Liu G, Zhang H, Yang M, et al. Robotic mitral valve repair: 7-year surgical experience and mid-term follow-up results. *J Cardiovasc Surg* 2019; 60:406–412.
11. Kim ER, Lim C, Kim DJ, Kim JS, & Park KH. Robot-assisted cardiac surgery using the da Vinci surgical system: a single center experience. *Kor J Thorac Cardiovasc Surg* 2015;48(2):99.

12. Morís C, Pascual I, Avanzas P. Will TAVI be the standard of care in the treatment of aortic stenosis? *Rev Español Cardiol (English Edition)* 2016;69(12):1131–1134.
13. Lange R, Bleiziffer S, Mazzitelli D, et al. Improvements in transcatheter aortic valve implantation outcomes in lower surgical risk patients: a glimpse into the future. *J Am Coll Cardiol* 2012;59:280–287.
14. Cao C, Wolfenden H, Liou K, et al. A meta-analysis of robotic vs. conventional mitral valve surgery. *Ann Cardiothorac Surg* 2015;4(4):305–314.
15. Cao C, Harris C, Croce B, Cao C. Robotic coronary artery bypass graft surgery. *Ann Cardiothorac Surg* 2016;5(6):594.

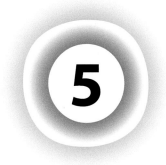

ANESTHESIA FOR MINIMALLY INVASIVE CARDIAC SURGERY

TI LIAN KAH, SOPHIA ANG BEE LENG, WEI ZHANG, LALITHA MANICKAM AND JAI AJITCHANDRA SULE

HISTORY AND INTRODUCTION

The definition of minimally invasive cardiac surgery (MICS) is not universally agreed upon. While traditional cardiac surgery involves median sternotomy, cardiopulmonary bypass (CPB) and cardioplegia, progress in technology has allowed cardiac surgery to be performed using smaller incisions with or without CPB. Therefore, MICS has been variously defined as the avoidance of CPB (e.g. off-pump coronary artery bypass grafting [OPCAB]), use of a thoracotomy to avoid median sternotomy on a beating heart (e.g. minimally invasive direct coronary artery bypass grafting [MIDCAB]) and minimal incision with CPB.

Since the 1960s, the development of cardiac anesthesia has supported the advances made in cardiac surgery practice based on necessity (Figure 5.1). With the advance of minimally invasive cardiac surgery, new challenges emerge in the development of cardiac anesthesia to facilitate the various operations this entails [1]. This chapter will focus on anesthesia for minimal-incision non-robotic cardiac surgery with and without CPB in adult heart surgery (Figures 5.2, 5.3 and 5.4).

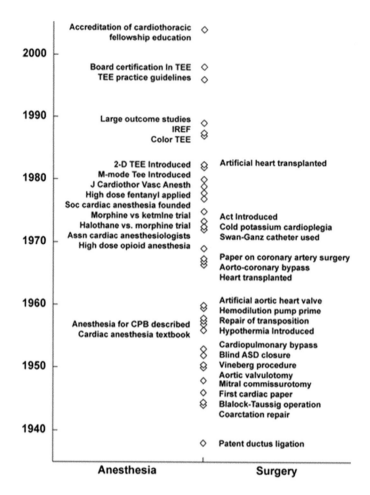

FIGURE 5.1 History of cardiac anesthesiology. (With kind permission from Springer Science+Business Media: Springer Nature, A History of Cardiac Anesthesiology, Edward Lowenstein, J. G. Reves © 2014.)

FIGURE 5.2 Anesthetic challenges in minimally invasive cardiac surgery.

FIGURE 5.3 The importance of the cardiac anesthesiologist.

FIGURE 5.4 Anesthesia implication of mics by Raghu Nalgikar.

FIGURE 5.5 The use of INVOS technology during cardiac surgery.

HOW TO DO IT/STEP BY STEP

MONITORING

Standard monitors are used including a five-lead electrocardiogram, capnograph, central venous pressure, oxygen saturation, core temperature and urine output. If balloon cardioplegia delivery is planned, invasive blood pressure should be measured via both right and left radial arteries. In our practice, pulmonary artery catheters are not routinely inserted. The Bispectral Index (BIS) may be useful to target a value of 50–60 to facilitate fast tracking. Near-infrared spectral (NIRS) analysis may be useful to guide adequate brain protection and leg perfusion in view of cannulation placement (Figure 5.5 and Figure 5.6).

ANESTHETIC PREPARATION

Preoperative discussion with the surgical team is essential to determine cardiopulmonary bypass cannulation, cardioplegia delivery and ventilation strategies. For most cases, only a single venous cannula via the femoral vein is required. The venous cannula is guided from the inferior vena cava (IVC) into the superior vena cava (SVC), and is large enough to allow adequate venous drainage by gravity alone, although a kinetic assist device may also be used. When the right atrium needs to be opened, e.g. for tricuspid valve surgery, or in the presence of an atrial septal defect, then an additional venous drain may be required through the right internal jugular vein to drain the SVC (Figure 5.7). Because of the size of the venous cannula, we typically induce general anesthesia before cannulation and the

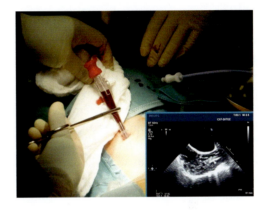

FIGURE 5.6 When neck cannulation is indicated, a Seldinger technique with transesophageal echo (bicaval view 90–120°) is used. (Republished with permission of Oxford University Press, from MMCTS on behalf of the European Association for Cardio-Thoracic Surgery, Nicholas W, Wolfgang H, Fitsum L et al. © 2015; permission conveyed through Copyright Clearance Center, Inc.)

FIGURE 5.7 Biomedicus™ next-gen demo.

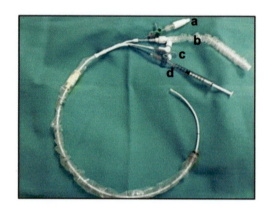

FIGURE 5.8 Percutaneous coronary sinus catheter (Endoplege; Edwards Lifesciences, Irvine, CA). a: Retrograde cardioplegia infusion port, b: Stylet, c: Coronary sinus pressure line, d: Balloon infusion port. (After Hanada S, Sakamoto H, Swerczek M, Ueda K. Initial experience with percutaneous coronary sinus catheter placement in minimally invasive cardiac surgery in an academic center. *BMC Anesthesiol.* 2016;16(1):33.)

cannula is inserted under transesophageal echocardiography (TOE) guidance.

Care must be taken not to shear the vein during insertion by providing for a generous skin cut. The cannula is immediately filled with heparinized saline to prevent clotting.

Depending on the size of the patient, the central venous line can then be inserted either through a double-puncture of the right internal jugular vein, or via the left internal jugular vein which is preferred. The introduction of newer femoral cannulas with perforating holes aligned to the SVC and IVC may obviate the need for a separate SVC cannula, as it allows the surgeon to isolate the right atrium with surgical tape ties.

Percutaneous placement of a coronary sinus catheter is required if retrograde cardioplegia is planned for (Figure 5.8). This may be required in the presence of significant aortic regurgitation or severe aortic atheroma. A dilated coronary sinus should raise the possibility of a persistent left superior vena cava (PLSVC), which would make retrograde cardioplegia ineffective. A bubble test may be performed if there is any suspicion of PLSVC (Figure 5.9).

The coronary sinus catheter should ideally be placed via the right internal jugular vein as this gives the best chance of successful cannulation. Guidance and confirmation of placement can be done with TOE and pressure measurements alone, although the use of fluoroscopy is commonly described

FIGURE 5.9 Initial experience with coronary sinus catheter.

in the literature. The placement success rate is about 90%, but it is time-consuming, adding as much as an hour to anesthesia preparation time [2].

MICS is typically performed with one-lung ventilation although lung isolation may be foregone over lung protection concerns [3]. For mitral, tricuspid and aortic valve surgeries, surgical access is through a right thoracotomy, requiring deflation of the right lung, while the converse is applicable for CABG where surgical access is through a left thoracotomy. We prefer double-lumen tubes

FIGURE 5.10 Management of one-lung ventilation.

FIGURE 5.11 Introduction to single-lung ventilation.

to bronchial blockers because they provide greater positional stability after insertion and allow the use of continuous positive airway pressure if needed (Figure 5.10).

Because of the greater potential of airway trauma associated with insertion of the double-lumen tube and bearing in mind the necessity of changing the tube to a single lumen tube before transfer to the intensive care unit, gentle intubation using a video-laryngoscope is desirable. If a video-laryngoscope is used, then a narrow blade model such as the CMAC is preferable to thicker disposable blades as it affords the most space to navigate the double-lumen tube (Figure 5.11).

External defibrillation pads need to be placed for all MICS procedures and their position should be modified according to the surgical incision planned. Bear in mind that defibrillation may not work well when the lung is deflated, and it may be necessary to reinflate the right lung when performing defibrillation.

TRANSESOPHAGEAL ECHOCARDIOGRAPHY (TOE)

Intraoperative transesophageal echocardiography is essential for guiding the placement and monitoring of lines, evaluating hemodynamic reserve and detecting aortic atheroma. A comprehensive pre-procedural TOE examination is initially performed to confirm the primary pathology, and to look for features that may influence the conduct of anesthesia and surgery [4].

For valvular pathology, the valves are assessed for severity of regurgitation, locating leaflet involvement and calcification of the annulus (Figure 5.12). Sizing of the annulus helps the surgeons decide on the size of the ring or prosthesis. In addition, for mitral valve repairs, potential for systolic anterior motion (SAM) post-repair must be assessed (Figure 5.13).

The left ventricle is assessed for overall function and size, and for regional wall motion abnormalities (RWMA), particularly in the territory of the circumflex artery (Figure 5.14).

The circumflex artery itself may be directly visualized in some patients, and sighting it should be attempted for all cases of mitral valve surgery because of the risk of circumflex artery injury (Figure 5.15).

Right ventricular function is assessed using tricuspid annular plane systolic excursion (TAPSE) (Figure 5.16).

Baseline pulmonary artery systolic pressure is estimated by adding the peak regurgitant pressure of the tricuspid

FIGURE 5.12 Flail P2 leaflet.

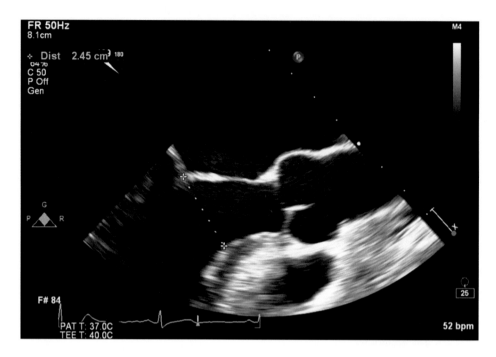

FIGURE 5.13 Assessment for potential for systolic anterior motion: C-Sept distance measurement.

FIGURE 5.14 Regional wall motion abnormality

FIGURE 5.15 Circumflex artery on TOE seen length-wise by rotating probe to the left

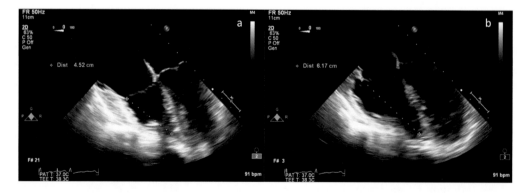

FIGURE 5.16 RV Function: TAPSE measurements in a: Systole and b: Diastole showing a normal value of 16.5 mm.

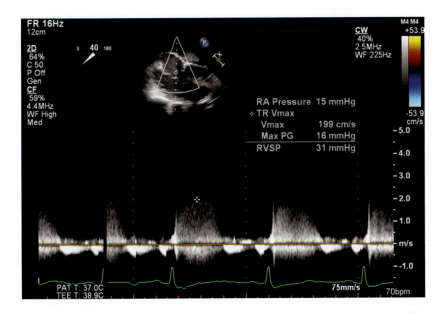

FIGURE 5.17 Pulmonary artery systolic pressure on TEE.

FIGURE 5.18 Wire to SVC

FIGURE 5.20 Cannula in RA/SVC.

FIGURE 5.19 Wire through patent foramen ovale (PFO)

regurgitation to the central venous pressure (Figure 5.17).

The presence of an atrial septal defect or large patent foramen ovale may necessitate placement of the SVC venous drain. Significant aortic atheroma should be highlighted to the surgical team. The bi-caval view is used for positioning of the venous drain. The wire should be visualized emerging from the IVC crossing the atrium to the SVC (Figure 5.18).

Misplacement of the wire across the intra-atrial septum or into the RV is not uncommon and should be looked out for (Figure 5.19). Once the wire is in position, the venous cannula is advanced until approximately 1–3 cm into the SVC (Figure 5.20). This position is ideal to adequately drain the heart. If there is difficulty in advancing the wire into the SVC, the surgeon has the option of leaving the venous drain in the right atrium and advancing it into the SVC by hand after initiation of CPB. The TOE is also used to assist de-airing of the heart. After separation from CPB, a comprehensive TOE examination is repeated.

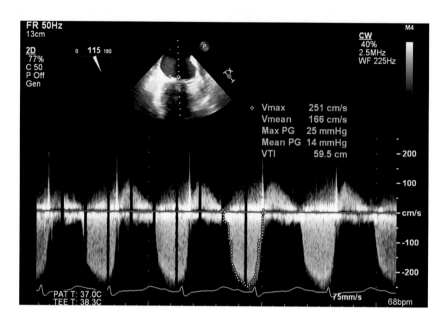

FIGURE 5.21   High gradient across mitral ring on TEE.

FIGURE 5.22   Systolic anterior motion (SAM) after mitral valve repair

FIGURE 5.23   New RWMA

For valvular repair, the presence of residual regurgitation needs to be carefully assessed. An adequate blood pressure (e.g. 130 mmHg systolic) should be achieved with vasopressors to test for residual regurgitation. The gradient across the valve is measured, particularly important when the annulus is downsized with a small ring (Figure 5.21).

For mitral valve repair, the function of the adjacent aortic valve, presence of SAM (Figure 5.22) and RWMA in the circumflex artery territory (Figure 5.23) need to be looked for. For valve replacement, the presence of para-valvular leaks should also be assessed (Figure 5.23) (Figure 5.24).

A para-valvular leak will usually necessitate going back on CPB. While two-dimensional (2D) TOE is useful in diagnosing the leak, three-dimensional (3D) echocardiography using full-volume color Doppler mode is the modality of choice to pinpoint the exact location of the leak (Figure 5.25).

FIGURE 5.24   Paravalvular leak

58   Minimally Invasive Cardiac Surgery

FIGURE 5.25 Paravalvular leak at posteromedial commissure

FIGURE 5.26 Basic perioperative transesophageal echocardiography.

VENTILATION STRATEGY

One lung ventilation is preferred for optimal surgical exposure. There will typically be two periods of one-lung ventilation. The period for surgical exposure prior to initiation of cardiopulmonary bypass is to establish surgical exposure. This period is typically short, and consequently is usually well tolerated. Ventilation is then stopped during cardiopulmonary bypass and resumed on two-lung ventilation for separation of bypass. After successful separation, a comprehensive TOE examination will be performed to assess the adequacy of surgical repair. Then one-lung ventilation will be resumed to allow for surgical hemostasis (Figure 5.26).

PRINCIPLES GUIDING CONDUCT OF ANESTHESIA

- ∞ Fast track and early extubation complement MICS.
- ∞ A low to moderate opioid technique with mild to moderate hypothermia is typically utilized.
- ∞ Full heparinization is employed, with an ACT target of >400 seconds.
- ∞ The potential for conversion to sternotomy should always be kept in mind (Figure 5.27).

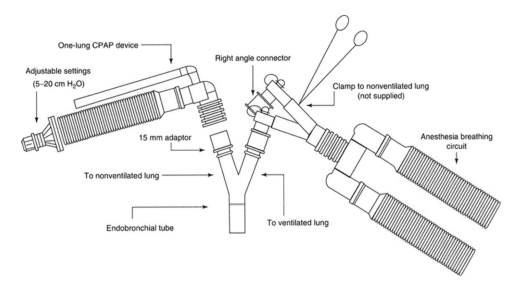

FIGURE 5.27 Application of CPAP to the non-ventilated lung. (With kind permission from Springer Science+Business Media, Springer Nature, Anesthesia for Robotic Cardiac Surgery, Gang, W. and Changqing, G. © 2014.)

TOOLS/INSTRUMENTS AND DEVICES

1. ***Shiley™ Endobronchial Tube (Medtronic, MN, USA)***
   To isolate the lungs physiologically and anatomically during a planned MICS procedure, a double-lumen tube (DLT) is used. DLT can provide selective ventilation to one lung and deflates the other to facilitate operative access (Figure 5.28).

2. ***Video Laryngoscope***
   Currently available video laryngoscopes are the C-MAC® (Karl-Storz, Tuttlingen, Germany) and McGrath™ (Medtronic, MN, USA) (Figure 5.29).

3. ***Transesophageal Echocardiography***
   The X8-2t xMatrix transesophageal transducer from Philips with acoustic design has an increased resolution and tissue filling in 2D and live 3D. The Vivid™ S70N from GE healthcare is a portable, robust cardiovascular ultrasound system with 4D capability (Figure 5.30, Figure 5.31 and Figure 5.32).

4. ***Near-Infrared Spectroscopy***
   Near-infrared spectroscopy (NIRS) is non-invasive and used for real-time monitoring of the oxygen content of

FIGURE 5.30 Vivid S70N Ultra Edition by GE Healthcare.

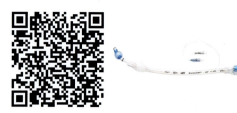

FIGURE 5.28 Shiley™ Endobronchial Tube. ©2020 Medtronic. All rights reserved. Used with the permission of Medtronic.

FIGURE 5.31 3D TEE imaging by Philips.

 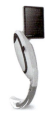

FIGURE 5.29 McGrath™ video laryngoscope. ©2020 Medtronic. All rights reserved. Used with the permission of Medtronic.

FIGURE 5.32 GE Healthcare cardiovascular ultrasound.

FIGURE 5.33 INVOS™ 5001C for cerebral/somatic oximetry.

FIGURE 5.36 On-Q pump from Avanos Medical.

FIGURE 5.34 NIRS from Nonin Medical, Inc.

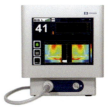

FIGURE 5.37 A. QR code for BIS™ monitor. B. BIS™ monitor. ©2020 Medtronic. All rights reserved. Used with the permission of Medtronic

FIGURE 5.35 FORE-SIGHT NIRS from CAS medical system.

cerebral tissue. INVOS™ (Somanetics Corporation, Troy, Michigan, USA) offers INVOS™ 5001C for cerebral/somatic oximetry. EQUANOX 7600 (Nonin Medical, Inc., Plymouth, Minnesota, USA) and EQUANOX 8004CA (Nonin Medical, Inc., Plymouth, Minnesota, USA) have strong sensors that minimize signal loss. Edward Lifescience has a precise, and tailorable tissue oximetry system and HemoSphere advanced monitoring platform (Figure 5.33, Figure 5.34 and Figure 5.35).

5. **Other tools**
The BIS™ monitor (Medtronic, MN, USA) and On-Q Pump (Avanos Medical Inc., Alpharetta, Georgia, USA) (Figure 5.36 and Figure 5.37).

PERIOPERATIVE CONSIDERATIONS

PRE-ANESTHETIC EVALUATION

The pre-anesthetic evaluation of patient undergoing minimally invasive cardiac surgery is generally similar to that for conventional surgery, including taking relevant history, doing physical examination, reviewing case notes and performing laboratory and imaging investigations. Consideration should be given to the use of TOE, including evaluations for gastric and esophageal diseases that may contraindicate TOE. History of dysphagia, chronic liver disease or upper gastrointestinal bleeding should be elicited and may suggest esophageal webs, esophageal varices and hiatus hernia, which may warrant further investigation.

Pulmonary function should be assessed in anticipation of single-lung ventilation. A history of heavy smoking, chronic cough and chronic pulmonary diseases indicates a need for pulmonary function tests and a baseline arterial blood gas assessment. Significantly abnormal pulmonary function tests, resting hypoxia and hypercapnia may be relative contraindications for single-lung ventilation [5,6] (Figure 5.38).

History of intermittent claudication, rest pain and risks factors for significant atherosclerotic disease such as dialysis dependence, cerebrovascular disease and ischemic heart disease should be elicited. Physical examination should be done to look for signs of peripheral vascular disease. Patients with risk factors may benefit from angiographic and echocardiographic evaluations of the ascending and thoracic aorta. Aortic cannulation may risk dislodging thrombus and atheromatous plaques in these patients.

Records of previous surgeries should be reviewed for airway management difficulties and adverse events. Medications should be reviewed, including antiplatelet and anticoagulant medications, and the patient advised on duration of cessation required before surgery. Airway should be assessed to look for predictors of difficult ventilation and intubation.

Attention should also be paid to factors and features that may affect the viability and success of the surgery, including the presence of pectus excavatum, breast implants, atheroma of the aorta and significant aortic regurgitation. These factors may necessitate changes in the surgical plan, which in turn will influence the anesthesia plan.

POSITIONING

For MICS of the mitral and tricuspid valves, the patient is positioned supine with the right side elevated and with the right arm allowed to fall to expose the lateral chest. The patient's right shoulder should be supported appropriately to avoid stress on the brachial plexus and neck, and head should be turned away from the incision site. Although this position appears to stretch the brachial plexus, we have not experienced any cases of nerve injury, and there have been no reports of injury in the literature. Pressure points should be padded to reduce risks of nerve compression. The Trendelenburg maneuver may be useful in reducing reduction in venous return and maintaining mean blood pressure during intraoperative cardiac manipulations.

For MICS of the aortic valve and MICS CABG (McGinn technique), the patient is placed supine or with the left side slightly elevated.

POSTOPERATIVE MANAGEMENT

Postoperatively, patients should be monitored for complications of peripheral cannulation following de-cannulation, including retrograde aortic dissection. Arterial cannulation sites are at risk for arterial thrombosis, whilst movement of the arterial catheter can dislodge atheromatous plaques resulting in systemic emboli that can produce damage to end organs such as the brain, kidneys and liver. Venous cannulation sites are at risk of thrombosis, putting patients at risk of pulmonary embolism [7].

FIGURE 5.38 Who should not have a mini-mitral procedure?

Adequate pain control with multimodal analgesia is important for faster recovery. Options include parenteral opioids, intercostals injections of local anesthetics, paravertebral blocks and thoracic epidural anesthesia. The use of paravertebral blocks avoids the potential problems of epidural abscess and spinal hematoma that are linked with epidural blocks, while providing similar pain relief with fewer complications [8]. In addition, paravertebral blocks facilitate extubation in the operating room if so desired [9].

Continuous paravertebral catheters such as the On-Q pump (Avanos Medical Inc., Alpharetta, Georgia, USA) inserted within the subpleural space during the time of surgery may alleviate the use of postoperative opioid analgesia and associated side effects (Figure 5.39).

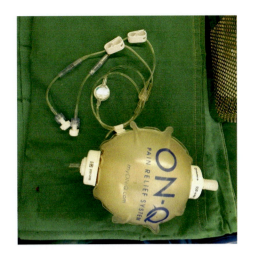

FIGURE 5.39 On-Q pump (Avanos Medical Inc., Alpharetta, Georgia, USA).

ALTERNATIVE APPROACHES

An alternative ventilation strategy, particularly for patients with poor lung function and right ventricular (RV) dysfunction, is to avoid the use of one-lung ventilation altogether. This can be achieved by lung retraction and intermittently stopping ventilation. However, the benefit of this strategy has to be balanced against the poorer surgical exposure as well as the necessity to commence CPB earlier to facilitate surgical dissection, adding to CPB time. Excessive lung retraction may also lead to mechanotrauma. These factors may negate the benefits of avoiding one-lung ventilation.

CAVEATS AND CONTROVERSIES

ONE-LUNG VENTILATION

The period of one-lung ventilation for hemostasis may be challenging. One-lung ventilation for MICS markedly reduces the PaO_2/FiO_2 ratio after termination of CPB [10]. Atelectasis, mechanotrauma from lung retraction and biotrauma from the inflammatory response to cardiopulmonary bypass all contribute to ventilation-perfusion imbalance, leading to desaturation [11]. The supine or minimally rotated position of the patient also accelerates the desaturation effect of one-lung ventilation. Acidosis, hypoxia and hypercarbia contribute to pulmonary hypertension and right heart strain. Myocardial stunning adds to right heart failure.

In our institution, we adopt lung-protective ventilation from the outset to reduce these complications. These include using small tidal volumes of 6 ml/kg, pressure-controlled ventilation, PEEP of 5–10 mmHg, increased FiO_2 as necessary and an increased respiratory rate. We tolerate a higher end-tidal CO_2, and accept a lower SaO_2 of >94% after cardiopulmonary bypass, rather than increasing tidal volume or airway pressure which may promote barotrauma and volutrauma to the lungs. In addition, minimizing the lengths of time that one-lung ventilation is used should be a priority for both anesthesia and surgery.

If ventilation difficulties occur during one-lung ventilation, the TOE can assist by providing information on pulmonary artery pressure and RV function. Ventilatory difficulties may quickly lead to hemodynamic instability and measures to reduce pulmonary pressures and increase RV function, such as the use of vasopressin to increase systemic pressure and milrinone or inhaled nitric oxide to reduce pulmonary vascular resistance, should be considered (Figure 5.40).

POSTOPERATIVE PULMONARY EDEMA

In the postoperative period, unilateral pulmonary edema has been reported to occur in up to 25% of patients [12]. This usually manifests in the first postoperative day, and it is hypothesized that this may be due to lung re-expansion injury or ischemic-reperfusion injury. Phrenic nerve injury which occurs more commonly in MICS than in conventional surgery may also play a role, but can be avoided by surgical identification and avoidance of the phrenic nerve [13]. In addition, gentle handling of the lung by the surgeon as well as gentle re-expansion may reduce the development of postoperative pulmonary edema. The use of Dexamethasone may also prevent it [14] (Figure 5.41).

SURGICAL TECHNIQUES IMPACTING ANESTHESIA

DEAIRING OF THE HEART

Surgical manipulation of the heart is limited, making deairing of the heart, particularly air trapped in the apex of the left ventricle, very difficult. In our practice, we routinely use carbon dioxide in the surgical field, and this has proved effective in markedly reducing the amount of air trapped in the heart. This is an essential part of the procedure because excessive air emboli have been implicated in poor neurological outcomes in early series of MICS [13].

MITRAL VALVE AND RIGHT MINI-THORACOTOMY

The surgeon's tactile feel is more remote due to the longer instruments. As such, there is greater potential for inadvertent damage to the circumflex artery or the leaflet of the aortic valve during sewing of the prosthetic mitral valve or annuloplasty ring, especially for a heavily calcified annulus, and injury to the left atrial appendage such as during cross clamping, which may cause profound bleeding necessitating emergent conversion. It is also imperative to be mindful of pericardial stay sutures prior to reinflating the right lung, as rapid inflation against

FIGURE 5.40   One-lung ventilation.

FIGURE 5.41   Pulmonary edema after MICS.

FIGURE 5.42 Long-acting cardioplegia.

taut sutures may result in catastrophic lung injury (Figure 5.42).

LONG-ACTING CARDIOPLEGIA

In MICS, surgeons may opt to use a long-acting cardioplegia solution such as Custodiol as it affords them a much longer time between runs of cardioplegia [15]. Custodiol provides myocardial ischemic protection for up to 3 hours. Unlike conventional cardioplegia, Custodiol hyperpolarizes the membrane of the cardiac myocytes, leading to arrest in diastole. Custodiol performs as well as conventional cardioplegia in the main outcomes of mortality, low cardiac output syndrome, inotrope use and hospital length of stay. However, it is associated with a higher rate of ventricular fibrillation, occurring as frequently as 20% of the cases, which needs to be aggressively addressed with defibrillation shocks, lidocaine and amiodarone. RV protection may also be inadequate, and patients with existing RV dysfunction are prone to worsening of their RV function. If large doses of Custodiol are given, it can potentially lead to hyponatremia, although the clinical effect of this is uncertain.

MICS CABG

PROXIMAL ANASTOMOSIS

During proximal anastomosis through the left anterolateral mini-thoracotomy, the stabilizer is placed over the pulmonary artery trunk or right ventricular outflow tract, depressing it in a left postero-inferior direction to create enough space for the anastomosis [16]. This may lead to acute RV strain. The use of milrinone has been advocated to support the RV during this period. A systolic blood pressure of 90–100 mmHg should be targeted as this makes the aorta more supple for the surgeon to work with. Occasionally, the surgeon may ask to check the SVC as the tape around the aorta may occlude it – this can easily be done by viewing the SVC inflow in the mid-esophageal bicaval TOE view.

REINFLATING THE LEFT LUNG

The use of moderately high PEEP and larger I:E ratios on the right lung pushes the heart to the left towards the surgeon, which facilitates surgery. It is therefore important to reinflate the left lung gently and under direct vision to prevent compromise of the left internal mammary to left anterior descending artery (LIMA-LAD) anastomosis by the expanding lung tissue.

RESEARCH, TRENDS AND INNOVATION

One of the main contributions of cardiac anesthesia to MICS is the use of intraoperative TOE, which is essential for the safe practice of modern cardiac surgery, let alone MICS, and even certain non-cardiac surgery. The increasing use of TOE by more qualified professionals warrants the development of updated clinical practice guidelines and training programs, especially in the era of MICS [17] (Figure 5.43).

With advancing TOE probe and software technology, the modern cardiac anesthetist is increasingly able to diagnose complications and residual cardiac defects. The role of the anesthetist will continue to grow with the increasing use of percutaneous technology

FIGURE 5.43 Intraoperative TEE review and evolution.

FIGURE 5.46 European Association of Cardiothoracic Anesthesiology.

FIGURE 5.44 Prevention of pulmonary edema after MICS.

FIGURE 5.45 The heart team of cardiovascular care.

and hybrid operating rooms [1]. The increasing use of advancing monitoring technology such as BIS and NIRS, and familiarity of the anesthetist with MICS techniques will also fuel new research into areas of safety and efficacy, including preventing specific complications associated with MICS. An example is the prevention of re-expansion pulmonary edema using a neutrophil elastase inhibitor [18] (Figure 5.44).

Another advancement since the SYNTAX trial and advent of transcatheter aortic valve implantation (TAVI) is the growing emphasis on the establishment of a "heart team" [19].

The inclusion of the cardiac anesthetist in this multidisciplinary team may be increasingly beneficial in the planning and implementation of MICS, and contribute to the growing future of cardiac anesthesia (Figure 5.45).

WHERE AND HOW TO LEARN

1. European Association of Cardiothoracic Anaesthesiology Courses: EACTA offers interactive cases i.e. case to case analysis; TOE training; an exchange training program and board-certified examination (Figure 5.46, Figure 5.47 and Figure 5.48).
2. Philips Live 3D TEE course: The education resources on the Philips product and clinical application.
    - ∞ Advanced Perioperative 3D TEE – Mitral Valve
    - ∞ Live 3D TEE in Structural Heart Disease
    - ∞ Comprehensive 3D Imaging and Interventions of the Mitral Valve
    - ∞ Perioperative 3D TEE
    - ∞ Live 3D Transesophageal Echo in the Operating Room
3. Open Anesthesia: This is an online learning platform sponsored by IARS. This platform consists of lectures, videos and presentations on TEE.

FIGURE 5.47 Philips Live 3D TEE course.

FIGURE 5.48 Open anesthesia course in basic TEE.

REFERENCES

1. Malik V, Jha AK, Kapoor PM. Anesthetic challenges in minimally invasive cardiac surgery: are we moving in a right direction? *Ann Card Anaesth.* 2016;19(3):489–97.
2. Hanada S, Sakamoto H, Swerczek M, Ueda K. Initial experience with percutaneous coronary sinus catheter placement in minimally invasive cardiac surgery in an academic center. *BMC Anesthesiol.* 2016;16(1):33.
3. Blank RS, Colquhoun DA, Durieux ME, et al. Management of one-lung ventilation: impact of tidal volume on complications after thoracic surgery. *Anesthesiology.* 2016;124(6):1286–95.
4. Jha AK, Malik V, Hote M. Minimally invasive cardiac surgery and transesophageal echocardiography. *Ann Card Anaesth.* 2014;17:125–32.
5. Wang JS. Pulmonary function tests in preoperative pulmonary evaluation. *Respir Med.* 2004;98(7):598–605.
6. Najafi M, Sheikhvatan M, Mortazavi SH. Do preoperative pulmonary function indices predict morbidity after coronary artery bypass surgery? *Ann Card Anaesth.* 2015;18(3):293–8.
7. Ramchandani M, Al Jabbari O, Abu Saleh WK, Ramlawi B. Cannulation strategies and pitfalls in minimally invasive cardiac surgery. *Methodist Debakey Cardiovasc J.* 2016;12(1):10–3.
8. Esper SA. Bottiger BA, Ginsberg B, et al. Paravertebral catheter-based strategy for primary analgesia after minimally invasive cardiac surgery. *J Cardiothorac Vasc Anesth.* 2015;29:1071–80.
9. Neuburger PJ, Ngai JY, Chacon MM, et al. A prospective randomized study of paravertebral blockade in patients undergoing robotic mitral valve repair. *J Cardiothorac Vasc Anesth.* 2015;29:930–6.
10. Kottenberg-Assenmacher E, Kamler M, Peters J. Minimally invasive endoscopic port-access intracardiac surgery with one lung ventilation: impact on gas exchange and anaesthesia resources. *Anaesthesia.* 2007;62(3):231–8.
11. Wang G, Gao C. Anesthesia for robotic cardiac surgery. In: Gao C, ed. *Robotic Cardiac Surgery.* Springer: New York, 2014:15–29.
12. Tutschka MP, Bainbridge D, Chu MW, Kiaii B, Jones PM. Unilateral post-operative pulmonary edema after minimally invasive cardiac surgical procedures: a case-control study. *Ann Thorac Surg.* 2015;99:115–22.
13. Cheng DCH, Martin J, Lal A, et al. Minimally invasive versus conventional open mitral valve surgery. a meta-analysis and systematic review. *Innovations.* 2011;6:84–103.
14. Keyl C, Staier K, Pingpoh C, et al. Unilateral pulmonary oedema after minimally invasive cardiac surgery via right anterolateral minithoracotomy. *Eur J Cardiothorac Surg.* 2015;47:1097–102.
15. Edelman JJB, Seco M, Dunne B, et al. Custodial for myocardial protection and preservation: a systematic review. *Ann Cardiothorac Surg.* 2013;2:717–28.
16. McGinn Jr JT, Usman S, Lapierre H, et al. Minimally invasive coronary artery bypass grafting. Dual-center experience in 450 consecutive patients. *Circulation.* 2009;120(Suppl 1):S78–S84.
17. Duque M, Machado HS. Intraoperative transesophageal echocardiography: review and evolution. *J Anesth Clin Res.* 2013;7:634.

18. Yamashiro S, Arakaki R, Kise Y, Kuniyoshi Y. Prevention of pulmonary edema after minimally invasive cardiac surgery with mini-thoracotomy using neutrophil elastase inhibitor. *Ann Thorac Cardiovasc Surg.* 2018;24(1):32–39.

19. Holmes DR Jr, Rich JB, Zoghbi WA, Mack MJ. The heart team of cardiovascular care. *J Am Coll Cardiol.* 2013;61(9):903–7.

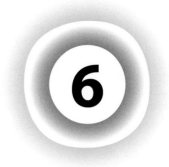

SURGICAL APPROACHES IN MINIMALLY INVASIVE CARDIAC SURGERY

FAIZUS SAZZAD AND THEO KOFIDIS

HISTORY OR INTRODUCTION

When given a choice, most patients are likely to choose minimally invasive heart surgery because of a number of benefits such as faster recovery, improved cosmesis, less blood loss and less arrhythmia. It is also a safe surgical option for patients with previous sternotomy. Although traditional median sternotomy has been the preferred approach for open heart surgery for years, the transition to minimally invasive cardiac surgery (MICS) after 1990 has altered this trend, and the degree of invasiveness has since switched from mini to micro over the years (Figure 6.1).

Despite concern over the duration of operation, technically demanding conduct, a steep learning curve, reproducibility of the innovative techniques, additional expenditure and uncertainty in the possibility of safe outcomes, a better picture of the present status of MICS is surely given by the lower degree of invasiveness in its current practice. Careful patient selection and an appropriate surgical plan and selection of surgical approach are the factors that determine the final outcome (Table 6.1).

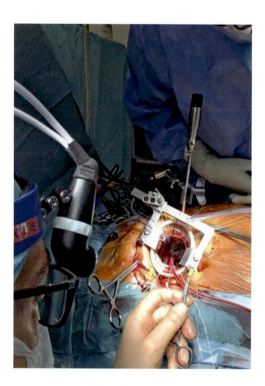

FIGURE 6.1 Minimally invasive heart valve surgery.

TABLE 6.1 Degrees of surgical invasiveness as proposed by Carpentier and Loulmet [1].
Carpentier–Loulmet Classification
Level I
Mini-incision (10–12 cm)
Direct vision
Level II
Micro-incision (4–6 cm)
Video-assisted
Level III
Micro or port incision (1–2 cm)
Video-directed
Level IV
Port incision with robotic instruments
Video-directed

FIGURE 6.2 Adopting an MICS platform by Joseph McGinn.

HOW TO DO IT/STEP BY STEP

PATIENT SELECTION, PREPARATION AND POSITIONING

Patient preparation varies according to the type of minimally invasive surgery. As of the current practice there are only a few limitations for overall MICS surgery [2]. A judicious way to select appropriate patients is to find patients NOT fit for MICS. A proper pre-surgical operative plan with viable alternatives and backup plans leads to a successful outcome [3] (Figure 6.2).

A. Pre-operative considerations

All patients should be assessed on an individual basis with a proper history and physical examination. Chest X-ray, CT-thorax/abdomen/pelvis (CT-TAP) and ECHO (TTE and TEE) should be carefully reviewed.

B. Patient positioning

Positioning of patient for heart valve surgery

The position for aortic and mitral valve surgery varies. Mostly the position is supine with some postural changes, namely supine position with leftward rotation of <15 degrees for MV/TV: Some degree of elevation of the right chest will expose the right axilla. This helps in placing a trans-thoracic cross clamp in the proper position. Supine with a roll under the shoulders for AVR: This is the

FIGURE 6.3 Minimal invasive aortic and mitral valve surgery (STS University).

FIGURE 6.4 Positioning and marking a thoracotomy.

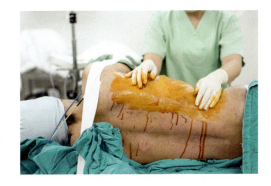

FIGURE 6.5 The lateral decubitus position.

FIGURE 6.6 MIS CABG by Joseph McGinn.

FIGURE 6.7 MMCTS tutorial for MIS CABG.

commonest position for most of the cardiac surgical procedures [4,5]. The video (Figure 6.3) provides a more in-depth discussion on the process of minimally invasive aortic and mitral valve surgery.

Positioning of patient for a trans-axillary approach

The trans-axillary approach requires a lateral decubitus with proper positioning of arm, waist and legs [6]. The link in Figure 6.4 contains a tutorial on positioning the patient in the lateral decubitus position and how to mark out the thoracotomy incision (Figure 6.5).

Positioning of patient for MIS CABG

A left thoracotomy approach for multivessel CABG or MIDCAB is usually used. The position is supine and exposes both lower extremities for vessel harvesting, as can be seen at the link in Figure 6.6, which provides a general insight into minimally invasive CABG. A substantial discussion has been provided in the MMCTS tutorial (Figure 6.7) with patient preparation, marking and required instruments for MIS CABG (Figure 6.8).

Positioning of patient for robotic surgery

The patient is usually positioned supine with varying degrees of rotation and exposed areas for the port accesses for robotic arms, as can be seen briefly in this introductory video on robotically assisted cardiac surgery (Figure 6.9).

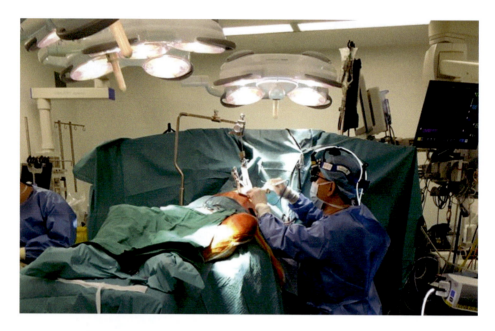

FIGURE 6.8   IMA harvesting and MIS CABG with patient's position on the surgical table.

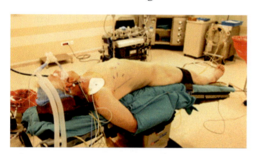

FIGURE 6.9   Position of patient prior to a robotic-assisted cardiac surgery. (After Gullu AU, Senay S, Alhan C. Robotic-assisted cardiac surgery: an overview. *OA Robotic Surgery* 2014 Feb 10;2(1):3, © 2014 OPAL).

Placement of external defibrillator pads

The use the self-adhesive external defibrillator pads is as described by Bojar [7]; just remember to modify according to the site of thoracotomy. Avoid placing them over the anticipated site of incision. Preferably the pads should be covered by transparent film dressing (e.g. Tegaderm™) (Figure 6.10 and Figure 6.11).

Patient selection

Surgical exposure can be difficult with obesity and chest wall abnormalities (e.g. pectus excavatum), and unusual cardiac orientation (left shift) and redo surgery (heart can't be completely mobilized). Concomitant procedures, such as CABG and/or additional valve procedures, may not be amenable to some or all minimally invasive approaches. The link in Figure 6.12 is to a discussion on who should not have MICS mitral valve surgery. The outcomes of minimally invasive mitral valve surgery, and the possible contraindications of minimally invasive approaches are presented.

PERIOPERATIVE CONSIDERATIONS

A. **Intraoperative Considerations and monitoring**

One-lung ventilation (OLV) and proper placement of the double lumen

FIGURE 6.10 Robotic cardiac surgery by Cleveland Clinic.

FIGURE 6.12 Indications and contra-indications for MiMVR.

FIGURE 6.11 Use of self-adhesive external defibrillator pads.

FIGURE 6.13 Double lumen ET tube training.

ET tube should be confirmed by bronchoscopy. Transesophageal echocardiography (TEE) is recommended for guiding cannulation, clearing intracardiac air and assessing the technical results (Figure 6.13).

I. **Placement of double lumen ET tube**: This is required for selective one-lung ventilation which facilitates the minimally invasive surgery approached via thoracotomy incisions.

II. **TEE-guided cannulation**: The cannulation is carried out by using Seldinger technique, i.e. a wire-mounted positioning of the cannula [5]. Transesophageal echocardiography is a direct guide for the placement of the wires and cannula in the correct and required position. The positions of the wire need to be seen in TEE, and then the venous cannula need to be ascertained in expected Position. Sometimes wires can be misplaced in the presence of oval foramen (Figure 6.14).

B. **Incisions and Exposure of the Aortic Valve**

Benefits of minimally invasive incision: Myth vs reality: Well-known benefits of minimally invasive incisions for aortic and mitral valve surgery have been described at the link in Figure 6.15, wherein an expert in the field (Robert J Wiechmann, Mayo Clinic) discusses and reviews the different treatment options that are available for minimally invasive heart surgery (Figure 6.16).

I. **Rationale for MiAVR**

Several minimally invasive techniques have been developed as an alternative to full sternotomy. The rationale for different incisions and the advantages of a right mini-thoracotomy over a mini-sternotomy, highlighted in Figure 6.17, include:

∞ Lower incidence of postoperative atrial fibrillation
∞ Shorter ventilation time, intensive care unit stay and hospital stay

FIGURE 6.14 TEE guided cannulation for peripheral CPB.

FIGURE 6.15 Minimally invasive aortic valve replacement myth vs fact.

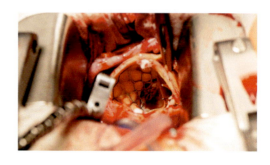

FIGURE 6.16 Exposure and implantation of sutureless aortic valve via minimally invasive approach.

FIGURE 6.17 The case of right thoracotomy by Mattia Glauber.

Additionally, the advantages of a right anterior mini-thoracotomy over conventional aortic valve surgery are:
- ∞ Lower incidence of postoperative atrial fibrillation and blood transfusion
- ∞ Shorter ventilation time and postoperative length of stay (Figure 6.18)

II. **Approaches for Minimally Invasive Aortic Valve Surgery (MiAVR)**
   i) **AVR via Upper Hemisternotomy**

   Upper hemisternotomy is one of the common approaches for AVR. Hemisternotomy offers a versatile access to supra-cardiac structures, with a shorter learning curve compared to anterolateral thoracotomy (Figure 6.19).

   a) **Upper J ministernotomy**: The cannulation technique and use of differently designed instruments can be applied for a similar hemisternotomy approach. A central cannulation with conventional instruments is also feasible (Figure 6.19). Alternatively, upper "J" hemisternotomy and manubrium limited sternotomy can be done with a fem-fem peripheral cannulation (Figure 6.20 and Figure 6.21).

   b) **Upper T ministernotomy**: The approach involving the use of an upper T mini-sternotomy in aortic valve surgery is a new minimally invasive technique for cardiac surgical procedures (Figure 6.22).

FIGURE 6.18 Different options in hemisternotomy.

FIGURE 6.20 Central cannulation, flexible cross clamp from Maimonides.

FIGURE 6.21 Upper "J" mini sternotomy, fem-fem cannulation, conventional clamp.

FIGURE 6.22 Upper "T" mini sternotomy.

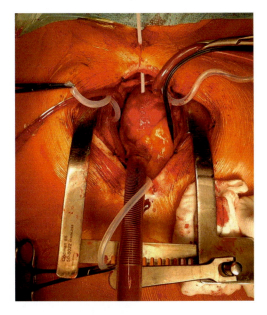

FIGURE 6.19 Operative set-up for surgical access to aortic valve via upper hemisternotomy.

ii) **AVR via Right Anterior Thoracotomy (RAT)**

Minimally invasive aortic valve replacement (MiAVR) performed through a right anterior thoracotomy (RAT) or upper hemisternotomy (UHS) is becoming a favored approach. Advantages, such as less bleeding and faster recovery due to the incision technique, make the right anterior thoracotomy a preferable approach, yet it is technically more challenging (Figure 6.23).

Ex-articulation of the second rib and ligation of the mammary artery (fem-fem cannulation) are achieved in the "Miami Method"; this was created by Joseph Lamelas [8] (Figure 6.24).

iii) **AVR via Right infra-axillary mini-thoracotomy**

Traditional minimally invasive approaches for aortic valve replacement (AVR) have not necessarily shown cosmetic superiority over standard median sternotomy. Right infra-axillary mini-thoracotomy for isolated AVR

FIGURE 6.23 RAT: Step by step by Marc Ruel.

FIGURE 6.26 Right infra-axillary mini-thoracotomy AVR (ACS).

FIGURE 6.24 Standard technique in RAT, "Miami Method".

has a more pronounced cosmetic outcome, especially in young adult woman. The scar is vertical and very lateral (Figure 6.26).

iv) **AVR via Supra-Sternal Approach**

Direct aortic deployment of a sutureless aortic valve eliminates the need for the sternotomy or thoracotomy and enables greater ease of placement of the epiaortic camera system, which is a new technology available for aortic valve surgery via the supra-sternal approach, and has been shown to be able to ensure a safe and successful surgical aortotomy closure [9]. In 2016, the initial experience and first clinical case on the use of the CoreVista® system was described by Dapunt et al., where the authors concluded that the technology was effective in achieving a successful direct aortic TAVR via a supra-sternal approach, with absence of procedural

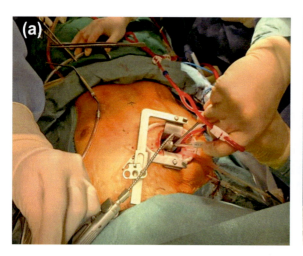
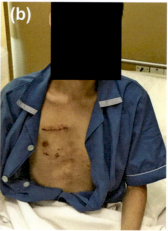

FIGURE 6.25 Illustration of the surgical field of a RAT AVR showing (A) the ascending aorta is crossed clamped with a flexible aortic clamp; (B) healed RAT incision.

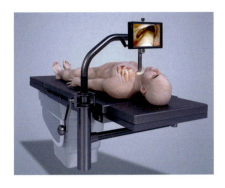

FIGURE 6.27 Exposure via supra-sternal approach by using The CoreVista® system. Reproduced with permission of CardioPrecision Ltd, UK.

FIGURE 6.29 AVR via right para-sternal approach.

FIGURE 6.28 Suprasternal approach for AVR.

FIGURE 6.30 Preparation of patient and cardio-pulmonary bypass.

or periprocedural mortality (Figure 6.27 and Figure 6.28).

v) **AVR via Right Para-sternal approach**

The right para-sternal approach is an old technique and nowadays not used for isolated aortic valve replacement [10]. AVR via right parasternal thoracotomy with moderate hypothermia is safe and effective for the avoidance of re-sternotomy-related complications. This approach is more challenging for the beginner; it can be greatly facilitated by new technology, such as COR-KNOT® and rapid-deployment heart valves (Figure 6.29).

C. **Incisions and Exposure of the Mitral Valve**

Approaches for minimally invasive mitral valve surgery (MiMVR): As alternatives to standard sternotomy, surgeons have developed innovative, minimally invasive approaches for conducting mitral valve surgery (Figure 6.30).

I. *MiMVR via Right Mini thoracotomy*
　i) **Preparation of the patient**
　　∞ Double lumen endotracheal tube
　　∞ US-guided insertion and TEE-guided positioned wire-reinforced right internal jugular/superior vena caval (SVC) cannula
　　∞ Trans-thoracic cross clamp or endoaortic balloon occlusion (Figure 6.30)
　ii) **Patient Positioning**
　　After anesthetic preparation, the patient is positioned

Chapter 6 – Surgical Approaches in Minimally Invasive Cardiac Surgery　　77

FIGURE 6.31 MiMVR – tips for safely negotiating the learning curve.

FIGURE 6.33 Robotic MiMVR animation.

FIGURE 6.32 MiMVR – step by step by Timothy H Williams.

supine with a small pillow under the right scapula to elevate the right hemithorax 15–20. The OR table is rotated moderately toward the left and placed slightly in reverse Trendelenburg position (Figure 6.31 and Figure 6.32).

iii) **Incision**

A small 4-cm right inframammary skin incision, when coupled with a few separate millimeter-sized stab incisions and a small groin incision, will provide sufficient access and visualization to perform complex mitral valve repair procedures [11]. In men, this incision should be placed just below the nipple and predominantly medially. In women, the incision is placed in the breast crease and soft tissue dissection is carried cephalad toward the chest wall. In general, a third/fourth intercostal space entry is optimal.

II. *Robotic MiMVR*

There are a number of potential benefits of robotic technology, including decreased morbidity and improved recovery; some have suggested a prohibitively high cost [12]. Patient selection and positioning are important factors for proper surgical access. A general robotic operating room outline is reflected in Figure 6.33, Figure 6.34 and Figure 6.35.

D. **Approaches for Minimally Invasive Coronary Artery Bypass Surgery (MiCABG)**

I. *MIDCAB*

Patient selection criteria for MIDCAB have been expanding since its inception. The commonest indication for MIDCAB is proximal LAD lesions, which are not suitable for angioplasty or failed catheter-based intervention [14]. Although there are no absolute contraindications for MIDCAB, relative contraindications are intramyocardial course of the vessel and small diffusely diseased vessel (Figure 6.36).

II. *Minimally invasive multivessel CABG*

There are five step in MICS CABG (please read detailed description in Chapter 12):

1. A small thoracotomy on the left side of the chest is placed just under the nipple.

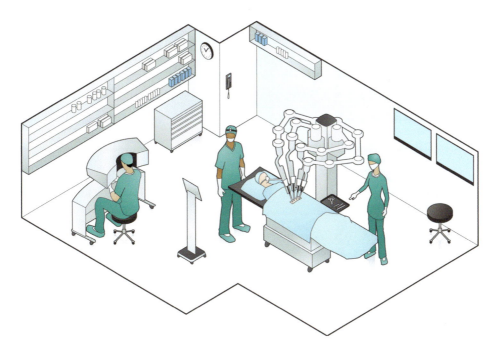

FIGURE 6.34　Operating room organization for robotic MiMVR.

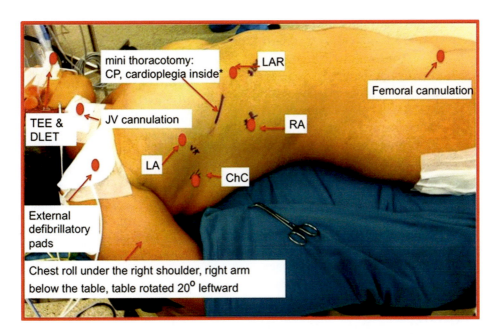

FIGURE 6.35　Patient positioning, marking and general set-up. LAR: Left atrial retractor; CP: Camera port; RA: Right arm; LA: Left arm; TEE: Transesophageal echocardiography; DLET: Double-lumen endotracheal tube; ChC: Chitwood clamp [13]. (Republished with permission of Oxford University Press, from *MMCTS* on behalf of the European Association for Cardio-Thoracic Surgery, Senay S, Gullu AU, Kocyigit M et al. © 2015.)

FIGURE 6.36 MIDCAB – step by step.

FIGURE 6.37 MiCABG technique overview, Medtronic.

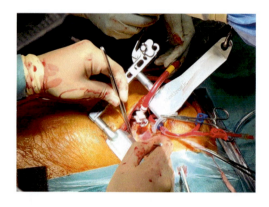

FIGURE 6.38 Mini-thoracotomy incision in MICS CABG in heart arrest. Use of the ThoraTrak® MICS Retractor System.

FIGURE 6.39 EVH – surgical approach.

2. The thoracotomy is usually at the left fourth intercostal space along the upper border of the lower rib to avoid the neurovascular injury. The ribs are retracted by using standard rib-retractors. A rib-resection usually not required.
3. Surgical approach step by step: LIMA is harvested through the thoracotomy. The LSV from the leg in this MICS CABG is usually harvested by endoscopic vein harvesting (EVH).
4. The bypass surgery is performed using all arteries or a combination of arteries and long saphenous veins (LSV).
5. The MiCABG surgical techniques (Figure 6.37 and Figure 6.38).

III. *Endoscopic vein harvesting (EVH)*
Traditionally, LSV is harvested using a lengthy incision in the lower limb. Concerns regarding wound morbidity and patient satisfaction led to the emergence of endoscopic vein harvesting (EVH) [15] (Figure 6.39).

IV. *Endoscopic Radial artery harvesting (ERH)*
The development and adoption of endoscopic minimally invasive saphenous vein harvesting prompted its application to the radial artery in an effort to minimize surgical trauma [16] (Figure 6.40).

V. *BITA harvesting using the ThoraTrak retractor system*
The ThoraTrak® MICS Retractor System has multiple interchangeable blades – including various lift blades and thoracotomy blades – to accommodate various patient anatomies.

VI. *Off-pump MICS CABG with BITA via left small thoracotomy under direct vision*

FIGURE 6.40   ERH – surgical steps.

FIGURE 6.41   BITA harvesting in MiCABG.

FIGURE 6.42   Multivessel minimally invasive coronary bypass by Mahesh Ramchandani.

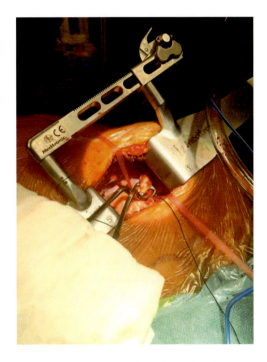

FIGURE 6.43   Construction of proximal anastomosis for MiCABG by using conventional side biting clamp.

This video (Figure 6.41) introduced techniques of minimally invasive cardiac surgery coronary artery bypass grafting (MICS CABG) via a single left thoracotomy for revascularization with bilateral internal thoracic arteries (BITA).

VII. **Construction of proximal anastomosis in MiCABG**

Top ends can be constructed by using conventional side biting clamp in MiCABG (Figure 6.42 and Figure 6.43).

VIII. **Aortic non-touch proximal anastomosis**

Proximal anastomosis can be performed without a partial clamp by using the Heartstring and or Passport device (Figure 6.42).

E. **Minimally invasive atrial ablation: Mini Maze**

The main principles of the maze procedure can be applied minimally invasively. A small incision is made and a videoscope is inserted through an incision to view the heart (read more in Chapter 13) (Figure 6.44 and Figure 6.45).

F. **Minimally Invasive LVAD implantation**

As LVADs device are being miniaturized, minimally invasive implantation of LVAD is being popularized. However, the current optimal approach and "standard of care" for the implantation of LVAD is still the full sternotomy [17], although this may change in future, given that minimally invasive techniques are becoming "smaller, yet safer", and may soon

FIGURE 6.44 Mini maze procedure for atrial fibrillation.

FIGURE 6.46 Minimally invasive off-pump implantation LAVD implantation.

FIGURE 6.45 Completely endoscopic microwave ablation of atrial fibrillation.

FIGURE 6.47 Sternotomy sparing LVAD.

replace the more invasive full sternotomy as the new norm for LVAD implantation in suitable patients (Figure 6.46 and Figure 6.47).

G. **Minimally Invasive ASD closure**

Atrial septal defects have usually been surgically closed via traditional sternotomy with low mortality. The technical ease of ASD closure has drawn the interest of surgeons in minimally invasive closure. The difficult part of the procedure is the technical challenge of the cannulation, strategy for cardioplegia, cross clamping and caval isolation (Figure 6.48).

This video (Figure 6.49) describes the steps of a minimally invasive ASD closure, and the relevant technical perils and pitfalls when resources are limited. There are also reported cases of 3D-video- and robot-assisted minimally invasive ASD closure using the port-access techniques [18].

H. **Minimally Invasive combined open heart procedure**

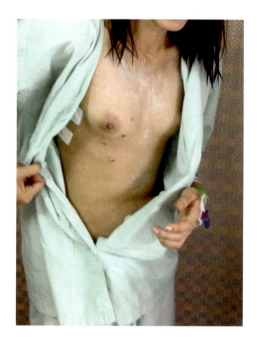

FIGURE 6.48 Postoperative photograph of a 27-year-old woman who was operated via a transaxillary approach.

One of the challenges of minimally invasive heart surgery is combined cardiac procedures. Examples: Right thoracotomy can provide access for multiple concomitant procedures, such as

FIGURE 6.49   MiASD – step by step, by CTS.net.

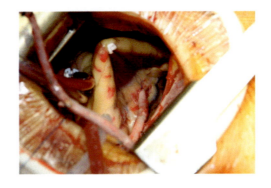

FIGURE 6.50   Minimally invasive combined open heart procedure using right thoracotomy.

On the mitral and tricuspid valve repair and/or replacement.

Mitral/tricuspid and a right sided bypass can be done via right thoracotomy (Figure 6.50).

TOOLS/INSTRUMENTS AND DEVICES

AtriClip® (Atricure Mason, Ohio, USA): To place the rectangular-shaped AtriClip device, the surgeon positions it around the left atrial appendage and then "closes" the device. This prevents blood from flowing into and out of the left atrial appendage, thereby reducing the risk of thromboembolism (Figure 6.51 and Figure 6.52).

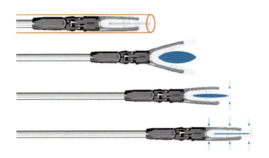

FIGURE 6.51   The AtriClip Pro-V Device application for LAA occlusion. Reproduced with permission of AtriCure, Inc. © 2020.

FIGURE 6.52   AtriClip Pro-V Device.

ALTERNATIVE APPROACHES

An alternative to all MICS surgical access is the conventional median sternotomy approach. Multiple co-morbidity and very high-risk patients, who are not fit for MICS surgery, are the potential candidates for the conventional approach. This can be evaluated by a proper pre-operative evaluation and planning. Seldom, an MICS may need to convert due to an emergency situation, which again requires conventional sternotomy access. However, there are some alternatives and modifications of the current

MICS practice. It varies from surgeon to surgeon and depends on institutional practice.

ALTERNATIVE CAVAL ISOLATION FOR RIGHT HEART

To overcome the challenges of right heart surgery, particularly in terms of caval isolation procedures in patients with enlarged and pressurized atria, alternative techniques can be used. The authors described (Figure 6.53) an alternative technique of caval isolation by using contralateral groin to place and occlude IVC with a Coda balloon (Cook Inc, Bloomington, IN).

TRANS-AREOLAR ENDOSCOPIC APPROACH

Trans-areolar mitral valve surgery can be done with endoscopic instrumentation. It gives an excellent cosmetic result (Figure 6.54).

FIGURE 6.53 Alternative caval isolation technique.

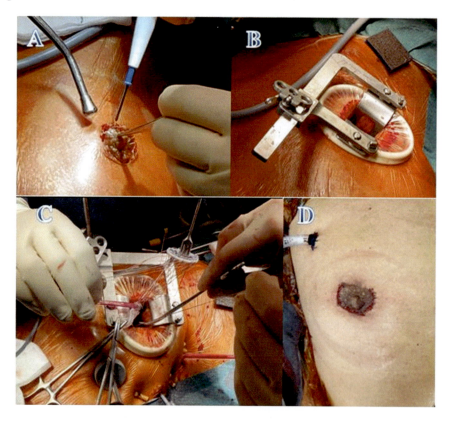

FIGURE 6.54 Photo panel showing trans-areolar MiMVr: A. Trans-areolar incision, B. Exposure, C. Mitral valve repair, D. Skin closure.

CAVEATS AND CONTROVERSIES

POTENTIAL COMPLICATIONS AND TROUBLESHOOTING

A. Saw injury: An oscillating saw is used for mini-sternotomy surgeries with smaller operating fields. The surgeon can feel a sudden "loss of resistance" when the blade has penetrated the posterior table.

B. Bleeding: During right anterior thoracotomy (RAT) for AVR, the right internal mammary artery (RIMA) can be divided and secured. Failure to identify RIMA during RAT may end up in its injury and profuse bleeding. Another potential source of continued bleeding is the pleural surface of the multiple puncture holes around the work port. An "angled dental mirror" or, better, an endoscope can be used to identify such source.

C. Phrenic nerve injury: Phrenic vessels and nerve are usually obvious on the pericardial surface. A 1-inch incision approximately above the phrenic bundle can prevent thermal and mechanical injury.

D. Cardiac injury: During pericardiotomy right atrial injury is not uncommon. The pericardiotomy should be performed after establishment of the CPB. The pacing wires should be in situ before the cross clamps are removed, or at least before coming off CPB. A superficial attachment or insertion is recommended, to avoid RV or RA injury at the time of removal.

E. Rib fracture: Usually, ribs can be detached from the costochondral junction. Re-fixation of the ribs: The best choice is with a screw and rib-plate, alternately thick absorbable suture materials.

F. Surgical emphysema (lung injury): Not common. Thoracotomy layers should be approximated properly (always cut the pericardial retraction stitches before you let the lungs come up at the end of the procedure. This is sometimes forgotten, resulting in potentially serious lung injury).

G. Postoperative pain: Common. Long-acting local anesthetic agents in the intercostal nerves are proven to be a better relief for the patients.

H. Pneumothorax and hemothorax: Small pneumo- or hemothorax are not uncommon. If patient is not symptomatic, they usually recover with conservative management. Rarely, re-exploration is required. Meticulous coagulation checks, clotting factor replenishment and/or increasing the PEEP to 8–10 for 4 hours postop may help cease or tamponade the generalized oozing.

REFERENCES

1. Ritwick B, Chaudhuri K, Crouch G, Edwards JRM, Worthington M, and Stuklis RG. Minimally invasive mitral valve procedures: the current state. *Minim Invasive Surg.* 2013; 2013: 679276. doi: 10.1155/2013/679276
2. Santana O, Xydas S, Williams RF, Wittels SH, Yucel E, and Mihos CG. Minimally invasive valve surgery in high-risk patients. *J Thorac Dis.* 2017; 9(Suppl 7): S614–S623. doi: 10.21037/jtd.2017.03.83
3. Ailawadi G, Agnihotri AK, Mehall JR, Wolfe JA, Hummel BW, et al. Minimally invasive mitral valve surgery I: patient selection, evaluation, and planning. *Innovations (Phila).* 2016; 11(4): 243–50. doi: 10.1097/IMI.0000000000000301

4. Kirmani BH, Jones SG, Malaisrie SC, Chung DA, and Williams RJ. Limited versus full sternotomy for aortic valve replacement. *Cochrane Database Syst Rev.* 2017; 10(4): CD011793. doi: 10.1002/14651858.CD011793.pub2
5. Rodriguez E, Malaisrie SC, Mehall JR, Moore M, Salemi A, Ailawadi G, Gunnarsson C, Ward AF, and Grossi EA. Economic workgroup on valvular surgery. Right anterior thoracotomy aortic valve replacement is associated with less cost than sternotomy-based approaches: a multi-institution analysis of 'real world' data. *J Med Econ.* 2014; 17(12): 846–52. doi: 10.3111/13696998.2014.953681
6. Ito T, Maekawa A, Hoshino S, and Hayashi Y. Right infra-axillary mini-thoracotomy for aortic valve replacement. *Ann Cardiothorac Surg.* 2015; 4(1): 57–58. doi: 10.3978/j.issn.2225-319X.2014.11.11
7. Bojar RM, Payne DD, Rastegar H, Diehl JT, and Cleveland RJ. Use of self-adhesive external defibrillator pads for complex cardiac surgical procedures. *Ann Thorac Surg.* 1988; 46(5): 587–8. DOI:10.1016/s0003-4975(10)64710-8
8. Lamelas J. Minimally invasive aortic valve replacement: the "Miami Method". *Ann Cardiothorac Surg.* 2015; 4(1): 71.
9. Dapunt OE, Luha O, Ebner A, Sonecki P, Spadaccio C, and Sutherland FW. New less invasive approach for direct aortic transcatheter aortic valve replacement using novel corevista transcervical access system. *JACC: Cardiovasc Interv.* 2016; 9(7): 750–753.
10. Nakayama T and Asano M. Aortic valve replacement via a right parasternal approach in a patient with a history of coronary artery bypass surgery and pericardiectomy: a case report. *Surg Case Rep.* 2019; 5: 39. doi: 10.1186/s40792-019-0598-5
11. Botta L, Cannata A, Bruschi G, Fratto P, Taglieri C, Russo CF, and Martinelli L. Minimally invasive approach for redo mitral valve surgery. *J Thorac Dis.* 2013; 5 (Suppl 6): S686–S693. doi: 10.3978/j.issn.2072-1439.2013.10.12
12. Lehr EJ, Guy TS, Smith RL, Grossi EA, Shemin RJ, Rodriguez E, Ailawadi G, et al. Minimally invasive mitral valve surgery III: training and robotic-assisted approaches. *Innovations (Phila).* 2016; 11(4): 260–267. doi: 10.1097/IMI.0000000000000299
13. Senay S, Gullu AU, Kocyigit M, Degirmencioglu A, Karabulut H, Alhan C, et al. Robotic mitral valve replacement. *Multimed Man Cardiothorac Surg.* 2014; 2014: pii: mmu016. doi: 10.1093/mmcts/mmu016
14. Cremer J, Schoettler J, Thiem A, Grothusen C, and Hoffmann G. The MIDCAB approach in its various dimensions. *HSR Proc Intensive Care Cardiovasc Anesth.* 2011; 3(4): 249–253. PMID: 23440055
15. Raja SG and Sarang Z. Endoscopic vein harvesting: technique, outcomes, concerns & controversies. *J Thorac Dis.* 2013; 5(Suppl 6): S630–S637. doi: 10.3978/j.issn.2072-1439.2013.10.01
16. Kim G, Jeong Y, Cho Y, Lee J, and Cho J. Endoscopic radial artery harvesting may be the procedure of choice for coronary artery bypass grafting. *Circ J.* 2007; 71(10): 1511–5.
17. Patil NP, Popov AF, and Simon AR. Minimally invasive left ventricular assist device implantation: at the crossroads. *J Thorac Dis.* 2015; 7(4): 564–565. doi: 10.3978/j.issn.2072-1439.2015.03.17
18. Reichenspurner H, Dieter HB, Armin W, Costas JS, Zwissler Bruno Reichart B, et al. 3D-video- and robot-assisted minimally invasive ASD closure using the port-access techniques. *Heart Surg Forum.* 1998; 1(2): 104–6.

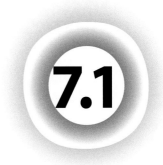

THE AORTIC VALVE
Minimally Invasive Aortic Valve Replacement. The Right Anterior Minithoracotomy

IGO B RIBEIRO AND MARC RUEL

INTRODUCTION

Aortic valve replacement (AVR) remains the gold standard for the treatment of aortic valve stenosis. AVR has traditionally been performed through a complete midline sternotomy. Alternative minimally invasive approaches have been developed not only to increase cosmesis, but also to allow for homeostasis disarrangements, faster recovery and an expedited return to daily activities. More recently, advances in catheter-based techniques have allowed the treatment of a stenotic aortic valve to be accomplished fully percutaneously. Transcatheter aortic valve implantation (TAVI) has been proved to be as effective as the standard midline sternotomy aortic valve replacement for selected candidates in many randomized clinical trials.[1–4] None of the trials, however, have compared the TAVI strategy to the minimally invasive aortic valve replacement (MICS AVR). Minimally invasive approaches have shown to decrease hospital length of stay, ICU stay, ventilation duration, time to return to work, blood transfusions and renal replacement therapy and increase overall patient satisfaction in comparison to standard AVR. [5–8] Moreover, MICS AVR allows for the

FIGURE 7.1.1 State of the art and future directions by Mattia Glauber.

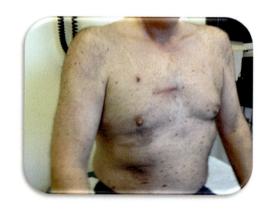

FIGURE 7.1.2 Right minithoracotomy incision: 5-cm transverse incision on the third right intercostal space. Take care to avoid any incision beyond the sternal border as this will not have any benefit on the exposure.

treatment of all-comers, which is not the case for TAVI. Aortic valve anatomic abnormalities such as bicuspid aortic valve, low implantation of coronary arteries and small roots are important limitations of the current TAVI technology. The best MICS AVR approach is a matter of discussion. The upper partial hemisternotomy (UPS) and the right anterior minithoracotomy (RAT) are the two most popular approaches that have survived the scrutiny of time. The UPS does not require the acquisition of advanced skills as it applies the standard skills set through a partial sternotomy with central cannulation and standard techniques. On the other hand, the RAT approach does not disrupt the sternum, being a total sternum-sparing technique. This chapter covers patient selection, the description of the technique and the outcomes of the RAT approach for minimally invasive aortic valve replacement (Figure 7.1.1).

HOW TO DO IT/STEP BY STEP

Our group has used a stepwise intraoperative approach to maximize exposure, decrease the need for specialized instrumentation and allow most patients to be operated on using this technique.

STEP 1: PATIENT PREPARATION AND EXPOSURE

The patient is in supine position on the operating table. Anesthesia is performed with TEE and use of single-lung ventilation through either an endotracheal right bronchial blocker or a double-lumen tube. After draping and prepping, a 5-cm-long skin incision is performed at the third intercostal space that ends at the right sternal border (Figure 7.1.2).

The right internal thoracic vessels are transected between hemoclips. Once the right pleura is entered, the fat tissue on the pericardium is removed through minimalist access between the ribs (Figure 7.1.3).

A small pericardiotomy is then performed to allow direct finger palpation of the level of the aortic valve annulus, which localizes the aortic valve plane in relation to the lower rib. This step is crucial for subsequent optimal visualization. In this regard, the ideal exposure consists of the creation of an operative field that is quadrangular and has the aortic annular plane at its most caudal border and the distal ascending aorta at its cephalad border. This is called "the box principle". Two scenarios are then possible

FIGURE 7.1.3 3cm right anterior thoracotomy AVR by Tristan D. Yan.

FIGURE 7.1.4 RAT-AVR – exposure and the creation of the box field by Mark Ruel.

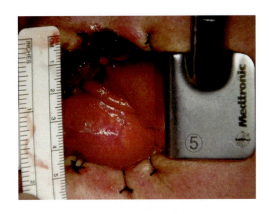

FIGURE 7.1.5 The box field: The box field consists of a quadrangular operative field that has the aortic annular plane at its most caudal border, the distal ascending aorta at its cephalad border, the pulmonary artery at its left side and the level of the right superior pulmonary vein on the right side. Please note the approximately 5-cm-long box field.

after direct finger inspection. First, the valvular plane is at the level of or less than 1 cm from the inferior rib. So, the caudal border of the box field is appropriate. The operative field should expand cephalad, and the upper costochondral joint should be dislocated. Second, the valvular plane is significantly lower than the inferior rib. The lower rib is dislocated to extend the box field caudally. We use electrocautery to luxate the rib at the costochondral joint. Once the rib is dislocated, a rib spreader is inserted. The small pericardial hole is extended proximally and distally, anterior to the ascending aorta and root. At this stage, single-lung ventilation with an increased PEEP on the left lung may improve visualization as it shifts the mediastinum towards the right side. Many, up to ten, pericardial stay sutures are applied at the skin edges and the pericardium to adjust the box field (Figure 7.1.4).

The role of these stay sutures is threefold. First, it allows mobilization of the distal ascending aorta and the aortic valve into the operative field, which defines the contour of the box field. Second, it pulls the aorta towards the incision and at the same pushes the skin edge towards the aorta, decreasing the anteroposterior distance. Third, it pulls the right superior pulmonary vein anteriorly, which facilitates its visualization for subsequent vent insertion. Upon completion of the pericardial stay sutures, the box field is optimized. The aorta is located at the center and displaced anteriorly. The aortic valvular plane and the ascending aorta are at its bottom and top, respectively. These maneuvers create the optimal exposure, the box field (Figure 7.1.5).

Next, the ascending aorta is inspected for calcification via direct palpation and epiaortic scanning, if desired. Table 7.1.1 depicts the key steps for the first part of the operation – exposure.

STEP 2: CPB INSTALLATION – CANNULATION, CARDIOPLEGIA AND LV VENTING

Arterial and venous cannulations are performed via groin cutdown. A 3-cm-long oblique incision is performed 2 cm below

TABLE 7.1.1 Patient preparation and the box field creation – key steps
• Endotracheal intubation with capability for single-lung ventilation. • Five-cm long transverse incision at the third intercostal space. Do not pass the sternal border. • Internal thoracic vessels are hemoclipped and transected. • Small pericardial opening to allow finger exploration to localize the aortic valvular plane. • Shingle the proper rib (third or fourth rib) according to aortic valve place. (See text – usually the third rib is shingled.) • Apply as many stay sutures as required to create the box field (box principle). They centralize the aorta and aortic valve, decrease the anteroposterior distance and expose the right superior pulmonary vein. (See text.) • Single-lung ventilation with increased left-lung PEEP may help optimal exposure pushing mediastinal leftward.

the inguinal ligament. This is usually at or above the inguinal crease. The dissection is carried out, and a single 5-0 polypropylene purse-string suture is placed on both femoral artery and veins. Heparin is given. Venous cannulation is achieved first as the procedure may have to be converted if venous cannulation is not established. Arterial cannulation is achieved next. TEE guides wire and cannula positioning in both cannulations. We use a #25 BioMedicus venous cannula (Medtronic, Inc, Minneapolis, Minn) for all cases, and a femoral arterial cannulation #17 or 19. Femoral arterial cannulation is abandoned in case of minimal resistance on cannula or guidewire placement. Alternative sites for arterial cannulation are direct aortic and axillary cannulation. Active vacuum-assisted venous drainage is used routinely. LV vent cannula is inserted directly through the right superior pulmonary vein in the standard fashion. An antegrade cardioplegia catheter is used in all patients. No retrograde cardioplegia catheter is inserted. Patients are kept normothermic. Once on full cardiopulmonary bypass, stable drainage and hemodynamics, a low-profile Cosgrove malleable shaft cross-clamp is applied in the distal ascending aorta (Figure 7.1.6).

One liter of 16:1 antegrade cold blood cardioplegia is delivered in patients who have less than 2+ AI. Cardioplegia is usually repeated at around 30 min. Some centers have used Custodiol® or Del Nido

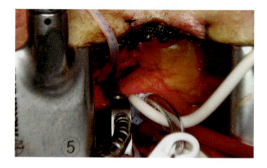

FIGURE 7.1.6 Aortic cross-clamp and cardioplegia catheter: Cosgrove malleable aortic cross-clamp has been applied. Note the cardioplegia catheter at the middle of the ascending aorta and LV venting catheter at the lower right corner.

cardioplegia solutions to allow for a single shot. However, we have used standard cold blood cardioplegia in all cases. For patients who have moderate to severe AI or in whom cardiac arrest was long, direct coronary ostial cardioplegia is delivered. Table 7.1.2 depicts the key steps for the second part of the operation – installation of cardiopulmonary bypass (Figure 7.1.7).

STEP 3: AVR – AORTOTOMY, AORTIC VALVE EXPOSURE AND REPLACEMENT

An oblique aortotomy is performed slightly higher than usual to facilitate closure. Aortic tear at the pulmonic side of the incision can be bothersome, mainly in low aortotomies. Therefore, a transverse arteriotomy should be avoided because of exposure difficulties

TABLE 7.1.2 Installation of cardiopulmonary bypass – key steps

- Right femoral cutdown.
- TEE-guided cannulation and guidewire positioning.
- #25 multistage venous cannulation first. (The inability to achieve proper vein cannulation requires conversion to full sternotomy.) Apply vacuum-assisted drainage.
- No-resistance femoral cannulation. Change cannulation strategy if any resistance.
- Central cannulation and axillary cannulation are alternative sites.
- Direct RSPV venting with malleable multihole cannula.
- Root cardioplegic cannula for induction. Ostial cardioplegia as required.
- Use low-profile Cosgrove malleable shaft cross-clamp at the distal ascending aorta.
- Aortic root cardioplegia for induction. Use direct ostial cardioplegia as needed. Make sure your induction cardioplegia allow an uneventful arrest.
- Before aortotomy, make sure the aorta is fully clamped and collapsed.

FIGURE 7.1.7 RAT-AVR – installation of cardiopulmonary bypass by Mark Ruel.

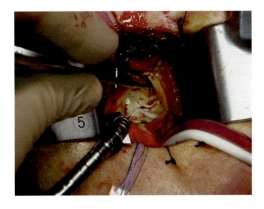

FIGURE 7.1.8 Valve exposure: Three commissure stay sutures are applied and tackled to the drapes to pull the valve up, optimizing the valve exposure.

in this area. Three 4-0 polypropylene sutures are passed in each commissure and tagged to the drapes. These sutures further bring the valve from the bottom of the incision upwards to the middle of the operative field (Figure 7.1.8).

We perform a standard AVR in all our patients, using conventional surgical instruments and standard aortic prosthesis. The aortic valve is removed, and the annulus is decalcified extensively in the usual fashion (Figure 7.1.9). Valve is sized.

Oversizing is a critical mistake. We use interrupted non-pledgeted 2-0 polyester suture technique in all patients (Figure 7.1.10). The valve suture knots are hand-made and tied in the standard fashion in all patients.

Very deep patients or small-handed surgeons may benefit from knot pushers or Cor-Knot®, mainly for the right coronary cusp. Some centers advocate for rapid deployment valves to minimize bypass time. This has not been our experience. The aorta is closed in the standard fashion, using 4-0 polypropylene. Before de-airing maneuvers and the aortic declamping, RV pacing wires are inserted while the heart is arrested. We use two soft peanuts (Lillehei's swab) to pull the RV into the field until a bare muscular free wall is visualized. A needle of adult size pacing wire is further curved to facilitate its insertion. The pacing wire is brought through the skin wherever is suitable. The LV is de-aired through the RSPV vent and the root. Hemostasis is checked. Both lungs are ventilated, and the cross-clamp removed. The patient is weaned from

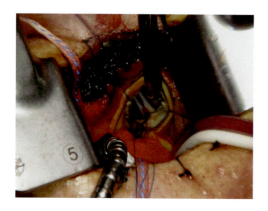

FIGURE 7.1.9 Valve removal and annular decalcification: The aortic cusps have been removed and annular decalcification was performed. See the anterior mitral valve underneath.

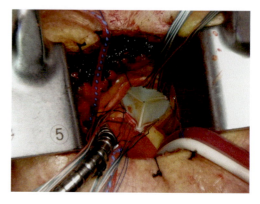

FIGURE 7.1.10 Aortic prosthesis implantation: Aortic bioprosthetic valve sits at the aortic annulus. It was implanted with single interrupted sutures.

cardiopulmonary bypass. A single Blake drain is inserted through the right chest into the pericardial over the aorta. We use a 4-cm-long titanium plate to re-attach the rib. However, suture-based rib re-attachment is likely to provide an acceptable result too. We tackle the pectoralis muscle to the periosteum to avoid bulging and lung herniation during deep respiration. Table 7.1.3 lists the key steps of the third part of the procedure (Figure 7.1.11).

TOOLS/INSTRUMENTS AND DEVICES

MEDTRONIC THORATRAK (MICS RETRACTOR SYSTEM)

The Medtronic ThoraTrak is a retractor used for minimally invasive cardiac surgery that adapts to the patient's anatomy (Figure 7.1.12).

The Cosgrove Quick BendT Flex Clamp is a flexible aortic cross-clamp used in minimally invasive surgery (Figure 7.1.13).

PERIOPERATIVE CONSIDERATIONS

Right anterior minithoracotomy has not gained as much popularity as the UPS approach mainly because of the perceived technical difficulty that requires advanced surgical skills, and tricky preoperative selection and special instrumentation advocated by some groups. However, the benefits of a sternal-sparing operation such as early mobilization, waiver of sternal precaution and lack of wound-healing issues stand out from the UPS approach. With careful patient selection, surgeons can build their experience and pass the learning curve related to this procedure smoothly. Table 7.1.4 lists the patient characteristics that increase the technical complexity of this approach, and, therefore, should be avoided during the learning curve.

These characteristics are not an absolute contraindication to the RAT approach; their absence, however, facilitates the procedure. Probably the only true contraindication at

TABLE 7.1.3 Aortic valve exposure and replacement – key steps

- High oblique aortotomy to facilitate closure. Transverse or low aortotomy should be avoided as bleeding at the pulmonic side may be bothersome.
- Standard decalcification and valve implantation with regular instrumentation. Rapid deployment valve system may be used to decrease pump time.
- Valve sutures on the right coronary cusps may be deep. Cor-Knot® or knot pushers may be required for patients with coronary cusps that are very deep.
- Aortic wall closure with 4-0 polypropylene suture in the usual fashion.
- Pacing wires and chest tube are placed BEFORE cross-clamp removal.
- Root and LV vent de-airing as usual with TEE guidance.
- Single chest tube is inserted through the right pleura into the pericardium, resting next to the aorta.
- Titanium plate or stainless-steel wire to re-attach the rib.
- Pectoralis major muscle is tackled to the periosteum to avoid paroxysmal bulging during deep respiration.

FIGURE 7.1.11 RAT-AVR – aortic valve exposure and replacement by Mark Ruel.

least to this technique is ascending aortic calcification to a more than mild degree, which is best dealt with via TAVI or, if unfeasible, full sternotomy.

Preoperative computed tomography (CT) is not mandatory in all-comers. However, many patients have preoperative chest and femoral CT as part of their eligibility for TAVI or other indication. The CT helps to delineate the atherosclerotic burden and ascending aorta calcification. Therefore, a high-risk patient with diffuse atherosclerosis warrants CT to rule out ascending aorta calcification and delineate the cannulation site strategy. Patients with the following characteristics are considered high risk – old age (>80 years old), heavy smoker, CKD, long-standing diabetes, chest wall radiation, chest X-ray with calcified aortic knob and any evidence of ascending aorta calcification during angiogram. Glauber and colleagues have proposed CT criteria for eligibility for the RAT approach

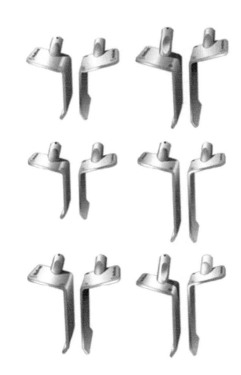

FIGURE 7.1.12A. Medtronic ThoraTrak™ MICS retractor. Reproduced with permission of Medtronic, Inc.

FIGURE 7.1.12B. QR code for Medtronic ThoraTrak.

Chapter 7.1 – The Aortic Valve

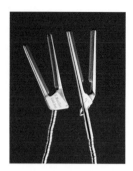

FIGURE 7.1.13A. Cosgrove QuickBend™ Clamp. [Reproduced with permission of Edwards Lifesciences LLC, Irvine, CA.]

TABLE 7.1.4 Challenging patient characteristics for RAT approach

- Previous chest surgery
- Severe COPD
- Documented PVD
- Morbid obesity
- LVOT size <2.0 cm
- Aortic root size <2.8 cm

FIGURE 7.1.13B QR code for Cosgrove flexible aortic clamp. Source: https://www.edwards.com/devices/accessories/atraumatic-occlusion.

FIGURE 7.1.14 RAT-AVR technique by the authors.

based on ascending aorta and valve position (towards the left) and depth.[9,10] However, other authors including our group have found that this should not be a contraindication or even a consideration,[11,12] as intraoperative maneuvers allow for aorta mobilization and proper exposure as described in the how-to-do-it section. This is also exemplified in our technique paper. Figure 7.1.14 has a link to it.[13]

ALTERNATIVE APPROACHES

Upper partial hemisternotomy or full sternotomy are the alternative approaches for surgical aortic valve replacement. The use of a sutureless valve (Perceval valve) can reduce cross-clamp time significantly. For patients who are at moderate or high risk of surgery or patients with severe ascending aorta calcification, TAVI is the alternative solution for aortic valve replacement.

CAVEATS AND CONTROVERSIES

To date, no randomized data has compared the right anterior minithoracotomy approach to either full sternotomy and upper partial hemisternotomy. However, three randomized clinical trials have shown no superiority of UPS over FS on hard endpoints.[14]-[16] In the only contemporary RCT, Nair and colleagues compared UPS to FS (222 patient). UPS did not result in shorter hospital stay, faster

FIGURE 7.1.15 Mini-Stern Trial.

FIGURE 7.1.16 The largest case series of RAT-AVR (Joseph Lamelas' experience).

recovery or improved survival compared to FS.[13] Therefore, in this context, RAT as a full sternum-sparing approach arises as a lesser minimally invasive alternative that may translate to better outcomes.

The Figure 7.1.15 is a link to the Mini-Stern Trial article by Nair et al., which is a randomized controlled clinical trial that compares the duration of postoperative hospital stay and the time to fitness for discharge from hospital after AVR between UPS and full sternotomy.

In a propensity-matched cohort (363 patients in each group), Del Giglio and colleagues compared RAT to FS. They showed similar outcomes in terms of major postoperative complications, including mortality, stroke and bleeding.[17] Phan and colleagues compared RAT to UPS through a network meta-analysis. They had similar results of 30-day mortality, stroke, reoperation for bleeding, wound complication and cross-clamp and CPB time.[6] Similarly, Deo and colleagues performed a contemporary meta-analysis with more than 10,000 pooled patients of high-volume centers (>50 patients) comparing the RAT and UPS to FS. They found that mortality and stroke were comparable between minimally invasive and conventional AVR. RAT had longer CBP time, less atrial fibrillation and shorter hospital stay compared to FS and UPS.[8]

Since the publication of Murzi and collegues[18] that showed an increased incidence of stroke in retrograde arterial perfusion compared to antegrade (5% vs. 1%), concerns about femoral cannulation for MICS have existed. However, this high incidence has not been seen in other publications. LaPietra and colleagues[19,20] reviewed 1501 patient who had minimally invasive valve surgery. Of those, 90.5% had femoral arterial cannulation. The incidence of stroke was only 1.53% (Figure 7.1.16).

Lamelas and colleagues have published their series on 1018 isolated aortic valve replacement via RAT and retrograde cerebral perfusion in 90% of the cases.[12] To date, this is the largest series of isolated RAT-AVR. The mean age of these patients was 72.5 ± 11.8 years and 60% were male. Stroke and mortality rates were 0.8% and 1.3%, respectively. Terwelp and colleagues[5] compared RAT to transfemoral TAVI in a propensity-matched study with 115 pairs. There was no difference in mortality. However, the stroke rate for this comparison favored RAT (0.4% vs. 3.6%) (Figure 7.1.17).

Our group has achieved excellent outcomes using this stepwise approach in all-comers.[13] We have not used special instruments, such as knot pushers and

FIGURE 7.1.17 Minimally invasive approaches to surgical aortic valve replacement: A meta-analysis.

FIGURE 7.1.18 Cardiac surgery, University of Ottawa, Canada.

FIGURE 7.1.19 Cardiac surgery, Cleveland Clinic, Cleveland, Ohio, USA.

rapid deployment valve systems. In 55 patients, there was no mortality or stroke. One (1.8%) patient required reoperation for bleeding through the same incision, one (1.8%) had a conversion to FS, and another one needed a permanent pacemaker. CPB time was 104.8 min ± 27.9, and cross-clamp time was 73.22 ± 22.8. The median length of stay was 6 days (Figure 7.1.18).

RESEARCH, TRENDS AND INNOVATION

Minimally invasive aortic surgery has shown to be safe and effective in the surgical treatment of aortic valve disease with at least equal results to full sternotomy. Full sternum-sparing operations such as the right anterior minithoracotomy have the advantage of early return to work and no need for sternal precautions. Also, the RAT approach has a better cosmesis compared to UPS and FS. Moreover, meta-analyses have shown less atrial fibrillation, shorter hospital stay and less bleeding in the minithoracotomy approach.[6,8] In those series, there is a lack of data on the outcomes of high-risk patients, though they will likely benefit the most from this procedure (Figure 7.1.19).

Right anterior minithoracotomy is a safe and effective approach for the surgical treatment of aortic valve replacement. It can be accomplished in all-comers and can be approached so that it does not require special imaging, a rapid deployment valve system or non-conventional instruments/knot pusher tools. Attention to technical details and the described stepwise approach allows most patients to benefit from this approach (Figure 7.1.20).

FIGURE 7.1.20 Cardiac surgery. University of Miami, FL, USA.

WHERE AND HOW TO LEARN

Department of Cardiac Surgery at University of Ottawa Heart Institute in Canada offers a Residency and Clinical Fellowship in Advanced Heart Surgery. The University of Miami Health System in the USA also provides a structured training on MiAVR. Also, in the USA, the Department of Cardiothoracic Surgery at Cleveland Clinic – Cleveland, Ohio, offers training through a Robotic and Minimally Invasive Cardiac Surgery Advanced Fellowship. NUHS, Singapore, also has a residency and clinical fellowship program on minimally invasive cardiac surgery (Figure 7.1.21).

FIGURE 7.1.21 NUHCS, Singapore.

REFERENCES

1. Adams DH, Popma JJ, Reardon MJ, et al. Transcatheter Aortic-Valve Replacement with a Self-Expanding Prosthesis. *N Engl J Med* 2014;370(19):1790–1798.
2. Leon MB, Smith CR, Mack MJ, et al. Transcatheter or Surgical Aortic-Valve Replacement in Intermediate-Risk Patients. *N Engl J Med* 2016;374(17):1609–1620.
3. Reardon MJ, Van Mieghem NM, Popma JJ, et al. Surgical or Transcatheter Aortic-Valve Replacement in Intermediate-Risk Patients. *N Engl J Med* 2017;376(14):1321–1331.
4. Smith CR, Leon MB, Mack MJ, et al. Transcatheter versus Surgical Aortic-Valve Replacement in High-Risk Patients. *N Engl J Med* 2011;364(23):2187–2198.
5. Terwelp MD, Thourani VH, Zhao Y, et al. Minimally Invasive Versus Transcatheter and Surgical Aortic Valve Replacement: A Propensity Matched Study. *J Heart Valve Dis* 2017;26(2):146–154.
6. Phan K, Xie A, Di Eusanio M, Yan TD. A Meta-Analysis of Minimally Invasive Versus Conventional Sternotomy for Aortic Valve Replacement. *Ann Thorac Surg* 2014;98(4):1499–1511.
7. Glauber M, Miceli A, Gilmanov D, et al. Right Anterior Minithoracotomy Versus Conventional Aortic Valve Replacement: A Propensity Score Matched Study. *J Thorac Cardiovasc Surg* 2013;145(5):1222–1226.
8. Chang C, Raza S, Altarabsheh SE, et al. Minimally Invasive Approaches to Surgical Aortic Valve Replacement: A Meta-Analysis. *Ann Thorac Surg* 2018;106(6):1881-1889.
9. Glauber M, Miceli A, Bevilacqua S, Farneti PA. Minimally Invasive Aortic Valve Replacement via Right Anterior Minithoracotomy: Early Outcomes and Midterm Follow-Up. *J Thorac Cardiovasc Surg* 2011;142(6):1577–1579.
10. Gilmanov D, Solinas M, Farneti PA, et al. Minimally Invasive Aortic Valve Replacement: 12-Year Single Center Experience. *Ann Cardiothorac Surg* 2015;4(2):160–169.
11. Lamelas J, Nguyen TC. Minimally Invasive Valve Surgery: When Less Is More. *Semin Thorac Cardiovasc Surg* 2015;27(1):49–56.
12. Lamelas J, Mawad M, Williams R, Weiss UK, Zhang Q, LaPietra A. Isolated and Concomitant Minimally Invasive Minithoracotomy Aortic Valve Surgery. *J Thorac Cardiovasc Surg* 2018;155(3):926-936.e2.

13. Ribeiro IB, Ruel M. Right Anterior Minithoracotomy for Aortic Valve Replacement: A Widely Applicable, Simple, and Stepwise Approach. *Innovations (Phila)* 2019;14(4):321–329.
14. Nair SK, Sudarshan CD, Thorpe BS, et al. Mini-Stern Trial: A Randomized Trial Comparing Mini-Sternotomy to Full Median Sternotomy for Aortic Valve Replacement. *J Thorac Cardiovasc Surg* 2018;156(6):2124-2132.e31.
15. Bonacchi M, Prifti E, Giunti G, Frati G, Sani G. Does Ministernotomy Improve Postoperative Outcome in Aortic Valve Operation? A Prospective Randomized Study. *Ann Thorac Surg* 2002;73(2):460–465; discussion 465–466.
16. Dogan S, Dzemali O, Wimmer-Greinecker G, et al. Minimally Invasive Versus Conventional Aortic Valve Replacement: A Prospective Randomized Trial. *J Heart Valve Dis* 2003;12(1):76–80.
17. Del Giglio M, Mikus E, Nerla R, et al. Right Anterior Mini-Thoracotomy vs. Conventional Sternotomy for Aortic Valve Replacement: A Propensity-Matched Comparison. *J Thorac Dis* 2018;10(3):1588–1595.
18. Murzi M, Cerillo AG, Miceli A, et al. Antegrade and Retrograde Arterial Perfusion Strategy in Minimally Invasive Mitral-Valve Surgery: A Propensity Score Analysis on 1280 Patients. *Eur J Cardiothorac Surg* 2013;43(6):e167–172.
19. LaPietra A, Santana O, Mihos CG, et al. Incidence of Cerebrovascular Accidents in Patients Undergoing Minimally Invasive Valve Surgery. *J Thorac Cardiovasc Surg* 2014;148(1):156–160.
20. Lamelas J, LaPietra A. Right Minithoracotomy Approach for Replacement of the Ascending Aorta, Hemiarch, and Aortic Valve. *Innovations (Phila)* 2016;11(4):301–304.

7.2

MINIMALLY INVASIVE AORTIC VALVE REPLACEMENT
Upper "J" Sternotomy

FAIZUS SAZZAD AND THEO KOFIDIS

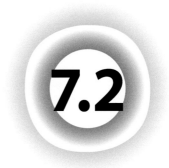

INTRODUCTION

The most common approach for minimally invasive aortic valve replacement is the J-shaped upper mini-sternotomy. Some of the reported results on the technique have demonstrated favorable long-term outcomes in elderly and redo patients when compared with conventional sternotomy, although right anterior mini-thoracotomy is steadily gaining in popularity [1,2]. This technique has its own benefit (Table 7.2.1) due to its similarity with the full sternotomy approach. Additionally, it is a safe and easy method for converting to a full sternotomy in an emergency scenario. There are several factors that determine a successful outcome in a J-shaped upper mini-sternotomy [3]. A brief description of these factors will follow in this chapter. With the advent of new technological innovations, a sub-group of J-shaped upper mini-sternotomy, "manubrium-limited" J-shaped upper mini-sternotomy, has developed over the years. This has subsequently paved the way for further advancements to the suprasternal MICS AVR approach as well (Figure 7.2.1).

TABLE 7.2.1 Benefits of Mini-sternotomy

- Stability – lower sternum intact
- Less sternal spreading
- Avoid intercostal nerves
- No muscle division
- Central cannulation (no retrograde flow to the brain)
- Direct access to aorta and aortic valve
- Easy to convert

FIGURE 7.2.1 Upper hemi-sternotomy by MMCTS.

HOW TO DO IT/STEP BY STEP

With a J-shaped upper mini-sternotomy the AVR can be done with different techniques. The additional exposure achieved from a conventional full sternotomy has little impact on the exposure of the aortic valve and proximal thoracic aorta. A minimally invasive approach with an upper hemi-sternotomy has an equivalent safety profile and has shown a significant difference in terms of reduced transfusion requirement, reduced respiratory complications, reduced postoperative pain and overall short length of hospital stay [4,5]. Upper J mini-sternotomy offers a great exposure of the superior mediastinal structures, and it is a viable option for performing MiAVR with the use of conventional instruments. Owing to its similarity to a full midline sternotomy, the process of achieving a J-shaped upper mini-sternotomy itself is relatively easy [6]. However, certain mandatory, recognized principles need to be followed in order to minimize complications Figure 7.2.2.

- **Patient positioning and draping**: Supine and standard draping with groin preparation.
- **Landmarks identification**: Supra sternal notch, angle of Louis, second to fourth intercostal space, xiphoid process.
- **Skin incision**: Usually, a 5-cm upper midline skin incision is performed in the midline extending from the second down to the fourth intercostal space. The third or fourth right intercostal space is then located and dissected laterally off the sternum. This is followed by the creation of a "J"-shaped periosteal mark Figure 7.2.3.
- **Sternotomy**: An oscillating saw is preferred to perform the sternotomy. A single-bladed "Finochietto" retractor is used for osteotomy. Care should be taken to locate and preserve the right internal mammary artery. If the retraction creates too much traction to the mammary artery, it would be better to ligate the vessel with large ligature clips and divide in-between.
- **Pericardiotomy**: A complete thymic dissection and removal of all thymic fat pads would be preferable for achieving good exposure. The pericardium is usually opened in the midline in an inverted-"T" fashion. Soft tissue retractors are not used in this approach. The pericardium is first pulled up with stay sutures that allow for excellent exposure. After complete pericardial retraction, the whole ascending aorta, SVC, most of the right atrium and the right superior pulmonary vein should be easy to approach. Visualization of the right

FIGURE 7.2.2 Upper J mini-sternotomy by Dr Natig Baku.

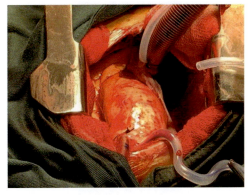

FIGURE 7.2.4 Operative field for MiAVR via Upper J mini-sternotomy (after pericardiotomy and pericardial retraction).

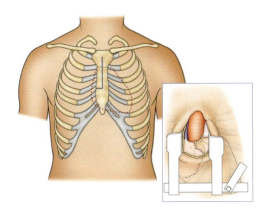

FIGURE 7.2.3 Schematic diagram of skin incision and access through upper mini-sternotomy. Division of the sternum is then either continued as a "J" or "T" to the fourth intercostal space. Inset: Exposure of epi-aortic structures. (Reprinted by permission from Taylor & Francis Group, LLC: CRC Press, Rob & Smith's Operative Cardiac Surgery, 6th Edition, Minimal access aortic valve surgery, Elizabeth HS, Michael AB, © 2019.)

FIGURE 7.2.5 Upper partial sternotomy by Yugal Mishra.

atrium is not necessary in a manubrium-limited approach Figure 7.2.4.

Cannulation: For the central cannulation approach, all cannulation can be carried out with the standard cannulation technique: Aortic cannulation, two-stage single venous cannulation, RSPV venting and non-selective cardioplegia cannulation. In the case of difficulty in establishing access for right atrium cannulation, or in manubrium-limited or supra-sternal approaches, femoro-femoral bypass can be performed Figure 7.2.5.

Cross clamps: Conventional aortic cross clamps can be used, but the use of flexible cross clamps like Cosgrove™ or Cygnet™ will allow for more space for the surgeon to operate.

Venting: RSPV or through aortotomy to left ventricle.

Cardioplegia: Non-selective or selective antegrade cardioplegia is preferred. Long-acting cardioplegia like Del Nido or Custodiol™ HTK can be used (Figure 7.2.6).

Choice of prosthesis: Conventional prostheses can easily be implanted like in the full sternotomy approach. The use of the automated suture knotting device (i.e. Cor-Knot™) is useful (Figure 7.2.7), but not mandatory. Sutureless valves are comparatively easier to implant in this case and have

FIGURE 7.2.6 Description of femoral cannulation technique during a mini-bentall surgery, CTS.net.

FIGURE 7.2.7 Corknot® (LSI Solution).

FIGURE 7.2.8 Perceval (LivaNova): Sutureless aortic valve replacement.

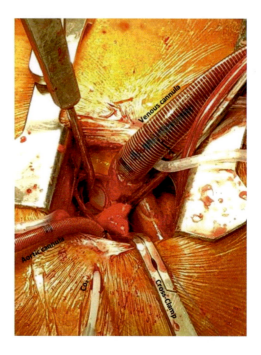

FIGURE 7.2.9 Bioprosthetic valve seen in situ, after MiAVR.

showed prominent results (Figure 7.2.8 to Figure 7.2.11).

Surgical procedure: The surgical procedures are performed in a standard fashion using standard methods, including curved aortotomy and standard exposure techniques of the aortic valve. Aortic valve repair or replacement can be carried out like in the full sternotomy approach. There are some reported cases of aortic root replacement and Bentall operation done via this approach, or even aortic valve repairs (Figure 7.2.18 and Figure 7.2.19).

AVR and ascending aorta (Bentall procedure) (Figures 7.2.12, 7.2.13), aortic root replacement, valve-sparing aortic root replacement (David procedure) (Figure 7.2.14) and a manubrium-limited aortic procedure can also be carried out by using the upper J mini-sternotomy approach (Figure 7.2.11, Figure 7.2.12, Figure 7.2.13 and 7.2.14).

SPECIAL CONSIDERATIONS

- ∞ Continuous CO_2 insufflation is used to minimize the risk of air embolism.
- ∞ Epicardial pacing wires are placed before the removal of the aortic cross clamp.
- ∞ Placement of one chest tube (if the right pleura is not opened) and one pericardial drain (Blake drains) is used.
- ∞ Sternal closure is achieved with three to four stainless-steel wires. The pectoral muscle, subcutaneous tissue and skin are closed in layers with absorbable running sutures. When performed properly, complications (conversion, bleeding and wound infection) are rare and easily managed.

FIGURE 7.2.10 Fast-track mini-AVR MiAVR, central cannulation technique with rapid deployment prosthesis (Edwards Intuity).

FIGURE 7.2.13 Bentall procedure via J mini-sternotomy.

FIGURE 7.2.11 Aortic valve repair – Ozaki technique.

FIGURE 7.2.14 David procedure through an upper partial sternotomy.

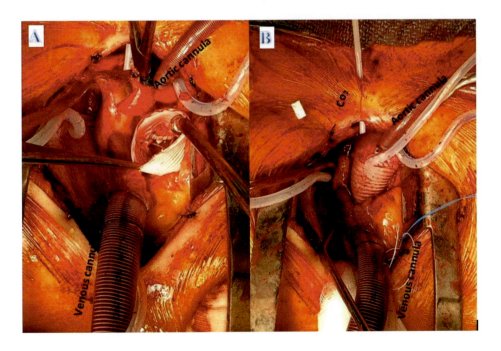

FIGURE 7.2.12 Aortic root and ascending aorta replacement via upper J mini-sternotomy. A. Operative view, B. Completion view.

Chapter 7.2 – The Aortic Valve 103

TOOLS/INSTRUMENTS AND DEVICES

SAW: OSCILLATING SAW

The oscillating saw can be used in "J-shaped" mini-sternotomy to achieve more precise and smaller cuts to the sternum that are suitable for a minimally invasive procedure. The oscillating saw can also be used in redo sternotomy patients (Figure 7.2.15).

AORTIC CANNULA: EOPA™

The EOPA (Medtronic) is an arterial cannula for aortic arch cannulation following mini-sternotomy. The newest version of this series is EOPA 3D®. (Figure 7.2.16)

AORTIC CROSS CLAMP

Cygnet™ from Péters Surgical is a flexible aortic cross clamp ideal for occluding the aorta in minimally invasive mini-sternotomy procedures (Figure 7.2.17).

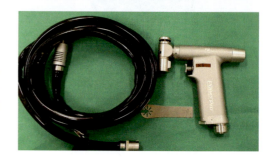

FIGURE 7.2.15   Oscillating saw.

AUTOMATED KNOT FASTENER

Cor-Knot® is an automated knot fastener used for knot security [7]. It has a variable length applicator, which is useful for deeply positioned or difficult to access valves. Its quick and easy aid makes MiAVR a time-saving procedure (Figure 7.2.18).

PERIOPERATIVE CONSIDERATION

PREOPERATIVE CT SCAN OF THE PATIENT (CT THORAX, ABDOMEN AND PELVIS)

CT TAP is an important and mandatory assessment tool for operative planning and evaluation of the patient. The location of the ascending aorta and its relationship with the manubrium play an important role. The groin vessels and condition of the thoracic aorta also need to be evaluated before a surgical decision can be made (Figure 7.2.19).

CHEST WALL DEFORMITY

Chest wall deformity is a limiting factor in the success of a mini-sternotomy procedure, particularly pectus excavatum and pectus carinatum. For an explanation of the differences between these two deformities, please see Figure (Figure 7.2.20)

SEVERE CALCIFIED ASCENDING AORTA

A severely calcified ascending aorta could make it difficult for a successful access

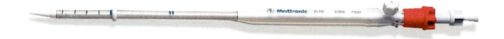

FIGURE 7.2.16   EOPA™ aortic cannula. Reproduced with permission of Medtronic, Inc.

104   Minimally Invasive Cardiac Surgery

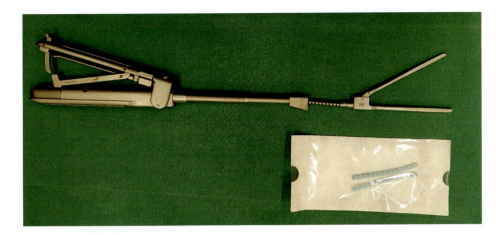

FIGURE 7.2.17   Cygnet™ aortic cross clamp.

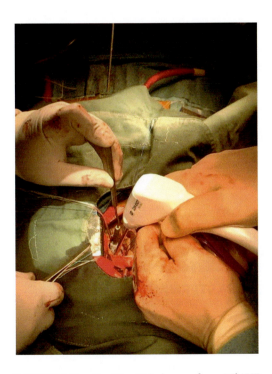

FIGURE 7.2.18   Cor-Knot® is in use for a MiAVR via upper J mini-sternotomy.

route through the vessel to be achieved and is hence an important perioperative consideration [8]. The linked video (Figure 7.2.21) demonstrates a case of dense calcification of the aorta visualized using fluoroscopic images during coronary angiographic examination.

FIGURE 7.2.19   Preoperative CT scan evaluation.

FIGURE 7.2.20   Chest wall deformities.

REOPERATIONS/REDO SURGERY

Another perioperative factor that needs to be taken into consideration is if the patient has undergone previous procedures that may result in potential complications to the current mini-sternotomy procedure (Figure 7.2.22).

STATUS POST-PNEUMONECTOMY

The status of the patient after a pneumonectomy is an important perioperative

FIGURE 7.2.21   Severely calcified aorta.

FIGURE 7.2.23   Manubrium limited MiAVR.

FIGURE 7.2.22   Redo MiAVR.

FIGURE 7.2.24   CoreVista by cardio precision.

consideration due to the possibility of the patient developing post-pneumonectomy syndrome.

OBESITY

Patient obesity is also another perioperative factor that could lead to complications during a mini-sternotomy procedure.

POST-RADIATION THERAPY

The status of the patient after radiation therapy is also a necessary perioperative consideration, owing to severe adhesions.

ALTERNATIVE APPROACHES

MANUBRIUM-LIMITED STERNOTOMY

The MAVRIC trial was conducted to evaluate the safety and efficacy of the manubrium-limited mini-sternotomy [9]. A presentation on the results of the MAVRIC trial can be found in Figure 7.2.23.

SUPRASTERNAL AVR

The presentation in Figure 7.2.24 allows for more detail on the suprasternal AVR approach, an alternative technique to the mini-sternotomy.

CAVEATS AND CONTROVERSIES

Mini- vs full sternotomy: A review on mini-sternotomy and its advantages and disadvantages compared to full sternotomy can be found in this video (Figure 7.2.25). An expert consensus came to a conclusion that sutureless and rapid deployment

FIGURE 7.2.25 Mini- vs full sternotomy – meta-analysis.

FIGURE 7.2.27 Options for treatment of aortic valve by Cleveland Clinic.

FIGURE 7.2.26 MiAVR via lower partial sternotomy.

FIGURE 7.2.28 Life expectancy after aortic valve replacement.

FIGURE 7.2.29 Valve-in-valve TAVI by Moninder Bhabra.

aortic valve replacement together with MICS offers an attractive option in AVR for patients requiring biological valve replacement [10].

Lower partial sternotomy: When the length of the patient's sternum is too short and the ascending aorta too long, lower partial sternotomy is preferred over an upper partial sternotomy. The link contains in Figure 7.2.26 contains a video essay describing the lower partial sternotomy technique.

AVR vs TAVI: For an expert opinion on the factors that qualify or disqualify a patient for TAVI, determining how TAVI should be used in lower risk patients and things that need to be taken into account in referrals for the treatment of aortic valve disease, reoperation and operating on younger patients, please access the link in Figure 7.2.27.

Outcomes after AVR: Figure 7.2.28 shows a video on the life expectancy and postoperative outcomes of AVR showing a general overview of the life expectancy after MiAVR surgery. The QUALITY-AVR trial was designed and aimed to determine if the minimally invasive approach improves quality of life [11].

Structural valve degeneration: TAVI is a choice of treatment option in high-risk patient >80 years old. The durability of TAVI valves is a valid question to ask. G Cosat et al. assessed SVD in TAVI and compared the 8-year durability is comparable to surgical replacement [12]. Although the early generation TAVI valve are more susceptible to structural valve deterioration and thus potentially less structurally durable than SAVR valves [13]. This presentation (Figure 7.2.29) highlights the importance of preoperative planning

FIGURE 7.2.30   Transapical TAVI by Edwards.

FIGURE 7.2.32 Professional education by LivaNova.

FIGURE 7.2.31   Valve-in-valve TAVI.

FIGURE 7.2.33   EACTS Academy.

before a valve-in-valve TAVI procedure and provides a guide on how to successfully deploy various TAVI valves. In general it's a procedural description for transcatheter implantation of a new valve in a previously replaced or repaired valve.

RESEARCH, TRENDS AND INNOVATION

TRANS-APICAL TAVI

An animation on how transcatheter aortic valve replacement valve is deployed and implanted via the transapical approach can be found in Figure 7.2.30.

VALVE-IN-VALVE

A clinical presentation on a case where valve-in-valve TAVR with a SAPIEN-3 valve was performed in a patient (Figure 7.2.31).

WHERE AND HOW TO LEARN

PROFESSIONAL EDUCATION: LIVANOVA

For information on a hands-on program on transcatheter valve replacement (Figure 7.2.32).

EACTS ACADEMY

Information on the EACTS Academy program is available in the link (Figure 7.2.33).

NATIONAL UNIVERSITY HEALTH SYSTEM (NUHS), SINGAPORE (ASTC)

More information on the procedure can also be found in the link in Figure 7.2.34 KHOO TECK PUAT advanced surgical training hub in NUH.

AORTIC VALVE AND ROOT BOOT CAMP

Details on the aortic valve and root boot camp by CryoLife can be found in Figure 7.2.35.

108   Minimally Invasive Cardiac Surgery

FIGURE 7.2.34 NUHS training hub: The Advanced Surgical Training Center (ASTC).

FIGURE 7.2.35 CryoLife boot camps.

REFERENCES

1. D. Gilmanov, M. Solinas, P. A. Farneti, A. G. Cerillo, E. Kallushi, F. Santarelli, M. Glauber, Department of Adult Cardiac Surgery, Gabriele Monasterio Tuscany Foundation, Pasquinucci Heart hospital. Minimally invasive aortic valve replacement: 12-year single center experience. *Ann Cardiothorac Surg* 2015; 4: 160–169.
2. D. Fudulu, H. Lewis, U. Benedetto, M. Caputo, G. Angelini, H. A. Vohra. Minimally invasive aortic valve replacement in high risk patient groups. *J Thorac Dis* 2017; 9: 1672–1696.
3. M. A. Amr. Evaluation of feasibility and outcome of isolated aortic valve replacement surgery through j-shaped upper mini-sternotomy: A comparative study versus full sternotomy. *J Egypt Soc Cardio-thorac Surg* 2016; 24: 123–130.
4. D. R. Merk, S. Lehmann, D. M. Holzhey, P. Dohmen, P. Candolfi, M. Misfeld, F. W. Mohr, M. A. Borger. Minimal invasive aortic valve replacement surgery is associated with improved survival: A propensity-matched comparison. *Eur J Cardio-thorac Surg* 2015; 47: 11–17.
5. B. Kirmani. *Minimally Invasive Versus Open Surgery for Aortic Valve Replacement.* February 2019. CTSnet. CTSNET, INC. Doi:10.25373/ctsnet.7771100.
6. V. Gaudiani, P. H. Tsau. *Upper Mini-Sternotomy, Aortic Valve Replacement, and Ascending Aortic Replacement.* January 2018. CTSnet. CTSNET, INC. Doi:10.25373/ctsnet.5801265.
7. Martin T. R. Grapow, Miroslawa Mytsyk, Jens Fassl, Patrick Etter, Peter Matt, Friedrich S. Eckstein, Oliver T. Reuthebuch. Automated fastener versus manually tied knots in minimally invasive mitral valve repair: Impact on operation time and short-term results. *J Cardiothorac Surg* 2015; 10: 146. Doi: 10.1186/s13019-015-0344-4. PMCID: PMC4632475
8. Daniel Fudulu, Harriet Lewis, Umberto Benedetto, Massimo Caputo, Gianni Angelini, Hunaid A. Vohra. Minimally invasive aortic valve replacement in high risk patient groups. *J Thorac Dis* 2017; 9(6): 1672–1696. Doi: 10.21037/jtd.2017.05.21. PMCID: PMC5506162
9. Enoch Akowuah, Andrew T. Goodwin, W. Andrew Owens, Helen C. Hancock, Rebecca Maier, Adetayo Kasim, Adrian Mellor, Khalid Khan, Gavin Murphy, James Mason. Manubrium-limited mini-sternotomy versus conventional sternotomy for aortic valve replacement (MAVRIC): Study protocol for a andomized controlled trial. *Trials* 2017; 18: 46. Published online 2017 Jan 28. Doi: 10.1186/s13063-016-1768-4. PMCID: PMC5273792
10. Mattia Glauber, Simon C. Moten, Eugenio Quaini, Marco Solinas, Thierry A. Folliguet, Bart Meuris, Antonio Miceli, Peter J. Oberwalder, Manfredo Rambaldini, Kevin H. T. Teoh, Gopal Bhatnagar, Michael A. Borger, Denis Bouchard, Olivier Bouchot, Stephen C. Clark, Otto E. Dapunt, Matteo Ferrarini, Theodor J. M. Fischlein, Guenther Laufer, Carmelo Mignosa, Russell Millner, Philippe Noirhomme, Steffen Pfeiffer, Xavier Ruyra-Baliarda, Malakh Lal Shrestha, Rakesh M. Suri, Giovanni Troise, Borut Gersak. International expert consensus on sutureless and rapid deployment valves in aortic valve replacement using minimally

invasive approaches. *Innovations (Phila)* 2016; 11(3): 165–173. Doi: 10.1097/IMI.0000000000000287. PMCID: PMC4996354

11. Emiliano A. Rodríguez-Caulo, Ana Guijarro-Contreras, Juan Otero-Forero, María José Mataró, Gemma Sánchez-Espín, Arantza Guzón, Carlos Porras, Miguel Such, Antonio Ordóñez, José María Melero-Tejedor, Manuel Jiménez-Navarro. Quality of life, satisfaction and outcomes after mini-sternotomy versus full sternotomy isolated aortic valve replacement (QUALITY-AVR): Study protocol for a andomized controlled trial. *Trials* 2018; 19: 114. Published online 2018 February 17. Doi: 10.1186/s13063-018-2486-x. PMCID: PMC5816540

12. Ravi K. Ghanta, Damien J. Lapar, John A. Kern, Irving L. Kron, Allen M. Speir, Edwin Fonner, Jr., Mohammed Quader, Gorav Ailawadi. Minimally invasive aortic valve replacement provides equivalent outcomes at reduced cost compared to conventional aortic valve replacement: A "realworld" multi-institutional analysis. *J Thorac Cardiovasc Surg* 2015; 149(4): 1060–1065. Doi: 10.1016/j.jtcvs.2015.01.014. PMCID: PMC4409485

13. Ashlynn Ler, Yeo Jie Ying, Faizus Sazzad, Andrew M. T. L. Choong, Theo Kofidis. Structural durability of early-generation Transcatheter aortic valve replacement valves compared with surgical aortic valve replacement valves in heart valve surgery: a systematic review and meta-analysis. *J Cardiothorac Surg* 2020; **15:** 127. (2020). Doi: 10.1186/s13019-020-01170-7

THE AORTIC VALVE
Sutureless Valves in the Setting of MICS AVR

THEODOR FISCHLEIN AND GIUSEPPE SANTARPINO

HISTORY AND INTRODUCTION

The conventional aortic valve replacement (AVR) has a relatively high success rate associated with a perioperative mortality risk of approximately 1–3% in patients younger than 70 years undergoing isolated AVR, increasing to 4–8% when combined with coronary artery bypass grafting [1]. However, not all patients are suitable for surgery, with several factors affecting a patient's suitability for surgery. Older age, left ventricle dysfunction or neurological dysfunction due to their high operative risk and a late outcome after surgery were listed as factors precluding surgery in a 2005 European Heart Survey on valvular heart study, which found that 33% of patients with severe aortic stenosis did not undergo surgery [2] (Figure 7.3.1).

On the other hand, there is a growing interest in minimally invasive access for aortic valve surgery, which reduces surgical trauma and pain to the patient and potentially allows a faster recovery [3].

There are two minimally invasive surgical options for AVR (Figures 7.3.2a, b): The upper hemisternotomy (ministernotomy) and right anterior minithoracotomy (RAT). Some surgeons remain skeptical about limited-access surgery because it is technically demanding, particularly in the case of RAT.

Given that prolonged ischemic and cardiopulmonary (CPB) times per se can affect

FIGURE 7.3.1 Percutaneous heart valve replacement for aortic stenosis.

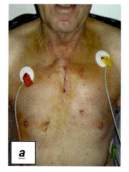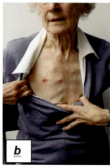

FIGURE 7.3.2 Postoperative MiAVR scar, a: Ministernotomy, b: Right anterior thoracotomy (RAT).

the clinical outcome of patients undergoing AVR, it can be hypothesized that an easier minimally invasive technique that enables shorter surgical times may result in an improved outcome [4, 5].

Sutureless aortic bioprostheses were developed to fulfil this niche and for use in high-risk patients undergoing surgical AVR due to severe aortic stenosis. In any case, as we will show later, these prostheses have also found space for use even in younger and lower-risk patients. In other words, they have become biological prostheses with the same indications and contraindications as the "conventional" biological aortic valve prostheses. Similar to transcatheter aortic valve implantation (TAVI) valves, sutureless valves are mounted on a stent and are self-anchoring within the aortic annulus. This results in shorter operative and, hence, ischemic times. Therefore, the use of these devices makes valve implantation easier and faster, which seems to improve postoperative outcomes.

The Perceval S (LivaNova, Plc, London, UK) was first implanted in humans in 2007 and the results were quite promising [6]. At present, the Perceval S is the only true commercially available sutureless valve, after Medtronic discontinued its 3F Enable valve in 2015 due to vague clinical results. However, the use of sutureless valves

TABLE 7.3.1 Key similarities and differences vs conventional prostheses and TAVI

	Sutureless valves
Conventional prostheses	
Similarity	Can be performed using full sternotomy or minimally invasive incisions
	CPB and crossclamping are mandatory
	Annulus is decalcified
Difference	Transverse aortotomy is performed ~1.5cm higher than ordinary (Perceval)
	Requiring three locking sutures for implantation (Intuity)
	Lower implant profile in the case of Perceval
TAVI	
Similarity	Similar principle of technology
Difference	Does not require crimping of the pericardium
	Provides direct visualization of implantation and target orifice
	Annulus is decalcified
	Diseased valve is excised

Abbreviations: Cardiopulmonary bypass. TAVI: Transcatheter aortic valve implantation. After Marco Di Eusanio and Kevin Phan. Sutureless aortic valve replacement. Ann Cardiothorac Surg. 2015 Mar;4(2):123–30 [7].

generally includes the rapid-deployment Intuity Elite (Edward Lifesciences, Irvine, USA) valve, which requires three locking sutures. Table 7.3.1 identifies the key features of sutureless valves in comparison to conventional prostheses and TAVI.

HOW TO DO IT/STEP BY STEP

A. PATIENT SELECTION

Indication for sutureless AVR should follow the European Society of Cardiology (ESC) or American Heart Association (AHA) guidelines [8–10]. Any patient with severe calcific aortic stenosis and suitable for bioprosthetic valve implantation can be considered for sutureless valve implantation. Patients with additional comorbidities and the elderly may benefit more from sutureless valve implantation [11–12]. Even in particular conditions, sutureless prostheses can represent an advantage in combination with a minimally invasive approach (e.g. redo) [13]. Peri-implantation steps for sutureless valves in terms of CPB and cross-clamping are the same as for conventional AVR.

B. PERCEVAL

1. A transverse aortotomy is performed approximately 1.5 to 2 cm higher than commonly for AVR. The reference point is the inferior margin of the Concato preaortic bundle or rim about 3.5 to 4 cm away from the aortic annulus.
2. The diseased native valve is completely excised and the aortic annulus thoroughly decalcified.
3. Sizing the valve: The valve sizer is designed so that the intra-annular head of the sizer (yellow) has the same external diameter as the supra-annular head (white) of the smaller size.
4. Three guiding 4-0 prolene sutures are placed at the nadir point of each valve sinus to act as a reference for accurate alignment of the inflow portion of the prosthesis into the aortic annulus.
5. The valve is collapsed using a specific device system.
6. The valve is connected to the guiding sutures through three eyelets placed on the midpart of the inflow ring.
7. The deployment system is parachuted down into the aortic root and the valve released into the aortic annulus. The inflow ring should completely cover the aortic annulus, such that no part of the native aortic annulus is exposed (Figure 7.3.3).

Although not recommended, it is still possible to adjust the valve position later or replace it again by using Debakey forceps applying a x-movement procedure as described elsewhere [14] (Figure 7.3.4).

8. Coaptation of the three leaflets is checked. Then, the inflating balloon is inserted into the inner orifice of sutureless valve and expanded with warm saline solution for 30 seconds at a pressure of 4 atm as described in the instructions for use (Figure 7.3.5).
9. Finally, the three guiding sutures are removed.
10. The valve is again checked for correct position, and the aortotomy is then closed using 4-0 or 5-0 running sutures.

Ministernotomy: In a standard operating room, general anesthesia and

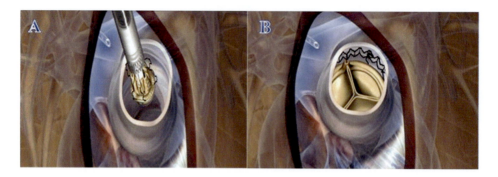

FIGURE 7.3.3 Schematic implantation technique of Perceval® S sutureless valve; A: Aortotomy and positioning of Perceval® S, B: Implanted prosthesis. Reproduced with permission of LivaNova USA, Inc.

FIGURE 7.3.4 Perceval® sutureless heart valve replacement implant animation.

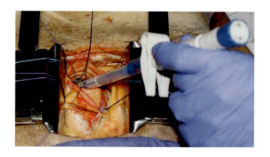

FIGURE 7.3.5 Positioning the Perceval® S in ministernotomy.

orotracheal intubation are carried out. The heart is exposed through an upper mini J-sternotomy extended to the fourth intercostal space. Sorin Perceval aortic valve implantation through a ministernotomy approach has been described in the linked video (Figure 7.3.6).

Right anterior thoracotomy (RAT): Perceval sutureless aortic valve prosthesis can also be implanted via a right anterior minithoracotomy MMCTS. Figure 7.3.7 shows positioning and implantation of Perceval S in RAT. Video link is in Figure 7.3.8, with description of a case.

C. INTUITY ELITE VALVE

1. A transverse aortotomy is performed approximately 1.5 to 2 cm higher than ordinary aortotomy for AVR. The reference point is the inferior margin of the Concato preaortic bundle.
2. The diseased native valve is completely excised and the aortic annulus thoroughly decalcified.
3. Sizing the valve: The cylindrical end of the sizer is first inserted. The proper valve size is one in which the operator feels some resistance when inserting the cylinder.
4. Once the proper valve size is chosen, valve preparation involves two 1-minute washes in saline solution (Figure 7.3.9).
5. Guiding sutures: Three braided 2-0 non-pledgeted sutures are placed at the nadir of each aortic sinus.
6. Each suture needle, which exits below the annulus, is then passed through the sewing ring of the Intuity Elite valve at the black markers and snared with a tourniquet.

FIGURE 7.3.6 Perceval® implantation via ministernotomy by G Santarpino.

FIGURE 7.3.8 Perceval® implantation via RAT Selim Isbir.

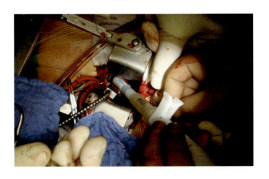

FIGURE 7.3.7 Positioning of the Perceval® in right anterior minithoracotomy (RAT).

FIGURE 7.3.9 INTUITY™ preparation.

7. The valve is then lowered down to the annulus and a standard shoehorn manipulation is employed to seat the valve with a gentle upward traction (Figure 7.3.10).
8. Once the valve system is seated, the balloon catheter is advanced into the valve holder and the inflation device is attached to the proximal end of the balloon catheter for 10 seconds (Figure 7.3.11).
9. The balloon is then fully deflated with negative pressure, and the inflation device is locked. The three polypropylene sutures on the valve holder are cut at the level of the stent posts and the entire valve system is gently removed.
10. The three annular guide sutures are then tied and cut.

Ministernotomy: Upper hemisternotomy MiAVR implantation of the Intuity valve with its rapid deployment system has been featured in the linked video (Figure 7.3.12).
Right anterior thoracotomy (RAT): The linked video (Figure 7.3.13) shows a sutureless bioprosthesis (Edwards Intuity) implantation via RAT for the treatment of calcific aortic stenosis. The prosthesis was implanted via a small 8-cm incision (Figure 7.3.14).

TOOLS/INSTRUMENTS AND DEVICES

1. PERCEVAL S (LIVANOVA GROUP, MILAN, ITALY)

The Perceval S device is a biologic prosthesis composed of bovine pericardium built on the Sorin Pericarbon (Sorin, Saluggia, Italy) and assembled on a nitinol stent. The self-expandable Nitinol stent fits the anatomy of the aorta and follows its movement during the entire cardiac cycle. It is designed to

FIGURE 7.3.10 INTUITY™ procedure animation.

FIGURE 7.3.12 INTUITY™ implantation via ministernotomy.

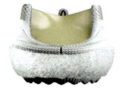 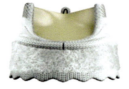

FIGURE 7.3.11 Rapid-deployment aortic valve: EDWARDS INTUITY™ valve system. Republished with permission of Elsevier Science & Technology Journals, from One-year outcomes of the Surgical Treatment of Aortic Stenosis With a Next Generation Surgical Aortic Valve (TRITON) trial: a prospective multicenter study of rapid-deployment aortic valve replacement with the EDWARDS INTUITY Valve System, Kocher AA, Laufer G, Haverich A, et al. *J Thorac Cardiovasc Surg.* 145(1):110-116, © 2013 The American Association for Thoracic Surgery; permission conveyed through Copyright Clearance Center, Inc.

FIGURE 7.3.13 MICS Edward INTUITY™ valve implant.

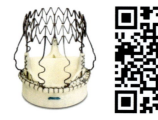

FIGURE 7.3.14 Perceval®: Sutureless aortic bioprosthesis. Reproduced with permission of LivaNova USA, Inc.

distribute the stresses in order to minimize the risk of damage to the aortic root. The reduced profile of the collapsed valve, when mounted in its dedicated holder, enhances visibility and control for the surgeon during positioning and is a big advantage especially during minimally invasive approaches.

2. INTUITY (EDWARDS LIFESCIENCES, IRVINE, CA)

The Intuity valve is built on the design platform of the Carpentier-Edwards Perimount Magna Ease aortic bioprosthesis. It is a trileaflet bovine pericardial device and has a balloon-expandable stainless-steel cloth-covered frame incorporated into the inflow aspect of the valve. The device is positioned and secured with three equidistant sutures which guide the placement of the valve frame into the native annulus. Given the need for three sutures, the Intuity bioprosthesis is more appropriately defined as a rapid deployment aortic valve, in that it enables a more rapid implantation compared with conventional prosthetic valves.

Characteristics of the Perceval and Intuity valves are illustrated in Table 7.3.2 (Figure 7.3.15).

TABLE 7.3.2 Characteristics of the sutureless Perceval S and rapid deployment Intuity valves

	Perceval (LivaNova)	Intuity (Edwards)
CE mark	2011	2012
Pericardial tissue	Bovine	Bovine
Rinsing	Not required	2 × 60 sec
Stent material	Nitinol	Stainless steel
Self-expandable	Yes	No
Collapsible	Yes	No
Sutures	0	3
Valve sizes (annular size)	S (19–21), M (21–23), L (23–25), XL (25–27)	19, 21, 23, 25, 27
Anti-calcification treatment	Yes	Yes
Tissue fixation	Glutaraldehyde	Glutaraldehyde

PERIOPERATIVE CONSIDERATION

Preoperative considerations and postoperative management for sutureless or rapid deployment valves should follow those of AVR via the chosen approach, whether it is via ministernotomy, RAT or conventional sternotomy. All patients should undergo an accurate preoperative transthoracic echocardiographic study for better evaluation of the aortic valve, diameters of the aortic annulus, sinuses, sinotubular junction and symmetry of the sinuses of Valsalva.

Patients undergoing minimally invasive AVR should undergo at least a non-contrasted computed tomography (CT) scan to evaluate aortic valve and root anatomy and extent of calcification. For patients undergoing RAT, this is necessary to evaluate the relationship among the aortic valve, sternum and intercostal spaces to determine feasibility as stated in the previous chapter. The patients are considered suitable for an RT approach if, at the level of the main pulmonary artery, the ascending aorta is rightward with respect to the right sternal border and the distance from the ascending aorta to the sternum does not exceed 10 cm [15].

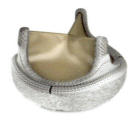 

FIGURE 7.3.15 INTUITY™: Sutureless aortic bioprosthesis. Reproduced with permission of Edwards Lifesciences LLC, Irvine, CA.

Choice of approach is also determined by center, preference and expertise, and the need for concomitant procedures. Appropriate training and experience of the team are vital to achieving desirable outcomes.

ALTERNATIVE APPROACHES

Although AVR is considered the only curative treatment known to improve symptoms and survival in patients with severe, symptomatic aortic stenosis, perioperative mortality increases among high-risk patients due to older age and comorbidities. TAVI is an advancing, catheter-based technology that is increasingly applied for patients with severe calcified aortic stenosis and intermediate to high Society of Thoracic Surgeons (STS) risk scores [8–9]. (See Chapter 8 on TAVI.) However, as TAVI devices are developing, sutureless AVR should be also considered in high-risk patients with a reasonable life expectancy, elderly patients and cases with difficult anatomical situations.

Patients requiring concomitant coronary artery bypass grafting (CABG) or other valve surgery form a special population that may benefit from the decreased CPB and crossclamp times offered by sutureless valve technology. They also form a unique group for sutureless AVR via a conventional sternotomy [16–17].

CAVEATS AND CONTROVERSIES

Contraindications to sutureless valve implantation include bicuspid aortic valve without a raphe (Sievers 0), sinotubular junction to aortic annulus ratio greater than 1:3 and endocarditis (Figure 7.3.16).

Specific caveats regarding sutureless valves are as follows [7]:

∞ Requires proctoring for the surgeon to traverse the learning curve.

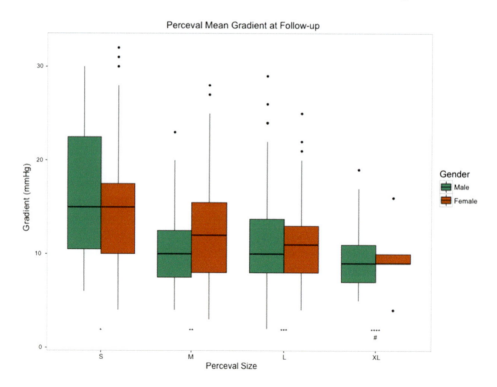

FIGURE 7.3.16 Improvement of mean transvalvular pressure gradient (mm Hg) related to higher prosthesis size. (Reprinted from *Ann Thorac Surg,* 105(1), Concistrè G, Chiaramonti F, Bianchi G, et al. Aortic Valve Replacement With Perceval Bioprosthesis: Single-Center Experience With 617 Implants, 40-46, © 2018 by The Society of Thoracic Surgeons, with permission from Elsevier.)

∞ Sizing is absolutely important to avoid paravalvular leaks, valve migration, root dehiscence and "stent creep", a permanent inward deflection of stent posts which may lead to valvular leak and insufficiency.

The surgical goal of applying minimally invasive techniques for AVR has been mooted for years [18]. Available data from recent systematic reviews and meta-analyses do not provide strong evidence of significant improvement in patient outcome to support abandoning conventional AVR through a full sternotomy, and significantly longer ischemic and CPB times have been reported with ministernotomy [19, 20]. It should be stressed that to date we do not have data with long-term follow-up on durability; therefore both models require some caution in implantation in young patients. However, the preliminary results even up to 10 years after implantation are very encouraging, and a new model more resistant to the risk of SVD has been developed for the Perceval model (Perceval plus) (Figure 7.3.17).

FIGURE 7.3.17 Short-term results of MiAVR with Intuity (ISMICS).

RESEARCH, TRENDS AND INNOVATION

PERCEVAL

Early postoperative observations confirmed implant safety with no risk of prosthesis migration and the benefit of short operative times – less than 20 minutes of aortic crossclamping via full sternotomy is possible [21]. Definitive early evidence of shorter operative times was provided by a study that included 100 patients undergoing minimally invasive isolated AVR by the same senior surgeon using the sutureless Perceval aortic valve (n = 50) versus conventional stented bioprosthesis (n = 50). Aortic crossclamp and CPB times were 39.4% and 34% shorter in the Perceval group respectively [22]. The Perceval sutureless prosthesis was developed to facilitate minimally invasive surgical AVR, showing optimal performance via both accesses, ministernotomy and RAT [11, 15, 23]. Early and mid-term results in large cohorts of patients showed favorable outcomes [16–17].

INTUITY

The prospective, multicenter, single-arm TRITON trial investigated the safety and performance of the Intuity device in 152 patients with aortic stenosis and reported a procedural success of 96%. In addition, mean aortic crossclamp time was reduced compared with that for conventional AVR [24].

The TRANSFORM trial showed excellent hemodynamic performance with the Intuity valve, but a permanent pacemaker rate of 11.9% [25].

PERCEVAL VERSUS INTUITY

A single-center analysis of 156 patients showed comparable good early clinical outcomes, low valve-related complications and excellent hemodynamic performance with both valves [26]. The largest multicenter study comparing the 2 valves in 911 patients at 18 institutions also revealed

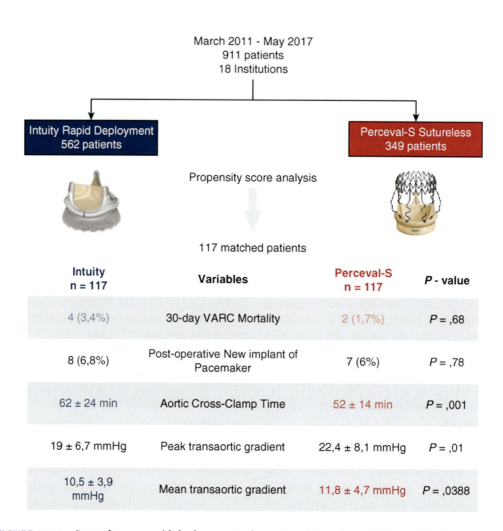

FIGURE 7.3.18 Sutureless vs rapid deployment valves. (Reprinted from *J Thorac Cardiovasc Surg*, S0022-5223(19), D'Onofrio A, Salizzoni S, Filippini C, et al. Surgical aortic valve replacement with new-generation bioprostheses: Sutureless versus rapid-deployment, 30977-8, © 2019 by The American Association for Thoracic Surgery, with permission from Elsevier.)

similar early clinical and hemodynamic outcomes. The Perceval S valve implantation required shorter crossclamp and CPB times, whereas the Intuity valve provided lower transaortic peak and mean gradients [27] (Figure 7.3.18).

For the second prosthetic model for Intuity (8300A), the scientific publications are fewer than those present on Perceval. After the publication of the main trial (TRANSFORM), there was a high incidence of pacemaker implants for which subsequent studies on the mechanisms underlying this risk have been published. In summary, to date this prosthesis is not recommended for patients "with risk factors" to implant a pacemaker [23, 28]. On the contrary, Perceval prostheses that initially showed high pacemaker rates, after appropriate suggestions and modifications of the implantation techniques, brought the incidence of this risk to the same values that can be recorded in patients with "conventional" prosthesis implants [29].

CURRENT EVIDENCE AND FUTURE PROSPECTS

Two European multicenter studies by Dalén et al. showed convincing evidence regarding ease of implantation of sutureless valves via ministernotomy. The first study evaluated 267 consecutive patients undergoing isolated AVR with the sutureless Perceval bioprosthesis through ministernotomy or full sternotomy at 6 European centers, and showed that although minimal invasive access surgery was more time-consuming, aortic crossclamp and CPB times did not differ between the groups [30]. In the second study, sutureless AVR via ministernotomy was associated with shorter operative times than stented AVR via full sternotomy [31]. The main contribution of sutureless AVR consists of making implantation more feasible through RAT even when the anatomical position of the aorta is unfavorable and suturing conventional prostheses would be difficult [12] (Figure 7.3.19).

The lack of prospective randomized trials comparing sutureless versus stented aortic bioprostheses is a major factor accounting for the exclusion of these devices from the therapeutic armamentarium recommended by current guidelines for the management of aortic valve disease. Because of that, an international multicenter randomized Perceval sutureless implant vs standard aortic valve replacement (PERSIST-AVR) trial was started in 2016 in order to test the safety and efficacy of the Perceval bioprosthesis against conventional sutured valves among patients undergoing surgical AVR (Figure 7.3.20).

It is our opinion that in the current TAVI era, isolated AVR – also using conventional prostheses – should always be performed via minimally invasive approaches. It is likely that, as definitive evidence is obtained to show long-term durability, and

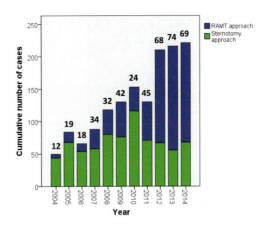

FIGURE 7.3.19 Proportion of AVR cases performed via RAMT over time, year by year (numbers above the bars indicate % of the total number of isolated AVR operations). Sternotomy approach (green bar) includes both full and partial sternotomy. Cases involving RAMT (blue bar) indicate that, since 2011, the overall number of AVR cases has increased, owing to the RAMT component. RAMT: Right anterior minithoracotomy. (Reprinted from *J Thorac Cardiovasc Surg*, 150(3), Glauber M, Gilmanov D, Farneti PA, et al. Right anterior minithoracotomy for aortic valve replacement: 10-year experience of a single center, 548-56.e2, © 2015 by The American Association for Thoracic Surgery, with permission from Elsevier.)

FIGURE 7.3.20 PERSIST-AVR Clinical Trial.

as the shorter implantation times are associated with improved clinical outcomes, the ease of implantation will make sutureless aortic valves the first-line treatment strategy for AVR in patients with suitable anatomy including minimally invasive AVR in younger patients (Figure 7.3.21).

FIGURE 7.3.21 Sutureless AVR by Di Eusanio.

FIGURE 7.3.22 The IVSSG – sutureless project.

WHERE AND HOW TO LEARN

INTERNATIONAL VALVULAR SURGERY STUDY GROUP (IVSSG)

The ongoing Sutureless Aortic Valve Replacement International Registry (SU-AVR-IR), undertaken by the International Valvular Surgery Study Group (IVSSG), including 36 expert valvular surgeons from 27 major centers across the globe, will provide new retrospective and prospective data on the safety, efficacy and durability of the Perceval and Intuity bioprostheses [32] (Figure 7.3.22).

REFERENCES

1. Authors/Task Force Members, Alec Vahanian, Ottavio Alfieri, Felicita Andreotti, Manuel J. Antunes, Gonzalo Barón-Esquivias et al. he Joint Task Force on the Management of Valvular Heart Disease of the European Society of Cardiology (ESC) and the European Association for Cardio-Thoracic Surgery (EACTS), *European Heart Journal*, 2012; 33 (19): 2451–2496 doi: 10.1093/eurheartj/ehs109.
2. Coeytaux RR, Williams JW Jr, Gray RN, Wang A. Percutaneous heart valve replacement for aortic stenosis: state of the evidence. *Ann Intern Med.* 2010;153(5):314-324. doi:10.7326/0003-4819-153-5-201009070-00267.
3. Shekar PS, Cohn LH. Minimally invasive aortic valve surgery. In Lawrence H. Cohn, David H. Adams (ed.), *Cardiac Surgery in the Adult*. New York: McGraw-Hill, 2008: 957–964.
4. Chalmers J, Pullan M, Mediratta N, Poullis M. A need for speed? Bypass time and outcomes after isolated aortic valve replacement surgery. *Interact Cardiovasc Thorac Surg* 2014; 19: 21–6.
5. Ranucci M, Frigiola A, Menicanti L, Castelvecchio S, de Vincentiis C, Pistuddi V. Aortic cross-clamp time, new prostheses, and outcome in aortic valve replacement. *J Heart Valve Dis* 2012; 21: 732–9.
6. Shrestha M, Khaladj N, Bara C, Hoeffler K, Hagl C, Haverich A. A staged approach towards interventional aortic valve implantation with a sutureless valve: Initial human implants. *Thorac Cardiovasc Surg* 2008; 56: 398–400.
7. Di Eusanio M, Phan K. Sutureless aortic valve replacement. *Ann Cardiothorac Surg* 2015; 4(2): 123–30.617.
8. Baumgartner H, Falk V, Bax JJ, et al. 2017 ESC/EACTS guidelines for the management of valvular heart disease. *Eur Heart J* 2017; 38(36): 2739–2791.
9. Nishimura RA, Otto CM, Bonow RO, et al. 2014 AHA/ACC guideline for the management of patients with valvular heart disease: A report of the American College of Cardiology/American Heart Association Task Force on practice guidelines. *Circulation* 2014; 129(23): e521–643.
10. Nishimura RA, Otto CM, Bonow RO, et al. 2017 AHA/ACC focused update of the 2014 AHA/ACC guideline for the management of patients with valvular heart disease: A report of the American College of

Cardiology/American Heart Association Task Force on Clinical Practice Guidelines. *Circulation* 2017; 135(25): e1159–e1195.

11. Gilmanov D, Miceli A, Ferrarini M, et al. Aortic valve replacement through right anterior minithoracotomy: Can sutureless technology improve clinical outcomes? *Ann Thorac Surg* 2014; 98: 1585–92.

12. Glauber M, Gilmanov D, Farneti PA, et al. Right anterior minithoracotomy for aortic valve replacement: 10-year experience of a single center. *J Thorac Cardiovasc Surg* 2015; 150: 548–56.

13. Santarpino G, Berretta P, Kappert U, et al. Minimally invasive redo aortic valve replacement: Results from a multicentric registry (SURD-IR). *Ann Thorac Surg.* 2020; 110(2): 553–557. doi:10.1016/j.athoracsur.2019.11.033.

14. Santarpino G, Pfeiffer S, Concistrè G, Fischlein T. A supra-annular malposition of the Perceval S sutureless aortic valve: The 'χ-movement' removal technique and subsequent reimplantation. *Interact Cardiovasc Thorac Surg* 2012; 15(2): 280–1.

15. Miceli A, Santarpino G, Pfeiffer S, et al. Minimally invasive aortic valve replacement with perceval S sutureless valve: Early outcomes and one-year survival from two European centers. *J Thorac Cardiovasc Surg* 2014; 148: 2838–43.

16. Laborde F, Fischlein T, Hakim-Meibodi K, et al. Clinical and haemodynamic outcomes in 658 patients receiving the perceval sutureless aortic valve: Early results from a prospective European multicentre study (the Cavalier Trial). *Eur J Cardiothorac Surg* 2016; 49(3): 978–86.

17. Concistrè G, Chiaramonti F, Bianchi G, et al. Aortic valve replacement with perceval bioprosthesis: Single-center experience with 617 implants. *Ann Thorac Surg* 2018; 105(1): 40–46.

18. Cooley DA. Minimally invasive valve surgery versus the conventional approach. *Ann Thorac Surg* 1998; 66: 1101–5.

19. Murtuza B, Pepper JR, Stanbridge RD, et al. Minimal access aortic valve replacement: Is it worth it? *Ann Thorac Surg* 2008; 85: 1121–31.

20. Brown ML, McKellar SH, Sundt TM, Schaff HV. Ministernotomy versus conventional sternotomy for aortic valve replacement: A systematic review and meta-analysis. *J Thorac Cardiovasc Surg* 2009; 137: 670–9.

21. Flameng W, Herregods MC, Hermans H, et al. Effect of sutureless implantation of the perceval S aortic valve bioprosthesis on intraoperative and early postoperative outcomes. *J Thorac Cardiovasc Surg* 2011; 142: 1453–7.

22. Santarpino G, Pfeiffer S, Concistré G, Grossmann I, Hinzmann M, Fischlein T. The perceval S aortic valve has the potential of shortening surgical time: Does it also result in improved outcome? *Ann Thorac Surg* 2013; 96: 77–81.

23. Fischlein T, Pfeiffer S, Pollari F, Sirch J, Vogt F, Santarpino G. Sutureless valve implantation via mini J-sternotomy: A single center experience with 2 years mean follow-up. *Thorac Cardiovasc Surg* 2015; 63: 467–71.

24. Kocher AA, Laufer G, Haverich A, et al. One-year outcomes of the surgical Treatment of aortic stenosis with a next generation surgical aortic valve (TRITON) trial: A prospective multicenter study of rapid-deployment aortic valve replacement with the EDWARDS INTUITY valve system. *J Thorac Cardiovasc Surg* 2013; 145: 110–5.

25. Barnhart GR, Accola KD, Grossi EA, et al. TRANSFORM (multicenter experience with rapid deployment Edwards INTUITY valve system for aortic valve replacement) US clinical trial: Performance of a rapid deployment aortic valve. *J Thorac Cardiovasc Surg* 2017; 153(2): 241–251.e2.

26. Liakopoulos OJ, Gerfer S, Weider S, et al. Direct comparison of the Edwards intuity elite and sorin perceval S rapid deployment aortic valves. *Ann Thorac Surg* 2018; 105(1): 108–114.

27. D'Onofrio A, Salizzoni S, Filippini C, et al. Surgical aortic valve replacement with new-generation bioprostheses: Sutureless versus rapid-deployment. *J Thorac Cardiovasc Surg* 2020; 159(2): 432–442. E1

28. Coti I, Schukro C, Drevinja F, et al. Conduction disturbances following surgical aortic valve replacement with a rapid-deployment bioprosthesis *J Thorac Cardiovasc Surg.* 2020; S0022-5223(20)30433-5. doi:10.1016/j.jtcvs.2020.01.083.

29. Vogt F, Moscarelli M, Nicoletti A, et al. Sutureless aortic valve and pacemaker rate: From surgical tricks to clinical outcomes. *Ann Thorac Surg* 2019; 108: 99–105.

30. Dalén M, Biancari F, Rubino AS, et al. Ministernotomy versus full sternotomy aortic valve replacement with a sutureless bioprosthesis: A multicenter study. *Ann Thorac Surg* 2015; 99: 524–30.
31. Dalén M, Biancari F, Rubino AS, et al. Aortic valve replacement through full sternotomy with a stented bioprosthesis versus minimally invasive sternotomy with a sutureless bioprosthesis. *Eur J Cardiothorac Surg.* 2016; 49(1): 220–227. doi:10.1093/ejcts/ezv014
32. Di Eusanio M, Phan K, Bouchard D, et al. Sutureless aortic valve replacement international registry (SU-AVR-IR): Design and rationale from the international valvular surgery study group (IVSSG). *Ann Cardiothorac Surg* 2015; 4: 131–9.

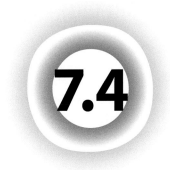

THE AORTIC VALVE
Endoscopic Aortic Valve Surgery

GIOVANNI DOMENICO CRESCE AND LORIS SALVADOR

HISTORY AND INTRODUCTION

Several minimally invasive approaches have been introduced in the past years for the surgical treatment of aortic valve disease [1]. Among them, currently the most popular are the partial sternotomy and the mini-right thoracotomy. The advantages of these approaches in terms of reducing the surgical trauma, the loss of blood, infections and the time of recovery are widely accepted, such as improved patient satisfaction [2]. However, these approaches still need either a sternal fracture or a rib resection and internal mammary vessel interruption.

We believe that surgical aortic valve replacement (AVR) can still offer some progress in the reduction of surgical trauma and surgical invasiveness. For these reasons, starting from our long experience in minimally invasive endoscopic mitral valve surgery, we decided to apply cardiac endoscopy also for aortic valve surgery.

Our technique is a completely video-guided operation using a miniaturized surgical approach. The surgical access is a 3–4-cm working port in the second right intercostal space with no rib spreading and without right mammary vessel sacrifice. Three additional 5-mm mini-ports are needed, for the introduction of a 30-degree thoracoscope, the trans-thoracic aortic clamp and the vent line.

OT SETUP AND INSTRUMENTATION

The operating theatre set-up for endoscopic AVR (E-AVR) is similar to standard AVR, except that a video column and specific long shaft instruments are needed. The use of 3D-video systems may speed up the procedure and provide better depth feedback. Its use anyway is not mandatory.

The patient is positioned supine with the right hemi-thorax elevated at an angle of 30°, in order to extend the intercostal spaces. The mechanical ventilation is achieved by a single-lumen endotracheal intubation, and a four-lumen central vein is placed. External plaques for direct current (DC) shock are applied. A transesophageal echocardiography (TEE) probe is placed, and its use is mandatory for this kind of operation.

HOW TO DO IT/STEP BY STEP

We start the operation with surgical exposure of the femoral vessels through a small skin incision (2 cm) and a limited dissection. Then, a 3- to 4-cm right mini-thoracotomy in the second or third intercostal space is done at the midclavicular line, representing our principal working port (Figure 7.4.1). Alternatively a right axillary artery cannulation can be done for peripheral CPB (Figure 7.4.2).

The surgical skin incision should be done just above the third rib, so that the second and the third intercostal spaces can be easily reached. A soft tissue retractor is then placed with no rib-spreading and without mammary vessel sacrifice. In obese or very muscular patients a self-retaining surgical retractor can be used in order to separate the tissue edges but not to spread the ribs, avoiding fractures and additional postoperative pain. Three additional 5-mm mini-ports are needed: In the fourth intercostal space to introduce the vent line; in the second intercostal space to introduce a 5-mm, 30° thoracoscope; in the first intercostal space to introduce the aortic cross clamp (Figure 7.4.3). A carbon dioxide line is connected to the trocar previously used to introduce the thoracoscope.

CARDIOPULMONARY BYPASS (CPB)

Since the limited working port does not enable direct central cannulation, CPB is achieved through femoral vessel cannulation under TEE guidance. The venous cannula has to be pushed into the superior vena cava to assure a good venous drainage. Vacuum-assisted venous drainage is

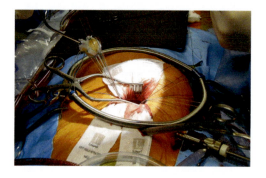

FIGURE 7.4.1 Mini-right thoracotomy. Working port detail.

FIGURE 7.4.2 Right axillary artery cannulation.

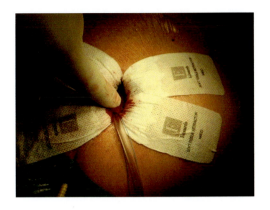

FIGURE 7.4.3　Operative setting.

FIGURE 7.4.4　AVR by using a completely video-guided approach.

needed, not exceeding −60 mmHg in the venous reservoir in order to avoid red blood cell damage.

AORTIC CROSS CLAMPING, CARDIOPLEGIA AND VENTRICULAR VENTING

Once the patient is under CPB the pericardium is opened under thoracoscopic vision, paying attention to avoid a phrenic nerve injury. The aortic cross clamping is achieved using a trans-thoracic Chitwood® clamp (Scanlan International, Inc, St Paul, MN, USA). It is very important to gently dissect the traverse sinus in order to avoid injury to the right branch of the pulmonary artery. A retroplegia catheter cannot be positioned through the working port, so the cardioplegia is delivered directly into the aortic root and then, after the aortotomy, directly into the coronary ostia if needed. Our preference of myocardial protection is the use of Bretschneider's histidine-tryptophan-ketoglutarate (HTK) cardioplegia solution, because a single dose provides a long period of myocardial protection. The vent line is placed through the superior right pulmonary vein and passed through the mini-port into the fourth intercostal space. Cardioplegia and ventricular venting can also be obtained by placing specific necklines (Propledge and Endovent, Edwards Lifesciences, Irvine, CA, USA). These lines keep the working port clear.

SURGICAL TECHNIQUE

The aortotomy should not be done toward the pulmonary artery, because this could be then difficult to manage if bleeding occurs. Moreover, it should be high enough if there is the intention to implant a sutureless or a rapid-deployment prosthesis. After the aortotomy, the aortic valve exposure is facilitated by using three retraction stitches placed at the aortic valve commissures. In addition, two or three stitches will keep the aortic wall away from the thoracoscope field. Then the aortic valve is normally excised and the annulus decalcified as necessary and the appropriate prosthetic valve implanted (Figure 7.4.4).

The aorta is normally closed using a double 4/0 prolene running suture. The ventricular pacing wire is placed on the inferior wall of the right ventricle after the closure of the aorta and before removing the aortic clamp or soon after, once the heart is empty. The de-airing of the left cavities is performed under TEE control, venting the ascending aorta and the left ventricle, without directly manipulating the heart. Two 24-Fr silastic chest tubes are positioned in the posterior pleural space and in the pericardial space passed through the mini-ports used to place the vent line and aortic clamp (Figure 7.4.5).

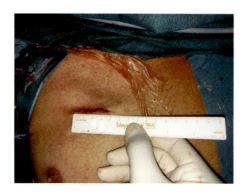

FIGURE 7.4.5 Final result (postoperative scar).

FIGURE 7.4.6 Minimally invasive endoscopic AVR: Operative results.

PROSTHETIC CHOICE

The choice of the prosthetic valve is made based on the characteristics and needs of the single patient and not influenced by the surgical exposure. In younger patients with good anatomy and in case of aortic regurgitation we implanted a standard stented bioprosthesis, which has a longer follow-up. In older patients, preferably with small aortic annulus, we implanted a sutureless valve. Rapid-deployment bioprostheses were preferred in younger patients with small annulus and "very left sided" aortic position, as well as in patients of any age with larger annulus but with mild ascending aorta dilatation.

SUMMARIZED EXPERIENCE

From July 2013 to October 2018, 165 consecutive patients (96 males, mean age 68.7 ± 11.4 years, mean EuroScore II 1.6 ± 1.4) underwent E-AVR at our institution. Thirty-four patients (20.6%) needed associated procedures: Septal miectomy in 8 cases, mitral valve surgery in 14 cases, combined mitral and tricuspid valve repair in 3 cases and ascending aorta surgery in 9 cases. Standard stented bioprostheses were implanted in 73 cases, rapid-deployment and sutureless bioprostheses in 34 and 58 cases respectively. In the 131 isolated E-AVR, mean aortic cross clamp and CPB times were 87.5 ± 22.6 and 126.6 ± 28.8 minutes respectively, and significant reduction was observed when a sutureless valve was implanted: 68.7 ± 14.7 and 105.6 ± 21.8 minutes (sutureless) vs 93.2 ± 15.1 and 135.5 ± 21.8 minutes (rapid deployment) and 100.6 ± 17.2 and 138.9 ± 21.9 minutes (stented). Mean ventilation, ICU time and hospital stay were 13.9 ± 39.3 hours, 45.6 ± 58.4 hours and 7.6 ± 7.8 days respectively. The overall mortality was 1.2%. In isolated AVR the mortality rate was 0.7%. Re-exploration for bleeding and new permanent pacemaker implantation occurred in 5 (3%) and 6 (3.6%) cases respectively. No major neurologic events were observed. No paravalvular leakage was detected at discharge. One conversion to sternotomy occurred (0.6%) (Figure 7.4.4).

CAVEATS AND CONTROVERSIES

Our setting allows working with indirect vision, to avoid rib spreading and mammary vessel sacrifice and to avoid preoperative CT scan screening and the preoperative patient selection.

A topic of discussion is the need for preoperative CT scan screening in minimally invasive AVR patients. We are aware that it is useful to assess the aortic anatomy and to identify the presence of potential contraindications. However, we did it not routinely, but only in cases where we wanted further investigation on patients with some dubious medical history or preoperative angiography images but not to assess the aortic anatomy, since the thoracoscopic vision does not limit the visual field and the ascending aorta can be easily reached. Nevertheless, we did not observe an increase in the embolic risk by avoiding routine CT scan as demonstrated by the lack of neurologic events in our experience.

Another controversy relates to the morbidity associated with peripheral cannulation. Murzi et al. [3] have shown that it may cause wound infection, pseudoaneurysms and neurological events, because the retrograde perfusion is an independent risk factor for neurological complications such as stroke and postoperative delirium. To avoid these complications, they suggest to cannulate the ascending aorta, which allows a more direct and physiological flow. The central cannulation is not feasible with our endoscopic approach. However, in our series we did not notice an increased neurological risk.

In the majority of previous reports, minimally invasive AVR is associated with longer operative times compared with standard sternotomy. Several studies have shown that the aortic cross clamp and cardiopulmonary bypass times are considered strong independent predictors of postoperative morbidity and mortality [4,5]. We are aware that building an endoscopic minimally invasive program requires a well-defined learning curve and so, at the beginning, the operative times are longer. We are confident that the operative times can be reduced over time with surgeons' growing experience and with the further development of sutureless or rapid-deployment valves. In our experience the Perceval valve required significantly shorter cross clamp and CPB times than the Intuity valve and the standard stented bioprosthesis. In E-AVR the Perceval valve seems to be the most comfortable prosthesis to implant, since it is collapsed on its holder and the visualization of the aortic annulus during positioning and deployment is maximized, even though its implantation requires a higher transverse aortotomy, reducing the space for proximal anastomoses.

WHERE AND HOW TO LEARN

Minimally invasive cardiac surgery is increasingly popular, and it is replacing the standard sternotomy technique to perform the majority of cardiac valvular operations. Nevertheless, all over the world most cardiac procedures are still performed by conventional standard sternotomy, which shows the need for proper training for minimally invasive techniques. The development and improvement of new surgical skills are challenging not only for residents and young surgeons, but also for more experienced consultants learning new techniques.

Nowadays there is a wide range of simulation-based training methods for surgeons starting or wanting to improve their learning curve in endoscopic cardiac surgery, such as "wet" and "dry" lab modules [6], which mainly reflects the use of synthetic or animal-model-based materials. At our institution we created a "wet" lab, where the basis of the simulation-based training method was a pig heart inserted into a

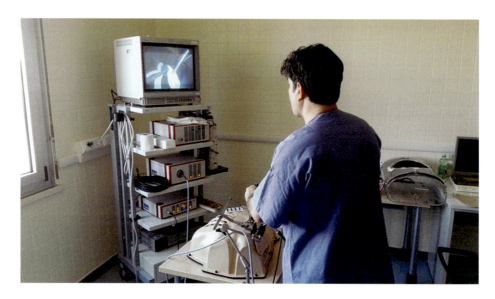

FIGURE 7.4.7 Wet lab.

chest model and a real video-column and the same long-shaft instruments were to simulate a real endoscopic heart operation (Figure 7.4.7).

After many hours of training and simulation in a wet lab, the learning process can be moved to the operating room. An initial period of supervision by a preceptor is essential, and it can be done using a fellowship or a residency model in specialized centers. Then a proctoring phase is needed, characterized by the presence of an observer who is responsible for the assessment of the skills and knowledge of the trainee during the initial learning curve.

CONCLUSIONS

Our experience shows that E-AVR is technically feasible and a safe procedure. The use of sutureless valves significantly reduces the aortic cross clamp and the CPB times. Concomitant procedures may be done through the same single working port. With further experience this approach may become the technique of choice for all patients undergoing AVR, and we can speculate that it may be the real alternative to TAVR in intermediate- and low-risk patients, but the advantage of this approach can be of benefit also for some high-risk patients.

REFERENCES

1. Ramlawi B, Bedeir K, Lamelas J. Aortic valve surgery: Minimally invasive options. *Methodist Debakey Cardiovasc J* 2016; 12(1): 27–32.
2. Glauber M, Ferrarini M, Miceli A. Minimally invasive aortic valve surgery: State of the art and future directions. *Ann Cardiothorac Surg* 2015; 4(1): 26–32. doi: 10.3978/j.issn.2225-319X.2015.01.01 2323
3. Murzi M, Cerillo AG, Miceli A, et al. Antegrade and retrograde arterial perfusion strategy in minimally invasive mitral-valve surgery: A propensity score analysis on 1280 patients. *Eur J Cardiothorac Surg* 2013; 43(6): e167–72.
4. Salis S, Mazzanti VV, Merli G, et al. Cardiopulmonary bypass duration is an independent predictor of morbidity

and mortality after cardiac surgery. *J Cardiothorac Vasc Anesth* 2008; 22: 814–22.
5. Al-Sarraf N, Thalib L, Hughes A, et al. Cross-clamp time is an independent predictor of mortality and morbidity in low- and high-risk cardiac patients. *Int J Surg* 2011; 9: 104–09.
6. Sardari Nia P, Daemen JHT, Maessen JG. Development of a high-fidelity minimally invasive mitral valve surgery simulator. *J Thorac Cardiovasc Surg* 2019; 157(4): 1567–1574.

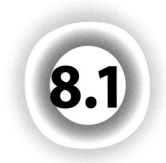

TRANSCATHETER AORTIC VALVE IMPLANTATION (TAVI)
Transapical Transcatheter Aortic Valve Replacement

AMALIA WINTERS, JESSICA FORCILLO AND VINOD H THOURANI

HISTORY AND INTRODUCTION

For decades, the standard of care for treating patients with aortic valvular pathology has required traditional surgical or minimally invasive aortic valve replacement (SAVR). However, in 2002 the future of treating these patients was changed when Dr. Alain Cribier performed the first transcatheter aortic valve replacement (TAVR) [1]. As we approach almost 15 years of experience with this technique, we have seen many variations of the initial technique described. While the first TAVR performed by Dr. Cribier was performed via an antegrade, transvenous, transseptal approach, more than 80% of TAVR procedures today worldwide are performed via a retrograde transfemoral (TF) approach. In the scenario when there is severe prohibitive peripheral vascular disease, alternative access procedures are performed including transapical (TA), transcarotid, subclavian, transcaval or transaortic approaches [2]. The most widely studied non-TF TAVR approaches include the transapical and transaortic TAVR. For this chapter, we will concentrate on the TA TAVR procedure (Figure 8.1.1).

The development of this new technology started with a few landmark clinical trials.

FIGURE 8.1.1 Round table on the future of aortic stenosis.

FIGURE 8.1.2 A discussion on the PARTNER 1A trial.

Published in 2010–2011, the Placement of Aortic Transcatheter Valves (PARTNER) trial was the world's first randomized controlled trial designed to study the safety and efficacy of the Edwards SAPIEN valve (Edwards Lifesciences, Irvine, California, USA), a balloon-expandable TAVR prosthesis. This device received FDA approval in 2011 for inoperable patients and in 2012 for high-risk patients. Transapical TAVR was first evaluated in the high-risk, PARTNER 1A study. This study randomized 699 high-risk patients to receive TAVR or SAVR and showed similar rates of survival between the procedures at 1 year. The results at 5 years maintain this trend and support TAVR as an alternative to surgery in high-risk patients [3,4]. In the PARTNER 1A study, both TAVR and SAVR offer a reduced mortality rate, reduction in symptoms and improved valve hemodynamics. However, the shortcomings of TAVR are the paravalvular regurgitation (PVRs), stroke rate and major vascular complications [4]. Device iterations have led to significant advances since the PARTNER 1 study (Figure 8.1.2). The PARTNER 2 study evaluated the SAPIEN XT and the SAPIEN 3 platforms, which have allowed significant reduction in complications associated with TAVR [5–8]. The two most notable advancements made since the original design include a skirt on the left ventricular portion of the valve to minimize PVR, and smaller access sheaths which have increased the number of eligible patients for TF TAVR from 55% to 90% (Figure 8.1.3).

HOW TO DO IT/STEP BY STEP

THE TRANSAPICAL APPROACH

The TA approach offers several advantages over its TF counterpart: (i) it is not limited by peripheral vascular anatomy and size, (ii) the valve is easily crossed in the antegrade direction (vs retrograde), (iii) the device does not cross the aortic arch, and (iv) there is improved fine adjustment prior to valve deployment. The TA approach allows for a more coaxial alignment of the stent-valve in the AV annulus and has been shown to have fewer paravalvular leaks than in those undergoing TF TAVR. Other potential advantages of the TA approach generally include shorter time for insertion and less contrast use. However, the effect of a thoracotomy on patient recovery, and the possibility of bleeding after direct cardiac cannulation make this a potentially higher-risk procedure than TF, which may not be suitable for those with significant parenchymal lung disease (for example forced expiratory volume in 1 second <35%) or low ejection fraction (<15–20%) [9].

FIGURE 8.1.3 A discussion on the PARTNER 2 trial.

OPERATIVE TECHNIQUE

TA-TAVR requires general anesthesia, and the procedure should be performed in a hybrid room with both fixed fluoroscopic imaging and TEE. Cardiopulmonary bypass should be readily available in case emergent conversion to open AVR is required. The patient is placed supine on the operating room table and femoral artery and vein access is achieved. A femoral transvenous pacer is placed in the right ventricle, and a pigtail catheter is placed in the aortic root via the femoral artery. Using fluoroscopic guidance, an anterolateral thoracotomy is made in the fifth or sixth intercostal space. A rib-spreading retractor is inserted, and the pericardium is incised and retracted with stay sutures to expose the left ventricular apex (Figure 8.1.4).

Two apical concentric pledgeted 2-0 prolene purse-string sutures are placed just cephalad to the apex and lateral to the LAD (Figure 8.1.5). The purse-string sutures must be deep into the myocardium as they are prone to tearing through the ventricular tissue.

The patient is heparinized to maintain an activated clotting time of 250 seconds. Fluoroscopy is used to position the aortic root and annulus perpendicular to each other, and to align all three aortic cusps in the same plane in a similar fashion to the TF approach. At our institution, we generally have performed this with the angled pigtail in the non-coronary cusp. The importance of achieving proper alignment cannot

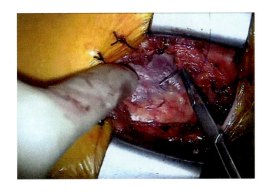

FIGURE 8.1.4 Exposure for transapical approach.

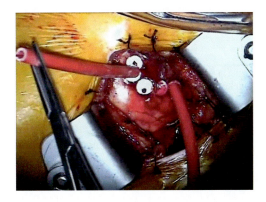

FIGURE 8.1.5 Purse-string sutures for transapical approach.

be overstated as this is crucial for accurate valve implantation. The LV cavity is punctured with a needle and a 0.035" wire is passed into the left ventricle, across the aortic valve and into the ascending aorta. The wire is maintained in the ascending aorta without entry into the carotid arteries as the needle is exchanged for a 7 French sheath. A catheter is then placed through the LV apex and across the aortic valve (Figure 8.1.6 and Figure 8.1.7). A right Judkins catheter is used to manipulate the 0.035" wire into the descending aorta. The 0.035" guide wire is exchanged for an Amplatz super stiff wire (Boston Scientific, Natick, MA) over which the valve will be delivered. The 7 French sheath is exchanged for the appropriate transapical delivery sheath

FIGURE 8.1.6　Transapical TAVI by Ahmed Ouda.

FIGURE 8.1.7 Transapical TAVI by Turki Albacker, Rajesh Ramankutty and Eric Roselli.

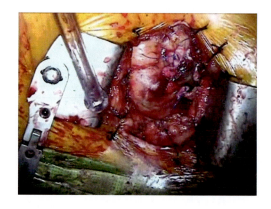

FIGURE 8.1.8 Ventriculostomy closure after transapical approach.

FIGURE 8.1.9　Hour-long documentary on TAVR team, technique and patients.

which is positioned 4 cm inside the LV. If a BAV is indicated, a valvuloplasty balloon is threaded over the wire and under rapid ventricular pacing of 180–200 beats per second the balloon is inflated. Most recently, we have not routinely performed a BAV in our TA cases, except in those circumstances where balloon sizing is required. Following BAV, the balloon is removed and the valve is delivered through the sheath and positioned across the valve.

Positioning of the valve is a critically important aspect of any TAVR procedure. Using both echocardiographic and fluoroscopic imaging, the valve is aligned parallel to the long axis of the aorta and perpendicular to the aortic annulus.[10] Both TEE and aortic root injection can be used to confirm the position of the valve and its spatial orientation. The SAPIEN valve, a balloon-expandable valve, is ideally positioned so that its upper margin covers the aortic leaflet tips, while the ventricular end covers the aortic annulus. Once the optimal position is established, the valve is deployed during rapid ventricular pacing. The valve delivery apparatus is then removed, leaving the stiff wire across the bioprosthesis. Echocardiography with color Doppler and angiography is employed to evaluate valve position and assess the amount of paravalvular leak. Repeat balloon dilation may be performed for ≥2+ paravalvular leak; however, most pericardial valves will have a small central aortic regurgitant jet.

Once satisfactory valve function and position are achieved, all catheters and wires are removed from the apex and purse-string sutures are tightened during rapid ventricular pacing. Protamine is administered and additional sutures may be placed in the LV apex to achieve hemostasis (Figure 8.1.8). The pericardium is closed loosely over the LV apex and a flexible chest tube is placed in the left pleural space. After hemostasis has been achieved, local anesthetic is injected into the intercostal bundle and the chest is closed in multiple layers (Figure 8.1.9).

TOOLS/INSTRUMENTS AND DEVICES

For transapical TAVI, standard transfemoral set is required. A thoracotomy set will be required for left anterior thoracotomy for accessing the apex.

PERIOPERATIVE CONSIDERATION

PREOPERATIVE ASSESSMENT AND PLANNING

In the U.S., TAVR is currently a suggested method of treatment for patients with a life expectancy greater than 1 year and severe AS, who are also considered intermediate-, high- or extreme-risk by a multi-disciplinary heart team. Under the current guidelines, these are patients who have a Society of Thoracic Surgeons (STS) predicted risk score of mortality (PROM) ≥3% or coexisting conditions that would be associated with a predicted 30-day surgical mortality of ≥15%. In August 2016, the SAPIEN 3 valve was approved in the U.S. for use in patients considered intermediate-risk for SAVR based on the PARTNER 2 S3i study.[6] (Figure 8.1.10).

Initial TAVR evaluation should include an assessment of the following patient variables: (i) severity of aortic stenosis, (ii) ileo-femoral vessel size, calcification and tortuosity, (iii) anatomic details of the aortic valve leaflets, (iv) annulus, sinotubular and sinus of Valsalva dimensions, (v) ventricular function and (vi) extent of coronary artery disease. Due to their accuracy and reproducibility, we utilize 3-D computed tomography (CT) of the chest, abdomen and pelvis, and echocardiography as the primary imaging modalities at our institution.

Echocardiography is primarily used to delineate the severity of aortic stenosis, aortic regurgitation and ventricular dysfunction. Measurements of the annulus as well as the sinus of Valsalva, the sinotubular junction and the coronary heights are commonly garnered from the CT scan (Figure 8.1.11 and Figure 8.1.12). Accurate measurement is essential, as failure to properly size the annulus may result in improper valve selection, with subsequent paravalvular leak or embolization. In addition, there is risk of coronary obstruction if the sinus of Valsalva is narrow, if there is a short distance between the annulus and the coronary ostia (<10 mm) or bulky leaflet calcification exists. In those who are unable to undergo a CT secondary to chronic kidney disease, accurate 3-D measurements of the annulus are obtained from a TEE. The use of supra-valvular aortography during balloon aortic valvuloplasty (BAV) may provide additional information when the aortic annulus size remains questionable.

FIGURE 8.1.10 Edwards transcatheter aortic valve system.

FIGURE 8.1.11 Role of 4D CT in TAVR.

In addition to valve measurements, the CT scan is also used for assessment of the femoral arteries and aorta. At our institution, CT measurements of the annular area and perimeter have supplanted two-dimensional echocardiography in guiding appropriate valve selection. If there are significant concerns with the size, calcification or tortuosity of the peripheral vessels, then alternative access is used. This is always a consensus decision among the dedicated heart valve team.

When a TF TAVR is contraindicated by preoperative imaging, alternative approaches are then considered. A TA approach, via an anterior left mini-thoracotomy, has traditionally been employed as the alternative in these patients. However, this approach comes with additional challenges, and may not be appropriate for all patients. In this scenario, a transcaval, transcarotid, subclavian or transaortic TAVR are possibilities[9].

ALTERNATIVE APPROACHES

Most TAVI procedures are performed under transfemoral approach. The following chapter focuses on a transfemoral approach for TAVI. Other possible accesses include transcaval, transcarotid, subclavian or transaortic TAVI.

CAVEATS AND CONTROVERSIES

The first feasibility studies were conducted in the early 2000s, and while they had procedural success, the patients had poor prognoses due to the inherent nature of their comorbid state. The first clinical series of transapical TAVR reported was from Walther et al. and included 50 patients successfully treated from 2006 to 2007[11]. Forty-seven of these patients received an Edwards SAPIEN valve via anterolateral thoracotomy, while three required conversion to a conventional sternotomy. During the follow-up period, which ranged from 6 to 18 months, 24 patients died due to non-valve-related causes.

The PARTNER trial was the first randomized controlled trial using TA TAVR. While this trial had a TF-first approach, transapical TAVR was performed in 30% of patients undergoing transcatheter valve replacement. Patients were grouped into two arms on the basis of whether transfemoral access was possible. In the TA arm of the PARTNER 1A trial, 207 high-risk patients were randomized to TA TAVR (n = 104) and 103 to SAVR. Thirty-day mortality was 3.8% in the TA-TAVR group compared to 7.0% in the surgical group in the intention to treat analysis, compared to the TF group where mortality was 3.3% and 6.2% in TF TAVR and SAVR groups, respectively. There were no significant differences in 1-year mortality in either group. The 5-year follow-up of the PARTNER trial showed a sustained benefit of TAVR in all-cause mortality,

FIGURE 8.1.12 Measurement of the aortic annulus on CT.

cardiovascular mortality, repeat hospitalization and functional status[12].

Since the analysis in the PARTNER study, there is some difficulty in assessing the optimal access, transfemoral vs transapical, as most trials have a TF TAVR-first policy. Therefore, it is common that TA patients are high-risk patients in terms of a higher incidence of iliofemoral disease and the associated cardiovascular co-morbidities when compared to TF patients. In a post-hoc analysis of the PARTNER 1 trial, a propensity-matched analysis of 501 TA and TF matches showed an increase in early mortality in the TA group, which equalized after 4 months. Transapical TAVR was associated with a longer hospital stay, and a slower, but equal after 6 months, improvement in NYHA status compared to TF TAVR. Stroke rates, pacemaker requirement and instance of post-operative MI were similar between the two groups[13]. From a cost-savings perspective, TF TAVR shows a modest decrease in cost, both in terms of cost index of hospitalization and costs in the first year after surgery, compared to SAVR, whereas TA TAVR is associated with a greater cost index of hospitalization as well as costs at 1 year[13].

In addition to the randomized trials with very experienced sites, the Society of Thoracic Surgeons (STS)/American College of Cardiology (ACC) Transcatheter Valve Therapies (TVT) database monitors the real-world experience in the United States. Holmes and colleagues have shown that from 2012 to end of 2014, the peak usage of TA TAVR was in 2013, with ~80% of cases performed using TF access, 10% as TA, and 10% as other[14]. In the largest study to date, Thourani and colleagues evaluated 4,085 patients undergoing TA TAVR in the U.S. national TVT database[2] They noted a mean age of 82 years and a median STS predicted risk of mortality of 8.8%. The 30-day mortality was 8.8% and 1-year was 25.6%. The in-hospital stroke rate was 2.2% and major vascular complications were 0.3%; while 1-year heart failure re-hospitalization was 15.7%. These outcomes, although not as robust as those in a clinical trial, do represent a real-world experience (Figure 8.1.13).

Over the past 15 years, the number of complications with TAVR has diminished dramatically. One of the devastating complications after any cardiovascular procedure is stroke. From the PARTNER I trial, rates of any neurologic event were higher in the TAVR group compared to SAVR at 30 days and 1 year (5.5% vs 2.4% at 30 days, and 8.3% vs 4.3% at 1 year). However, with device iteration and operator experience, the risk of stroke has significantly decreased. In the most recent PARTNER 2 study, the overall stroke rate at 30 days was as low as 1.5% in high-risk patients.

Other complications for TAVR include the need for a new pacemaker which varies widely from approximately 4% to 40% depending on the device used. The most common conduction abnormality seen after TAVR is complete AV block, but symptomatic brady-arrythmias have been reported. The majority of cases of heart block occur within the first 7 days after TAVR, so careful monitoring in the immediate post-operative period is important. Generally, TAVR with a self-expandable valve requires a longer assessment for conduction abnormalities, compared with the balloon-expandable valves[15,16]

The reported incidence of AKI after cardiac surgery varies widely but has been reported to be as high as 30%, with approximately 1–5% of patients requiring renal replacement therapy[17]. Therefore, it is no surprise that AKI is seen after TAVR as well. Reported rates of AKI in the PARTNER trials were low, and there was no significant difference in AKI between the TAVR and SAVR groups (Figure 8.1.14).

While major bleeding complications are more common in SAVR patients compared to TAVR patients, bleeding complications cannot be ignored. In the PARTNER trial, the incidence of major bleeding complications was 8.8% in the TA group compared to 11.3% in the TF group and 22.7% in the SAVR group. Major bleeding had an adverse effect on 1-year mortality in the total population, but in the sub-analysis of both TA and TF patients, there was no difference in 1-year mortality between patients who had, and those who had not, experienced a major bleeding complication[18].

RESEARCH, TRENDS AND INNOVATION

Nearly 15 years after this operation was pioneered, we have seen a major change in direction in treatments for valvular disease, with all four heart valves being treated via transcatheter procedures, as well as the valve-in-valve TAVRs for failing bioprosthetic valves. TAVR has become the standard of care for patients with severe symptomatic AS deemed high- or extreme-risk and is now approved for those who are at intermediate risk. The PARTNER 3 trial will give us more insight on moving TAVI towards low-risk patient groups. While most procedures are performed via a transfemoral or transapical approach, the access options such as transaortic, transcaval, transcarotid and subclavian approaches are narrowing the list of anatomic exclusions to TAVR and have served to make this procedure more accessible to a wide variety of patients. Now that the learning curve has been passed in most large centers, future studies may be better able to elucidate differences between the different access options for TAVR.

WHERE AND HOW TO LEARN

Prof Alain Cribier workshop in Rouen France: The program known as "Minimalist TF-TAVI Workshop". Hands-on experience is provided with work on an electronic simulator, on CT-imaging in our radiology lab, on TAVI devices and closure devices. This program is accredited by the European Board for Accreditation in Cardiology (EBAC) for 10 hours of external CME credits (Figure 8.1.15).

Medtronic TAVI workshop for cardiac surgeons: The Medtronic Training and Education TAVI program gives participants a better understanding of TAVI best practices. The TAVI Training Programme features a blended learning curriculum, combining online training, live cases, case discussions, simulation and updates on new developments in the treatment of aortic stenosis and patient environment best practices (Figure 8.1.16).

FIGURE 8.1.13 Physicians respond to intermediate-risk TAVR approval.

FIGURE 8.1.14 Explant of a migrated TAVR valve.

FIGURE 8.1.15 Minimalist TF-TAVI Workshop.

FIGURE 8.1.16 Medtronic Training and Education TAVI programme.

REFERENCES

1. Cribier A, Eltchaninoff H, Bash A, Borenstein N, Tron C, Bauer F, Derumeaux G, Anselme F, Laborde F, and Leon M. Percutaneous transcatheter implantation of an aortic valve prosthesis for calcific aortic stenosis: first human case description. *Circulation*. 2002;106:3006–3008.
2. Thourani VH, Li C, Devireddy C, Jensen HA, Kilo P, Leshnower BG, Mavromatis K, Sarin EL, Nguyen TC, Kanitkar M, Guyton RA, Block PC, Maas L, Simone A, Keegan P, Merlino J, Stewart JP, Lerakis S, and Babaliaros V. High-risk patients with inoperative aortic stenosis: use of transapical, transaortic, and transcarotid techniques. *The Annals of Thoracic Surgery*. 2015;99:817–25.
3. Smith CR, Leon MB, Mack MJ, Miller DC, Moses JW, Svensson LG, Tuzcu EM, Webb JG, Fontana GP, Makkar RR, Williams M, Dewey T, Kapadia S, Babaliaros V, Thourani VH, Corso P, Pichard AD, Bavaria JE, Herrmann HC, Akin JJ, Anderson WN, Wang D, and Pocock SJ. Transcatheter versus surgical aortic-valve replacement in high-risk patients. *The New England Journal of Medicine*. 2011;364:2187–98.
4. Mack MJ, Leon MB, Smith CR, Miller DC, Moses JW, Tuzcu EM, Webb JG, Douglas PS, Anderson WN, Blackstone EH, Kodali SK, Makkar RR, Fontana GP, Kapadia S, Bavaria J, Hahn RT, Thourani VH, Babaliaros V, Pichard A, Herrmann HC, Brown DL, Williams M, Akin J, Davidson MJ, and Svensson LG. 5-year outcomes of transcatheter aortic valve replacement or surgical aortic valve replacement for high surgical risk patients with aortic stenosis (PARTNER 1): a randomised controlled trial. *The Lancet*. 2015;385:2477–84.
5. Leon MB, Smith CR, Mack MJ, Makkar RR, Svensson RG, Kodali SK, Thourani VH, Murat Tuzcu E, Miller DC, Herrmann HC, Doshi D, Cohen DJ, Pichard AD, Kapadia S, Dewey T, Babaliaros V, Szeto WY, Williams MR, Kereiakes D, Zajarias A, Greason KL, Whisenant BK, Hodson RW, Moses JW, Trento A, Brown DL, Fearon WF, Pibarot P, Hahn RT, Jaber WA, Anderson WN, Alu MC, and Webb JG for the PARTNER 2 Investigators. Transcatheter or surgical aortic-valve replacement in intermediate-risk patients. *The New England Journal of Medicine*. 2016;374:1609–1620.
6. Thourani VH, Kodali S, Makkar RR, Herrmann HC, Williams M, Babaliaros V, Smalling R, Lim S, Malaisrie SC, Kapadia S, Szeto WY, Greason KL, Kereiakes D, Ailawadi G, Whisenant BK, Devireddy C, Leipsic J, Hahn RT, Pibarot P, Weissman NJ, Jaber WA, Cohen DJ, Suri R, Tuzcu EM, Svensson LG, Webb JG, Moses JW, Mack MJ, Miller DC, Smith CR, Alu MC, Parvataneni R, D'Agostino Jr RB, and Leon MB. Transcatheter aortic valve replacement versus surgical valve replacement in intermediate-risk patients: a propensity score analysis. *The Lancet*. 2016;387:2218–2225.
7. Kodali S, Thourani VH, White J, Malaisrie SC, Lim S, Greason KL, Williams MW, Guerrero M, Eisenhauer AC, Kapadia S, Kereiakes DJ, Herrmann HC, Babaliaros V, Szeto WY, Hahn RT, Pibarot P, Weissman NJ, Leipsic J, Blanke P, Whisenant BK, Suri RM, Makkar RR, Ayele GM, Svensson LG, Webb JG, Mack MJ, Smith CR, and Leon MB. Early clinical and echocardiographic outcomes after SAPIEN 3 transcatheter aortic valve replacement in inoperable,

high-risk and intermediate-risk patients with aortic stenosis. *European Heart Journal.* 2016;21(28):2252–62.
8. Herrmann HC, Thourani VH, Kodali SK, Makkar RR, Szeto WY, Anwaruddin S, Desai N, Lim S, Malaisrie SC, Kereiakes DJ, Ramee S, Greason KL, Kapadia S, Babaliaros V, Hahn RT, Pibarot P, Weissman NJ, Leipsic J, Whisenant BK, Webb JG, Mack MJ, and Leon MB for the PARTNER Investigators. One-year clinical outcomes with SAPIEN 3 transcatheter aortic valve replacement in high-risk and inoperable patients with severe aortic stenosis. *Circulation.* 2016;134:130–140.
9. Thourani VH, Gunter RL, Neravetla S, Block P, Guyton RA, Kilgo P, Lerakis S, Devireddy C, Leshnower B, Mavromatis K, Stewart J, Simone A, Keegan P, Nguyen TC, Merlino J, and Babaliaros V. Use of transaortic, transapical, and transcarotid transcatheter aortic valve replacement in inoperable patients. *The Annals of Thoracic Surgery.* 2013;96:1349–57.
10. Walther T, Dewey T, Borger MA, Kempfert J, Linke A, Becht R, Falk V, Schuler G, Mohr FW, and Mack M. Transapical aortic valve implantation: step by step. *The Annals of Thoracic Surgery.* 2009;87:276–83.
11. Walther T, Falk V, Kempfert J, Borger M, Fassl J, Chu M, Schuler G, and Mohr F. Transapical minimally invasive aortic valve implantation; the initial 50 patients. *European Journal of Cardio-thoracic Surgery.* 2008;33(6):983–988.
12. Kapadia S, Leon MB, Makkar RR, Tuzcu EM, Svensson LG, Kodali S, Webb JG, Mack MJ, Douglas PS, Thourani VH, Babaliaros VC, Herrmann HC, Szeto WY, Pichard AD, Williams MR, Fontana GP, Miller DC, Anderson WN, and Smith CR for the PARTNER Trial Investigators. 5-year outcomes of transcatheter aortic valve replacement compared with standard treatment for patients with inoperable aortic stenosis (PARTNER 1): a randomised controlled trial. *The Lancet.* 2015;385(9986):2485–2491.
13. Kappetein P, Head SJ, Treede H, Reichenspurner H, Mohr F, and Walther T. What is the evidence allowing us to state that transcatheteraortic valve replacement via the femoral artery is a more attractive option compared to transapical valve replacement? Early clinical and echocardiographic outcomes after SAPIEN 3 transcatheter aortic valve replacement in inoperable, high-risk and intermediate-risk patients with aortic stenosis. *EuroIntervention.* 2011;7(8):903–4.
14. Holmes DR, Nishimura NA, Grover FL, Brindis RG, Carroll JD, Edwards FH, Peterson ED, Rumsfeld JS, Shahian DM, MD, Thourani VH, Tuzcu M, Vemulapalli S, Hewitt K, Michaels J, Fitzgerald S, Mack MJ, for the STS/ACC TVT Registry. Annual outcomes with transcatheter valve therapy: from the STS/ACC TVT Registry. *The Annals of Thoracic Surgery.* 2016;101:789–800.
15. Erkapic D, De Rosa S, Kelava A, Lehmann R, Fichtlscherer S, and Hohnloser SH. Risk for permanent pacemaker after transcatheter aortic valve implantation. *Journal of Cardiovascular Electrophysiology.* 2012;23(4):391–397.
16. Rivard L, Schram G, Asgar A, Khairy P, Andrade JG, Bonan R, Dubuc M, Guerra PG, Ibrahim R, Macle L, Roy D, Talajic M, Dyrda K, Shohoudi A, le Polain de Waroux JB, and Thibault B. Electrocardiographic and electrophysiological predictors of atrioventricular block after transcatheter aortic valve replacement. *Heart Rhythm.* 2015;12(2):321–9.
17. Mao H, Katz N, Ariyanon W, Blanca-Martos L, Adýbelli Z, Giuliani A, Danesi T, H, Kim J, C, Nayak A, Neri M, Virzi G, M, Brocca A, Scalzotto E, Salvador L, and Ronco C. Cardiac surgery-associated acute kidney injury. *Cardiorenal Medicine.* 2013;3:178–199.
18. Généreux P, Cohen DJ, Williams MR, Mack M, Kodali SK, Svensson LG, Kirtane AJ, Xu K, McAndrew TC, Makkar R, Smith CR, and Leon MB. Bleeding complications after surgical aortic valve replacement compared with transcatheter aortic valve replacement: insights from the PARTNER I trial (placement of aortic transcatheter valve). *Journal of the American College of Cardiology.* 2014;63(11):1100–1109.

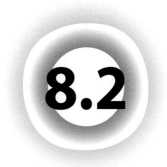

TRANSFEMORAL TRANSCATHETER AORTIC VALVE IMPLANTATION

IVANDITO KUNTJORO AND EDGAR TAY

HISTORY AND INTRODUCTION

Transcatheter aortic valve implantation (TAVI), a percutaneous treatment for severe aortic valve stenosis, is increasingly performed worldwide. It is the standard of choice for patients who are deemed inoperable and a good alternative for patients who are at high surgical risk. While adoption of the technology has been rapid, it is interesting to note that the success story of TAVI is quite recent [1].

The first percutaneous implantation of expandable aortic valve was performed by Andersen et al. in an animal model in 1992 [2]. The technique of implanting a stented valve mounted on a balloon over a delivery catheter was thus proven to be feasible (Figure 8.2.1).

The early development stage of TAVI was done by the anterograde approach by performing trans-septal catheterization from the right femoral vein which was used as an access route for delivering the percutaneous heart valve (PHV) to the stenotic native valve [3,4]. The first human case description of a successful TAVI by this method was reported by Cribier et al. in 2002 [3].

From April 2002 to August 2003, the team successfully performed the procedure in six patients who had severe calcific aortic stenosis (AS) [4]. Despite showing positive short-term results, the steep learning curve with regards to positioning difficulties of the PHV from this anterograde approach

FIGURE 8.2.1 Development of TAVR: an ongoing odyssey.

has prompted substantial modification of the technique. A different approach by a retrograde route of implantation was pioneered by Webb et al. in 2006 and displayed initial procedural success of 78% [5].

Using the Cribier Valve (Edwards LifeSciences Inc, Irvine, CA), the delivery sheath was inserted from the femoral artery (instead of vein) and then advanced to reach the aortic valve retrogradely from aorta. This "retrograde" approach is now the preferred route access in carrying out transfemoral TAVI. Procedure outcomes continued to get better as the implantation techniques, the PHV modification, the delivery sheath and patient selection improved. The first randomized trial of TAVI in inoperable and high-risk patients with symptomatic severe AS, the Placement of Aortic Transcatheter Valve (PARTNER) trial, demonstrated the safety and efficacy of this treatment, and cemented TAVI's role in high-risk and inoperable symptomatic severe AS patients [6].

Currently TAVI is indicated for the treatment of severe AS patient with very high surgical mortality (inoperable) and an alternative for patients with high and intermediate surgical risk. This recommendation was endorsed by both the American College of Cardiology (ACC) and the European Society of Cardiology (ESC). Both however emphasized the importance of a multidisciplinary "heart team" involving cardiologists and cardiac surgeons to make conjoint decisions for the optimal treatment. The PARTNER 2 study demonstrated the safety and efficacy of TAVI in intermediate surgical risk patients, which resulted in TAVI being a reasonable alternative to surgery for this group of patients [7].

HOW TO DO IT/STEP BY STEP

PATIENT SELECTION

Patient risk undergoing cardiac surgery is most commonly assessed by using either the Society of Thoracic Surgery Predicted Risk of Mortality (STS-PROM) or the EuroSCORE. These calculations can help provide the objective quantification of the surgical risk. In general, a patient is considered to have high surgical risk if they have STS-estimated 30-day mortality of >8% or a logistic EuroSCORE >20%. However certain patient characteristics such as porcelain aorta, prior chest radiation and other factors such as patient frailty, nutritional status and mobility status are not included as part of the risk score assessment, and may result in underestimation of the patient overall surgical risk. It is also becoming clearer that some patients may be at such high risk that therapy may be futile (e.g. patients with metastatic cancer, bedbound patients or those with severe advanced lung disease).

SETUP AND EQUIPMENT

The procedure can be performed in either the cardiac catheterization laboratory or hybrid operating room with the capability of providing high-quality fluoroscopic images. For high-risk patients the cardiopulmonary bypass (CPB) machine should be

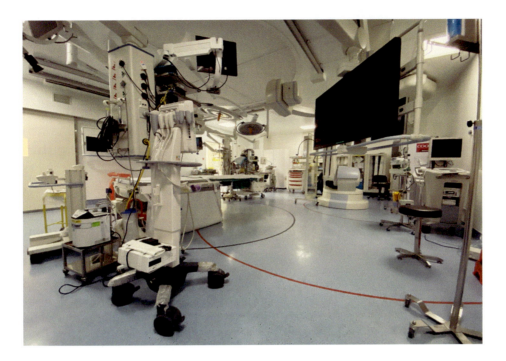

FIGURE 8.2.2 Hybrid operating room.

made available for emergencies. Equipment for emergency coronary and peripheral or vascular intervention should also be available. Transesophageal echocardiography (TOE) can be used for imaging if the patient is under general anesthesia, while transthoracic echocardiography (TTE) is used for patients treated under sedation and local anesthesia. The room should be adequately sized to accommodate the team members including the operators, cardiac imaging team, cardiac anesthetic team, supporting nurses and radiographers (Figure 8.2.2).

VASCULAR ACCESS

The preferred site for procedural access should ideally be decided before the procedure based on the data obtained from computed tomography (CT) angiography. The access can be obtained by direct percutaneous cannulation approach or surgical cutdown. In order to minimize complication and increase safety, our unit uses a 4F micro puncture needle and sheath in which an 18G needle is used initially to obtain arterial and venous access and upsized to a 5Fr or 6Fr sheath respectively. For calcified vessels around the puncture site, vascular access will be performed under ultrasound guidance. Via the venous sheath, the temporary pacemaker wire would be inserted. Note that alternative sites for this could be from the internal jugular veins.

The arterial access will allow passage of a pigtail catheter for aortic root angiogram. A cross-over angiogram is performed to delineate the ideal puncture site for the site of TAVI delivery sheath access. This can be done using a pigtail, Judkins right (JR) or internal mammary artery (IMA) catheter. In our unit we usually place a 0.018" V-18 ControlWire Guidewire (Boston Scientific, Marlborough, MA, USA) from the contralateral side to act as a safety wire (Figure 8.2.3), which allows ease of intervention for vascular complications. The wire also helps localize the femoral artery

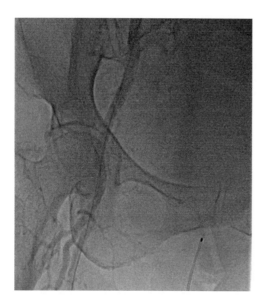

FIGURE 8.2.3 Control wire V18 positioned on the contralateral side of the femoral artery access.

FIGURE 8.2.4 Assessment of ideal implantation angle.

and assists in cannulation of the femoral artery site chosen for TAVI access. Once arterial access is obtained, a 6F sheath is inserted, then the access is "pre-closed" with two Perclose ProGlide® (Abbott, Chicago, IL, USA) or Prostar (Abbott, Chicago, IL, USA) vascular closure devices. For larger-size artery with no significant calcification or tortuosity, the access site can be alternatively closed with a Manta® vascular closure device.

TEMPORARY PACEMAKER PLACEMENT

The pacemaker wire position has to be stable (the balloon should be deflated when balloon tipped wires are used) and then tested for adequate capture. The pacemaker should be able to perform overdrive pacing which is essential to reduce cardiac output and transvalvular blood flow which are critical during balloon aortic valvuloplasty (BAV) and valve deployment of the balloon-expandable valve.

AORTIC ROOT ANGIOGRAM

The pigtail catheter is inserted from the contralateral arterial access. This is ideally positioned on the non-coronary cusp. The pre-determined angle of implantation based on the CT angiography is tested to make sure that all the inferior aspects of the three aortic cusps are aligned and lie along a single line (Figure 8.2.4). Minor adjustment may be needed for ideal positioning, but importantly this has to be done before valve implantation.

DELIVERY SHEATH INSERTION

The femoral artery is sequentially dilated to facilitate placement of the larger TAVI delivery sheath. It is important to ensure that the large sheaths are inserted and advanced over a stiff wire (usually the Amplatz super stiff or extra stiff wire). The sheath should be secured with sutures and flushed.

AORTIC VALVE CROSSING

Prior to the valve crossing, patient has to be fully anticoagulated with heparin to achieve an activated clotting time (ACT) of >250s. The native aortic valve can be crossed using the Amplatz left 1 (AL1) with a straight tip 0.035" polytetrafluoroethylene (PTFE) or hydrophilic (Terumo) wire. Other catheters that can be used are the Judkins right (JR4), AL2 or rarely JL6 or multipurpose catheter.

The wire should be advanced gently to probe the aortic orifice. Once the valve is crossed, the catheter can be advanced into the left ventricle guided by the wire. This wire can then be exchanged with a stiffer exchange length wire. The standard wire that can be used is the Amplatz Extra-Stiff 0.035" wire (Cook Medical, Bloomington, IN, USA) or the Amplatz Super Stiff™ wire (Boston Scientific, Marlborough, MA, USA), which can be manually shaped to conform to the LV cavity. Other alternatives are the pre-shaped TAVI guidewires such as the Confida Guidewire (Medtronic, Fridley, MN, USA) and the Safari Guidewire (Boston Scientific, Marlborough, MA, USA).

Good wire positioning can allow easy valve delivery and reduces the risks of excessive premature ventricular ectopics (PVCs) and left ventricular (LV) perforation. In some cases, this can be achieved by insertion of a pigtail catheter to the LV. The operator must pay attention and maintain the wire position inside the LV at all times until the valve is successfully deployed.

BALLOON AORTIC VALVULOPLASTY (BAV)

Predilation with BAV is occasionally done to facilitate the insertion and deployment of the valve (Figure 8.2.5). This is no longer a routine and is used for selected cases (such as for patients with critically stenosed valves with very high gradients, bicuspid aortic valve for assisted sizing or assessment of coronary obstruction risk in some patients). The annular size is used as guidance to choose the balloon size. The size of the valvuloplasty balloon selected should not exceed the minor axis dimension of the annulus. Once the balloon crosses the valve, rapid pacing is initiated to achieve adequate reduction of the pulse pressure before the balloon can be inflated.

VALVE IMPLANTATION

The delivery system with the mounted valve is introduced into the sheath and inserted over the stiff wire. Each prosthetic valve has its unique delivery system. However, the objective is to deliver the valve with minimal trauma across the aortic arch and to finally position it at the annulus.

Prior to final valve deployment, the position of the crimped valve in relation to the aortic cusp has to be assessed with aortic root angiogram and adjusted if necessary. There are again differences in the deployment steps for each valve. For the balloon-expandable valve, the deployment is done under rapid pacing (Figure 8.2.6).

The self-expandable valves however do not require rapid ventricular pacing. After the valve is fully deployed in a satisfactory position, the delivery system can be removed while still maintaining the stiff wire in the LV cavity in anticipation of post-balloon dilation. The removal of the delivery system must be done cautiously under fluoroscopy to ensure that the nose cones of the devices do not interact with the valve or

FIGURE 8.2.5 Rapid pacing during BAV.

FIGURE 8.2.6 Valve deployment under rapid pacing.

FIGURE 8.2.7 TAVI animation, PARTNER trial video link.

cause trauma to the aorta (Figure 8.2.7 and Figure 8.2.8).

POST-VALVE IMPLANTATION ASSESSMENT

It is crucial to immediately assess the hemodynamic function of the valve following valve deployment. This can be achieved using echocardiography to assess the valve stability, mean gradients and presence of aortic regurgitation (AR). Invasive assessment can also be done by placing a pigtail catheter into the left ventricle.

The Sinning index as well as mean gradients can be calculated. Aortic root angiography can also be performed to assess for aortic regurgitation. After satisfactory valve function is confirmed, the stiff wire can be removed from the LV cavity (this is done by exchanging the stiff wire with a pigtail catheter). The pre-deployed sutures are then tightened.

It is important to perform a contralateral angiogram to assess the femoral artery flow on the TAVI access site and rule out any vascular complications such as dissection or perforation. Over the V-18 wire, a multipurpose catheter can be used to perform the angiogram. If vascular complication is identified on the access site, the wire can also be used to track a peripheral angioplasty balloon to tamponade the bleeding site while considering definitive measures such as percutaneous treatment with a covered stent or surgical repair (Figure 8.2.9 and Figure 8.2.10).

TOOLS/INSTRUMENTS AND DEVICES

SAPIEN 3 (EDWARDS LIFESCIENCES, IRVINE, CA, USA)

The Edwards Sapien 3 transcatheter heart valve is a biological valve that replaces diseased aortic valve. It is available in four sizes, 20 mm, 23 mm, 26 mm and 29 mm in diameter. Approved for valve-in-valve for both aortic and mitral position (Figure 8.2.11).

∞ Commander and Certitude delivery systems.

EVOLUT R (MEDTRONIC, FRIDLEY, MN, USA)

The Evolut™ R valve was built on the CoreValve™ system. The Evolut R features a supra-annular positioning and it has a low delivery profile. The latest iteration is the Evolut Pro which has an external pericardial wrap to reduce paravalvular leak (Figure 8.2.12).

∞ EnVeo PRO delivery system; Confida Brecker Guidewire (CBG).

LOTUS EDGE (BOSTON SCIENTIFIC, MARLBOROUGH, MA, USA)

The Lotus Edge Aortic Valve System is a controlled-expansion TAVR valve designed to provide unmatched freedom from paravalvular leak (PVL) (Figure 8.2.13).

∞ Lotus Introducer set; Safari Guidewire.

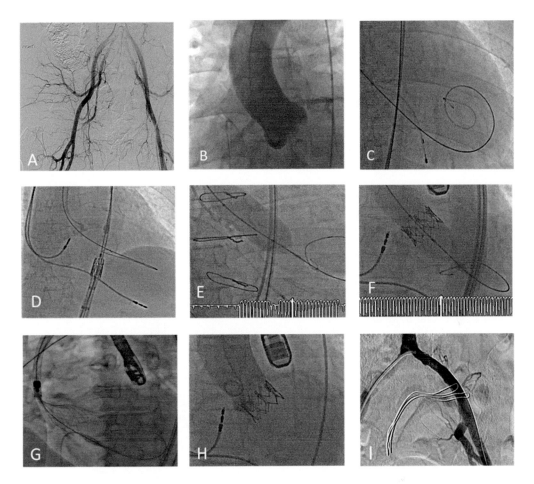

FIGURE 8.2.8 Crucial steps in valve deployment during transfemoral TAVI. (A) Contralateral femoral artery angiogram using digital subtraction angiography (DSA) to assess the femoral artery patency, calcification, stenosis and ideal puncture position in relation to the femoral head. (B) Aortic root angiogram to assess the optimal implantation angle during valve deployment in which all three aortic cusps can be seen on the same plane. (C) Crossing of the native aortic valve followed by stiff wire placement on the LV cavity. (D) Advancement of the crimped valve and delivery catheter on the descending aorta. (E) BAV under rapid pacing. (F) Balloon-expandable valve deployment under rapid pacing. (G) Slow valve deployment for self-expandable valve. (H) Post-deployment angiogram to assess valve position, stability and degree of aortic regurgitation. (I) Iliofemoral angiography using DSA to assess for vascular complication; two pre-deployed Perclose ProGlide® wires can be seen on the left femoral artery.

FIGURE 8.2.9 TF-TAVI Linköping, Sweden.   FIGURE 8.2.10 TF-TAVI by Guilherme Attizzani.

Chapter 8.2 – Transfemoral Transcatheter Aortic Valve Implantation   149

FIGURE 8.2.11   Sapien 3, Edwards.

FIGURE 8.2.14   Portico, Abbott.

FIGURE 8.2.12   Evolut R, Medtronic.

FIGURE 8.2.15   Micropuncture® Access Set, Cook.

FIGURE 8.2.13   Lotus Edge, Boston Scientific.

FIGURE 8.2.16   V-18 Control Wire Guidewire, Boston Scientific.

PORTICO (ABBOTT, CHICAGO, IL, USA)

Portico is a self-expanding valve. Intra-annular position, gradual-controlled deployment and no rapid pacing is usually required during deployment (Figure 8.2.14).

Accessories

Cook (Cook Medical, Bloomington, IN, USA) offers a portfolio of procedure-specific accessories to support your endovascular procedures, i.e. Micropuncture® Access set. Cook Medical also provides Amplatz Extra-Stiff 0.035" Support Wire, Royal Flush® Catheter. Access more details via link provided in Figure 8.2.15.

Boston Scientific, Marlborough, MA, USA, provided the V-18 Control Wire Guidewire (Figure 8.2.16). Other accessories include Perclose ProGlide® (Abbott, Chicago, IL, USA); Prostar XL (Abbott, Chicago, IL, USA); TriGuard 3 (Keystone Heart Inc., Tampa, FL, USA), Sentinel® Cerebral protection device (Boston Scientific) – the latter two devices are used to reduce the risks of cerebral embolism – True® Dilatation (Bard Inc., New Providence, NJ, USA) and True® Flow Valvuloplasty perfusion catheter (Bard Inc., New Providence, NJ, USA).

PERIOPERATIVE CONSIDERATIONS

PREOPERATIVE ASSESSMENT AND SCREENING

Patients who are considered for TAVI should undergo a complete clinical assessment. Basic clinical evaluations including a comprehensive clinical history, physical examination and laboratory investigation should be performed during the initial visit. In some centers, frailty assessment as well as various surrogates such as grip strength, walk distances or questionnaires have been used. There is however no consensus on the role of specific frailty assessment.

Assessment of the baseline kidney function is essential. TAVI has been associated with varying degrees of post-procedural acute kidney injury (AKI). The development of AKI post-procedure has been associated with negative prognostic outcomes [8,9].

Other routine laboratory investigations may unmask clinically significant problems especially in the elderly population, e.g. iron deficiency anemia caused by gastrointestinal pathologies. Such incidental findings occasionally affect the decision for procedure timing and whether to proceed with TAVI.

ECHOCARDIOGRAM

TTE is the gold standard for the diagnosis of severe aortic stenosis. It is essential to assess the severity of AS and document the essential parameters such as the aortic jet peak velocity, mean and peak gradient, aortic valve area (AVA) based on continuity equation and planimetry, velocity ratio/dimensionless index and energy loss index (ELI). The morphology of the aortic valve, number of aortic cusps, presence and distribution of valvular calcification and restricted motion of the valve are important to note (Figure 8.2.17).

Other essential information such as LV function, size and presence of hypertrophy can also be obtained during the initial echocardiogram (Figure 8.2.18 and Figure 8.2.19). In conditions where "paradoxical" low-flow, low-gradient aortic stenosis is identified, specific parameters such as the Stroke Volume Index (SVI), Systemic Arterial Compliance (SAC) and Valvulo Arterial Impendence (Zva) can be helpful to refine the diagnosis.

Although TTE can provide measurement of the aortic annulus diameter, contemporary measurement by ECG gated CT scan is considered the current gold standard. Prominent hypertrophic interventricular septum near the left ventricular outflow tract (LVOT), which potentially can interfere valve deployment, can be recognized during echo study. In addition, TTE can detect the presence of other significant valvular stenosis or regurgitation.

In most cases, TTE is sufficient to confirm the etiology and diagnosis of severe aortic stenosis. Transesophageal echocardiogram (TOE) is only performed when there is doubt about valve anatomy, number of cups and aortic root anatomy or whenever imaging from TTE is insufficient. Other tests such as exercise stress test or low-dose dobutamine stress echocardiography may be performed to distinguish true from pseudo aortic stenosis, or to assess contractile reserve in severe AS patients with reduced LV ejection fraction.

CARDIAC CATHETERIZATION

Coronary artery disease (CAD) is often co-existent in patients with severe AS. This is not surprising since the risk factors for AS

TABLE 8.2.1 Some of the commercially available bioprosthetic valves for TF-TAVI

Valve	Bioprosthetic valve	Valve Sizes, mm	Sheath sizes, Fr	Minimum Access Vessel Diameter, mm	Leaflet Tissue	Delivery System	Sheath
Sapien XT Valve (Edwards Life sciences)		23/26/29	16/28/20	6/6.5/7	Bovine	Novaflex	eSheath
Sapien 3 valve (Edwards Life sciences)		20/23/26/29	16/16	5.5/6	Bovine	Commander	eSheath
CoreValve (Medtronic)		23/26/29/31	18	6	Porcine	Delivery Catheter System	Introducer Sheath
CoreValve Evolut R (Medtronic)		23/26/29/34	14	5	Porcine	EnVeo R Delivery Catheter System	In line sheath
CoreValve Evolut Pro (Medtronic)		23/26/29	16	5.5	Porcine	EnVeo R Delivery Catheter System	In line sheath

(Continued)

152   Minimally Invasive Cardiac Surgery

TABLE 8.2.1 (CONTINUED) Some of the commercially available bioprosthetic valves for TF-TAVI

Valve	Bioprosthetic valve	Valve Sizes, mm	Sheath sizes, Fr	Minimum Access Vessel Diameter, mm	Leaflet Tissue	Delivery System	Sheath
Portico (St Jude Medical)		23/25/27/29	18/19	6/6.5	Bovine Pericardial valve; Porcine Pericardial Sealing cuff	Portico	Ultimum™ or Terumo SoloPath™
Lotus (Boston Scientific)		23/25/27	18/20	6/6.5	Bovine	Lotus valve system	Introducer sheath
Direct Flow Medical (Direct Flow Medical) Company closed in Dec 2016		25/27/29	18	6	Bovine	Direct flow medical delivery system	Introducer sheath

Chapter 8.2 – Transfemoral Transcatheter Aortic Valve Implantation

TABLE 8.2.2 Predictors of acute kidney injury

Variables	Univariate OR (95% CI)	p-value	Multivariate OR (95% CI)	p-value
Chronic renal insufficiency*	1.92 (1.23-3.00)	0.004	11.2 (5.12-23.73)	<0.001
Transfusion ≥3 Units¶	1.78 (1.11-2.87)	0.017	1.65 (1.02-2.68)	0.041
Female	1.42 (1.06-1.09)	0.020	1.37 (1.01-1.87)	0.045
General anesthesia	1.38 (1.01-1.87)	0.043	1.37 (1.00-1.87)	0.050
Second CoreValve deployed	1.72 (0.93-3.20)	0.086	1.83 (0.97-3.42)	0.061
Prior CABG	0.69 (0.54-1.06)	0.087	0.71 (0.45-1.12)	0.141
Age (years)	0.99 (0.97-1.01)	0.415	0.99 (0.96-1.01)	0.179

* Defined as eGFR rate <60ml/min. ¶ Within 72 hours of the procedure.
Abbreviations: AKI: Acute kidney injury; CABG: Coronary artery bypass grafting; CI: Confidence interval; OR: Odds ratio.
Source: Republished with permission of Europa Group from EuroIntervention on behalf of the EuroPCR and EAPCI, Barbanti M, Latib A, Sgroi C, et al. Acute kidney injury after transcatheter aortic valve implantation with self-expanding CoreValve prosthesis: results from a large multicentre Italian research project, 10(1):133-140, © 2014.

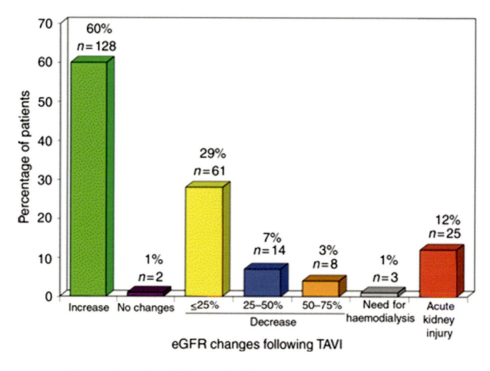

FIGURE 8.2.17 Changes in estimated glomerular filtration rate (eGFR) at 48 h following transcatheter aortic valve implantation (TAVI). (Republished with permission of Oxford University Press, from *Eur Heart J* on behalf of the European Society of Cardiology, Bagur R, Webb JG, Nietlispach F, et al. Acute kidney injury following transcatheter aortic valve implantation: predictive factors, prognostic value, and comparison with surgical aortic valve replacement, 31(7):865-874, © 2010.)

FIGURE 8.2.18 Short axis view showing severe AS with aortic cusp calcification and restricted motion.

FIGURE 8.2.19 Parasternal long axis view of severe aortic stenosis. This patient has left ventricular hypertrophy as a consequence of chronic pressure overload from AS.

are quite similar to those of atherosclerosis [10]. Significant numbers of patients undergoing TAVI have prior history of myocardial infarction (MI) (12% to 51%), prior percutaneous (16% to 34%) or surgical revascularization (14% to 48%) [11]. As reported by Dewey et al., patients with CAD had higher 30-day and 1-year mortality compared with patients without CAD. They are also 10 times more likely to die within 30 days after TAVI compared with those without CAD [12].

Coronary angiogram is routinely performed to assess the presence of significant CAD. The risk of ischemia and hemodynamic instability for these patients is highest during episodes of hypotension such as during induction of general anesthesia, rapid ventricular pacing during BAV and valve implantation for the balloon-expandable valve (Figures 8.2.5 and 8.2.6).

Revascularization should preferably be performed before TAVI if one is found to have significant coronary stenosis that translates to a large area of myocardium at risk. The indications for revascularization in such circumstances have not been clearly defined by evidence, and practice remains heterogeneous (Figure 8.2.20).

During coronary angiogram, evaluation of the anatomy, size and tortuosity of the femoral and iliac vessels can be performed with angiography (Figure 8.2.21) although access site assessment has now been mainly replaced by CT angiography.

COMPUTED TOMOGRAPHY (CT) ANGIOGRAPHY

Anatomical assessment is a critical part of TAVI procedure planning. The role of multi-detector CT is pivotal in providing detailed assessment of the aortic root, aortic valve and aortic annulus size and shape. In addition, it can accurately assess the size, tortuosity and presence of calcification of the femoral and iliac arteries to determine the ideal access route for transfemoral TAVI. CT can also help to predict the ideal implantation angle during valve implantation and deployment.

The most vital measurement obtained from CT is aortic annular size. This measurement will help in selecting the ideal size of the prosthesis to suit the patient. Undersizing of the prosthetic valve will result in paravalvular leak and increases the risk of valve embolization. On the other hand, oversizing will increase the risk of conduction disturbances needing pacemaker implantation and the risk of annular rupture, especially in the presence of heavy and eccentric calcification around the annulus and LVOT [13]. The aortic valve annulus is an imaginary

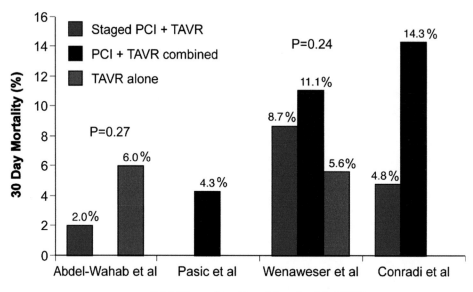

FIGURE 8.2.20 Thirty-day mortality in published studies including patients undergoing staged or combined percutaneous coronary intervention (PCI) with transcatheter aortic valve replacement (TAVR). (Reprinted from *J Am Coll Cardiol*, 62(1), Goel SS, Ige M, Tuzcu EM, et al. Severe aortic stenosis and coronary artery disease–implications for management in the transcatheter aortic valve replacement era: a comprehensive review, 1-10, © 2013 American College of Cardiology Foundation, with permission from Elsevier.)

virtual ring with three anatomical anchor points at the base of each of the attachments of the aortic valve (Figure 8.2.22). This virtual ring represents the narrowest part of the aortic root where the percutaneous prosthetic valves anchor and should be used as guidance for choosing the proper valve size [14].

This may differ somewhat in bicuspid valves where the anchoring of the prosthetic valves occurs at the level of the leaflets (supra annular). Finally, CT provides crucial information of the coronary ostia and helps to predict the risks of coronary artery occlusion. These risks are highest when the coronary ostial heights are low, the sinuses of Valsalva are narrow and where there is heavy bulky calcification of the valve leaflet tips.

ASSOCIATED CO-MORBIDITIES

Routine screening of TAVI patient includes carotid Doppler and pulmonary function tests. The presence of significant stenosis or a flow-limiting lesion on carotid Doppler may predict higher risks of stroke. Severe abnormalities on the spirometry test may impact treatment choices. Extreme severity of lung abnormalities may preclude TAVI if longevity is limited.

FIGURE 8.2.21 Femoral and iliac artery angiogram using digital subtraction angiogram (DSA).

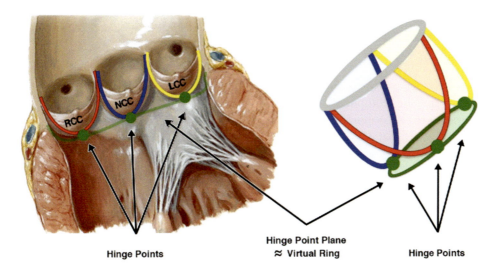

FIGURE 8.2.22   Normal anatomy of the aortic annulus. The aortic annulus accounts for the tightest part of the aortic root (A) and is defined as a virtual ring (green line) with three anatomical anchor points at the nadir (green points) of each of the attachments of the three aortic leaflets (B). LCC = left coronary cusp; NCC = noncoronary cusp; RCC = right coronary cusp. (Reprinted from *JACC Cardiovasc Imaging,* 6(2), Kasel AM, Cassese S, Bleiziffer S, et al. Standardized imaging for aortic annular sizing: implications for transcatheter valve selection, 249-262, © 2013 American College of Cardiology Foundation, with permission from Elsevier.)

ALTERNATIVE APPROACHES

TAVI can be performed under conscious sedation, which may be favored over general anesthesia especially in the case of severe lung abnormalities to reduce the risks of prolonged mechanical ventilation and severe carotid disease to mitigate the risks of stroke.

BAV is not routinely performed. Valves which are heavily calcified with very severe stenosis and high gradients should be considered for BAV.

The alternative approaches to transfemoral TAVI are transapical TAVI (see chapter for transapical TAVI) or trans-subclavian which is presently useful for high-risk patients with severe peripheral arterial disease. Transcarotid TAVI is also an alternative approach in patients without significant carotid disease and unsuitable for transfemoral access due to small-sized vessels or severe peripheral vascular disease (Figure 8.2.23). Transcaval accesses have also been proposed in cases where there are no other options for access. Any patient who is potentially operable however should be counselled for SAVR rather than to persist on a suboptimal access choice, and the decision on treatment choice should be made by a structural heart team.

FIGURE 8.2.23   TAVI by MMCTS.

CAVEATS AND CONTROVERSIES

PARAVALVULAR REGURGITATION (PVR)

PVR is a specific complication for the TAVI procedure. As reported initially by the PARTNER trial and 2-year follow up, the incidence of moderate or severe aortic regurgitation was more prevalent in the TAVI group compared to the surgical group (12.2% vs 0.9% at 30 days, 6.8% vs 1.9% at 2 years, $p < 0.001$ for both comparisons) [6,15]. Transvalvular regurgitation usually results from the interaction of the valve leaflet and the guidewire across the valve and disappears after wire removal.

The occurrence of PVR is clinically important because the effect on survival is directly related to the degree of regurgitation, and even mild PVR may be associated with increased mortality as reported by the 2-year follow up on PARTNER trial and vice versa [15].

In a meta-analysis of TAVI performed between 2008 and 2012 the presence of moderate to severe PVR has been associated with a 3-fold increase in mortality at 30 days and 2.3-fold increase in mortality at 1 year [16]. Several factors have been identified as causes for PVR such as undersizing of prosthetic valve size relative to the aortic annulus size, presence of calcium on the aortic root which can interfere with uniform valve expansion and sealing and finally implantation depth which can affect the ability of the skirt portion of the valve to provide adequate seal around the annulus (Figure 8.2.24).

Several methods can be used to assess PVR. The most frequently used modality is echocardiography which can identify, localize and grade the severity of PVR. Cineangiography can also be done but is highly subjective and has wide interobserver variability. Other methods include

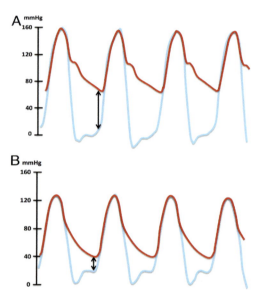

FIGURE 8.2.25 Calculation of the AR Index. Simultaneous determination of left ventricular end-diastolic pressure (LVEDP) (blue line) and diastolic blood pressure (DBP) in the aorta (red line) in a patient without peri-prosthetic aortic regurgitation (periAR) (A) and in a patient with moderate periAR (B) for the calculation of the aortic regurgitation (AR) index: ([DBP − LVEDP]/SBP) × 100. (A) AR index = ([65 − 10]/160) × 100 = 34.4. (B) AR index = ([40 − 20]/130) × 100 = 15.4. (Reprinted from *J Am Coll Cardiol*, 59(13), Sinning JM, Hammerstingl C, Vasa-Nicotera M, et al. Aortic regurgitation index defines severity of peri-prosthetic regurgitation and predicts outcome in patients after transcatheter aortic valve implantation, 1134-1141, © 2012 American College of Cardiology Foundation, with permission from Elsevier.)

FIGURE 8.2.24 Treatment of PVR after TAVI.

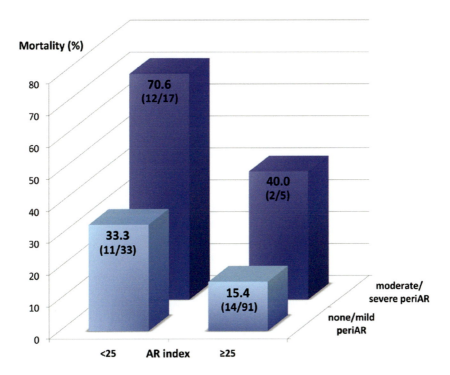

FIGURE 8.2.26 One-year all-cause mortality (%) according to the severity of periAR (none/mild vs moderate/severe) and the AR index cutoff value. (Reprinted from *J Am Coll Cardiol*, 59(13), Sinning JM, Hammerstingl C, Vasa-Nicotera M, et al. Aortic regurgitation index defines severity of peri-prosthetic regurgitation and predicts outcome in patients after transcatheter aortic valve implantation, 1134-1141, © 2012 American College of Cardiology Foundation, with permission from Elsevier.)

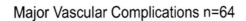

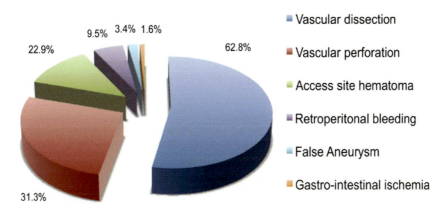

FIGURE 8.2.27 Distribution of type of major vascular complications after transcatheter aortic valve replacement. (Reprinted from *J Am Coll Cardiol*, 60(12), Généreux P, Webb JG, Svensson LG, et al. Vascular complications after transcatheter aortic valve replacement: insights from the PARTNER (Placement of AoRTic TraNscathetER Valve) trial, 1043-1052, © 2012 American College of Cardiology Foundation, with permission from Elsevier.)

hemodynamic measurement. An objective measurement of PVR severity called the aortic regurgitation index was proposed by Sinning et al. This is a simple, reproducible method to assess AR, calculated by the following formula: [(DBP − LVEDP)/SBP] ×100 (DBP = diastolic blood pressure, LVEDP = left ventricular end diastolic pressure, SBP = systolic blood pressure) [17] (Figure 8.2.25).

Patients with AR index <25 had a significantly increased 1-year mortality compared with patients with AR index ≥25 (46.0% vs 16.7%, p < 0.001) (Figure 8.2.26).

CARDIAC ATRIOVENTRICULAR CONDUCTION ABNORMALITIES

Patients undergoing TAVI are susceptible to cardiac conduction problems with the consequence of needing a permanent pacemaker implantation. This is due to the close relationship and location of the valve implantation site and the atrioventricular (AV) node. The risk of developing AV conduction problems may vary depending on valve type. Certain valve designs which apply higher radial forces to the aortic annulus at the level of the frame skirt adjacent to the LVOT area will have a higher rate of conduction problems [18]. In one study comparing these valves, the rate of implantation of new permanent pacemakers was significantly lower in the balloon-expandable valve group compared to the self-expandable group (17.3% vs 37.6%, RR 0.46, 95% CI: 0.28–0.74) [19]. Other factors that have been associated with a higher occurrence of cardiac conduction abnormalities following TAVI procedures are male gender (RR 1.23), pre-procedure first-degree AV block (RR 1.52), pre-procedure left anterior hemi-block (RR 1.62), intra-procedural AV block (RR 3.49), baseline right bundle branch block (RBBB) (RR 2.89) and the use of self-expandable valves (RR 2.54) [20].

STROKE

Stroke is a serious complication after TAVI and can occur due to dislodgement of the emboli during the valve advancement through the aortic arch, valve positioning and deployment. Based on the PARTNER cohort A trial, the rate of all neurologic events including strokes and transient ischemic attacks (TIA) was higher in the TAVI group compared to the surgical group stroke at 30 days (5.5% vs 2.4%, p = 0.04) and at 1 year (8.3% vs 4.3%, p = 0.04). Rates of major stroke were 3.8% in the transcatheter group and 2.1% in the surgical group at 30 days (p = 0.20) and 5.1% and 2.4%, respectively, at 1 year (p = 0.07) [6]. The risks of stroke have significantly improved in more contemporary trials which show that early stroke risks following TAVI are lower than those of surgery in the low-risk TAVI trials.

The incidence of neurological events may be higher if we include the occurrence of subclinical brain injury detected by transcranial Doppler (TCD) or diffusion-weighted magnetic resonance imaging (MRI). In one study looking at the embolic load during TAVI procedures using TCD to measure high-intensity transient signals, they found that the highest load of cerebral embolism happened during valve deployment [21]. Asymptomatic new ischemic brain lesions have been reported to occur even more frequently in up to 84% who underwent transfemoral TAVI. These lesions are typically multiple and can be seen in both cerebral hemispheres but are not associated with clinically significant neurological deficit and cognitive impairment during 3-month follow up [22].

The use of an embolic protection device during the procedure has been proposed to decrease the incidence of embolic events. Our center uses the Sentinel cerebral protection device. This deploys two filters in the innominate and left common carotid artery. The safety of the device was confirmed in the SENTINEL trial. The DEFLECT III trial using the TriGuard™ HDH Embolic Protection Device (TriGuard) during the procedure was associated with fewer new ischemic brain lesions (26.9% vs 11.5%), and fewer new neurologic deficits detected by the National Institutes of Health (NIH) Stroke Scale (3.1 vs 15.4) at discharge and 30-day follow up [23].

Patients undergoing TAVI have a higher prevalence of atrial fibrillation due to their advanced age and cardiac co-morbidities. Based on a study by Amat-Santos et al., new onset of atrial fibrillation was detected in 31.9% of patients within 30 days following the procedure. The majority of these occurred during the procedure (36.3%) or within 24 hours post-procedure (4.6%). Although there were no differences in mortality, the incidence of new onset atrial fibrillation was associated with higher rate of stroke or systemic embolism [24].

VASCULAR COMPLICATIONS

Vascular complication (VC) is frequent after transfemoral TAVI. Based on the Valve Academic Research Consortium-2 (VARC-2) consensus document published in 2013, there is now a standardized definition for major or minor VC [25]. With the first-generation devices, as reported by the PARTNER trial, the rates of major VC and minor VC were 15.3% and 11.9%,

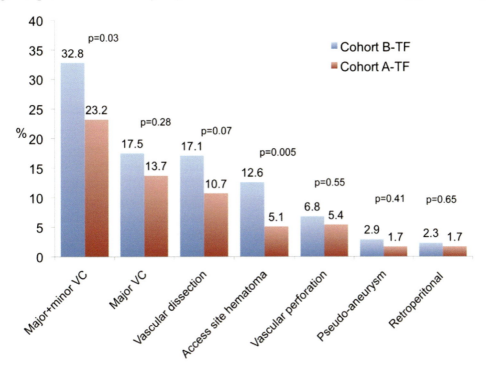

FIGURE 8.2.28 Difference in rates of VC from cohort 1B to cohort 1A. The rates of all vascular complications (VC), vascular dissection and access site hematoma decreased from cohort 1B to cohort 1A, suggesting improved outcomes in a lower-risk population and with more experienced operators. TF = transfemoral. (Reprinted from *J Am Coll Cardiol*, 60(12), Généreux P, Webb JG, Svensson LG, et al. Vascular complications after transcatheter aortic valve replacement: insights from the PARTNER (Placement of AoRTic TraNscathetER Valve) trial, 1043-1052, © 2012 American College of Cardiology Foundation, with permission from Elsevier.)

respectively. Major VC, but not minor VC, was associated with significantly higher 30-day rates of major bleeding, transfusions and renal failure requiring dialysis, and a significantly higher rate of 30-day and 1-year mortality [26] (Figure 8.2.27).

Most VCs are largely preventable by careful planning and assessment of vessel diameter, tortuosity and calcification before the procedure. In Asian populations, vascular access is more likely due to the smaller diameter of the vessels compared to Western patient populations. Independent predictors of smaller iliofemoral dimensions were female gender, lower body surface area, diabetes mellitus (DM), dyslipidemia and smoking history [27] (Figure 8.2.28).

SPECIFIC CAVEATS

- ∞ The decision for TAVI should be made by a dedicated dynamic "heart team" comprising cardiologists, cardiac surgeons and possibly including imaging specialists and anesthetists.
- ∞ Accurate preoperative imaging and anatomical assessment are critical for appropriate valve choice and sizing, and safe positioning and deployment.
- ∞ Cardiopulmonary bypass machine backup should be readily available for emergencies, especially for high-risk patients.
- ∞ Equipment for emergency coronary and peripheral vascular intervention should be readily available.
- ∞ It is essential that, prior to performing BAV, the prosthetic valve is ready for deployment. This is in anticipation of hemodynamic instability from severe AR that can ensue after BAV. Rapid pacing can be initiated if the patient develops severe AR while waiting for the valve to be deployed.
- ∞ Annular rupture is a potential life-threatening complication. Emergency pericardiocentesis followed by conversion to open surgery needs to be immediately performed to save the patient. Small aortic annulus size and heavy and eccentric calcification around the aortic annulus are associated with this complication. The oversized balloon-expandable valve and aggressive post-balloon dilatation are also considered risks.
- ∞ Coronary obstruction, although rare, will result in high mortality during the procedure. Risk factors are low coronary ostia height with small aortic sinus and heavy calcification.
- ∞ Subclinical leaflet thrombosis has been a concern recently when CT imaging following TAVI showed reduced aortic-valve leaflet motion (Figure 8.2.29). Fortunately, there were no overt clinical sequelae. Treatment with anticoagulation was associated with reduced incidence but more research has to be performed before a definitive management strategy can be proposed [28].

RESEARCH, TRENDS AND INNOVATION

CURRENT STATUS OF TAVI

TAVI has rapidly evolved from experimental to an established procedure of choice for patients with severe AS. The first multicenter PARTNER trial published in 2011 established the benefit of TAVI. As reported in PARTNER Cohort B (TAVI vs medical therapy in inoperable severe AS patients), the mortality rate at 1 year was reduced with TAVI.

FIGURE 8.2.29 Leaflet thrombosis in bioprosthetic valves? NEJM.

A recently published study suggested that the benefit was maintained 5 years after the treatment in which the risk of all-cause mortality at 5 years was 71.8% in the TAVR group vs 93.6% with standard treatment (hazard ratio 0.50, 95% CI: 0.39–0.65; p < 0.0001). The majority of patients who survived at 5 years had reported New York Heart Association class 1 or 2 symptoms [29].

In a separate publication, the 5-year follow up on PARTNER Cohort A (high-risk surgical patients) treated with TAVI showed no significant differences in all-cause mortality, cardiovascular mortality, stroke or need for repeat hospital admission compared to the surgical AVR patients [30].

Durability of the valve has been one of the concerns since the procedure was first introduced. While the valve platform was derived from the time-proven bioprosthetic surgical valve, there are differences in the way the valve is mounted. Potential valve leaflet damage during the crimping process and asymmetric and incomplete expansion can be a potential concern [30]. However, echocardiography assessment on 5-year follow-up results for both PARTNER trial patient cohorts reassuringly showed no structural valve deterioration or migration, and more importantly the improvements in valve area and gradient were maintained [29,30].

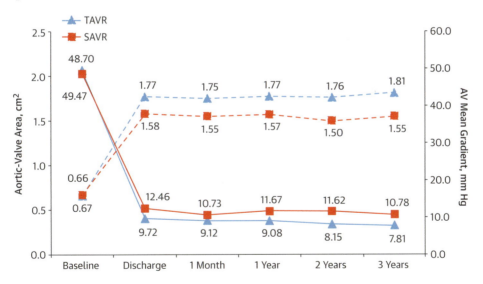

FIGURE 8.2.30 Echocardiographic findings over time: paired analysis. Reduction in aortic valve (AV) mean gradient and increased AV area are maintained through 3 years. Data reported on the basis of site-reported echocardiographic findings in patients with echocardiographic measurements at all time points reported. Paired sets of mean AV gradient data were available for 174 TAVR and 113 SAVR patients; AV area was available for 126 TAVR and 85 SAVR patients. TAVR was associated with significantly lower gradients and larger aortic valve areas at each time point (all p < 0.05). (Reprinted from *J Am Coll Cardiol*, 67(22), Deeb GM, Reardon MJ, Chetcuti S, et al. 3-Year Outcomes in High-Risk Patients Who Underwent Surgical or Transcatheter Aortic Valve Replacement, 2565-2574, © 2016 American College of Cardiology Foundation, with permission from Elsevier.)

Since the first-generation valves and early procedure experience, device technology and operator experience have significantly improved, resulting in better outcomes. The multicenter randomized trial of the self-expanding valve in the United States showed that TAVI had superior survival and lower all-cause mortality at 1 year compared to surgical AVR [31]. A study on 2-year outcomes consistently showed lower all-cause mortality in the TAVI group than in the surgical group (22.2% vs 28.6%; p < 0.05) with an absolute reduction in risk of 6.5% [32]. Interestingly, the 3-year data suggested that aortic valve mean gradients and effective orifice areas were better with TAVI patients although the rate of moderate and severe residual AR was still higher compared to surgery [33] (Figure 8.2.30).

Although the current approved indication for TAVI is for degenerative aortic stenosis patients, off-label use of TAVI to treat a few conditions such as pure aortic regurgitation, anatomical abnormality (e.g. bicuspid valve, annulus diameter out of the recommended range), very low ejection fraction (EF) <20% and concomitant severe mitral regurgitation has been reported with good outcomes. Nonetheless, the 30-day mortality for off-label use is higher (off-label vs on-label mortality 14.7% vs 7.9%, p = 0.01) [34].

The subgroup of patients with lowest mortality is the Valve-in-Valve (ViV), suggesting the potential value of TAVI as a treatment option for degenerated aortic bioprosthetic valves. Subsequent studies confirmed these findings, resulting in expanded CE certification for CoreValve (in 2013) and Edward Sapiens XT (in 2014) as new options to treat degenerated bioprostheses [35–37]. The JenaValve (JenaValve Technology GmbH, Munich, Germany), with its unique mechanism of anchoring to the native aortic valve, has shown excellent results for the treatment of pure aortic regurgitation [38] (Figure 8.2.31).

BALLOON VALVULOPLASTY CATHETER

Rapid pacing during BAV can cause a drop in blood pressure and cardiac output, which might cause hemodynamic instability, particularly in patients with significant CAD or LV dysfunction. New balloon valvuloplasty catheters have been designed to overcome these issues. True Dilatation™ Balloon Valvuloplasty Catheters (Bard Inc., New Providence, NJ, USA) provide faster inflation and deflation times, resulting in a shorter time needed for rapid pacing. This non-compliant and fiber-based balloon ensures accurate and controlled size of dilatation with minimal risk of rupture or tear.

The True™ Flow Valvuloplasty Perfusion Catheter (Bard Inc., New Providence, NJ, USA) has a unique design that allows continuous cardiac blood flow even during full inflation. The eight individual balloon chambers will retain the balloon integrity for the duration of maximal inflation while maintaining the central lumen for continuous blood flow.

DELIVERY SHEATH DESIGN

Vascular complication has been closely associated with the delivery sheath size. The first-generation devices required up to 24F sheaths. Dramatic reductions in sizes have been made over the past decade. Most TAVI valves currently can be placed via 18-19Fr sheaths. The Evolut R (Medtronic, MN, USA) inline sheath results in an overall sheath size of 14F. Significant strides have also been made in the use of expandable sheaths which may reduce vascular injury. Access and delivery sheath refinement will result in further size reduction, thus increasing safety and reducing complications.

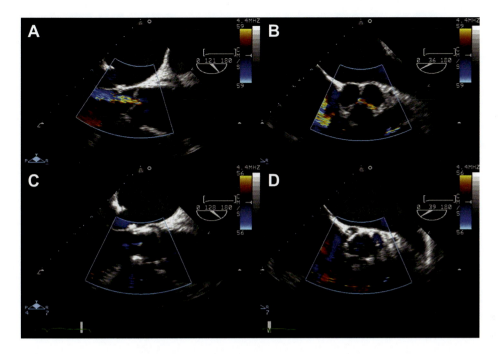

FIGURE 8.2.31 TAVI and concomitant LVAD implantation. Moderate central aortic regurgitation prior to implantation of a left ventricular assist device (LVAD) (A, B). In anticipation of worsening aortic regurgitation and hemodynamic compromise during LVAD support, a 27-mm JenaValve prosthesis was implanted transapically beforehand. Color Doppler confirms optimal function of the implanted transcatheter heart valve (C, D). (Reprinted from *JACC Cardiovasc Interv*, 6(6), Seiffert M, Diemert P, Koschyk D, et al. Transapical implantation of a second-generation transcatheter heart valve in patients with noncalcified aortic regurgitation, 590-597, © 2013 American College of Cardiology Foundation, with permission from Elsevier.)

FUTURE OF TRANSFEMORAL TAVI

TAVI has developed into an established treatment alternative to surgical AVR for patients with aortic stenosis. With more published clinical data confirming its efficacy, safety and more importantly the long-term bioprosthetic valve durability, the TAVI clinical indication will expand over time. The randomized trial comparing TAVI to surgical AVR for intermediate-risk patients, defined as having an STS score at least 4.0% up to 8.0%, or less than 4% with co-existing medical conditions, showed that the rate of death from any cause and stroke was similar in both groups (p = 0.001 for noninferiority). In the subgroup with transfemoral access, TAVI resulted in a lower rate of death and stroke compared to the surgical group [7].

The most recent PARTNER 3 trial comparing transfemoral TAVI with surgery in low-risk patients showed excellent results in both groups, and better primary composite endpoints in the TAVI group (Figure 8.2.32). Complications that were more frequent with TAVR than with surgery in

FIGURE 8.2.32 TAVI in low-risk patients.

FIGURE 8.2.33 Implications of low-risk TAVR for the future of cardiothoracic surgery.

FIGURE 8.2.35 PCR Online TAVI Atlas.

FIGURE 8.2.34 Medtronic TAVI course.

FIGURE 8.2.36 ESC courses.

previous trials, including major vascular complications, new permanent pacemaker insertions, moderate or severe PVR and coronary-artery obstruction, occurred with similar frequency in the two groups in this trial [39].

With this positive result, it is expected that transfemoral TAVI will become a viable option for selected low-risk patients. With the next generation of transfemoral TAVI devices incorporating better valve designs and improved sheath profiles, the outcomes are poised to improve further with this approach (Figure 8.2.33).

WHERE AND HOW TO LEARN

1. MEDTRONIC TAVI COURSE

The program features a selection of courses tailored to meet the needs of individuals and teams with different levels of knowledge and experience in TAVI procedures (Figure 8.2.34).

2. PCR ONLINE TAVI ATLAS

This new website section focusing on TAVI. This educational tool embraces all facets of transcatheter aortic valve therapies: anatomy of the aortic valvar complex, imaging, transcatheter aortic valve devices, procedural concepts, complications and bailout procedures, meet the team and more (Figure 8.2.35).

3. ESC COURSES

These courses focus on transcatheter therapies for valvular heart disease. PCR London Valves is an EAPCI official annual course. It takes place every year at ExCeL, London, UK (Figure 8.2.36).

REFERENCES

1. Cribier A. The development of transcatheter aortic valve replacement (TAVR). *Glob Cardiol Sci Pract*. 2016;4:e201632.
2. Andersen HR, Knudsen LL, Hasenkam JM. Transluminal implantation of artificial heart valves: description of a new expandable aortic valve and initial results with implantation by catheter technique in closed chest pigs. *Eur Heart J*. 1992;13:704–708.
3. Cribier A, Eltchaninoff H, Bash A, et al. Percutaneous transcatheter implantation of an aortic valve prosthesis for calcific aortic stenosis. *Circulation*. 2002;106:3006–3008.
4. Cribier A, Eltchaninoff H, Tron C, et al. Early experience with percutaneous transcatheter implantation of heart valve prosthesis for the treatment of end-stage inoperable patients with calcific aortic stenosis. *J Am Coll Cardiol*. 2004;43:698–703.
5. Webb JG, Chandavimol M, Thompson CR, et al. Percutaneous aortic valve implantation retrograde from the femoral artery. *Circulation*. 2006;113:842–850.
6. Leon MB, Smith CR, Mack M, et al. for the PARTNER Trial Investigators. Transcatheter aortic-valve implantation for aortic stenosis in patients who cannot undergo surgery. *N Engl J Med*. 2010;363(17):1597–607.
7. Leon MB, Smith CR, Mack MJ, et al.; PARTNER 2 Investigators. Transcatheter or surgical aortic-valve replacement in intermediate-risk patients. *N Engl J Med*. 2016;374(17):1609–20.
8. Barbanti M, Latib A, Sgroi C, et al. Acute kidney injury after transcatheter aortic valve implantation with self-expanding CoreValve prosthesis: results from a large multicentre Italian research project. *EuroIntervention*. 2014;10:133–40.
9. Bagur R, Webb JG, Nietlispach F, et al. Acute kidney injury following transcatheter aortic valve implantation: predictive factors, prognostic value, and comparison with surgical aortic valve replacement. *Eur Heart J*. 2010;31(7):865–74.
10. Stewart BF, Siscovick D, Lind BK, et al. Clinical factors associated with calcific aortic valve disease. Cardiovascular health study. *J Am Coll Cardiol*. 1997;29:630–4.
11. Goel SS, Ige M, Tuzcu EM, et al. Severe aortic stenosis and coronary artery disease--implications for management in the transcatheter aortic valve replacement era: a comprehensive review. *J Am Coll Cardiol*. 2013;62(1):1–10.
12. Dewey TM, Brown DL, Herbert MA, et al. Effect of concomitant coronary artery disease on procedural and late outcomes of transcatheter aortic valve implantation. *Ann Thorac Surg*. 2010;89:758–67.
13. Kasel AM, Cassese S, Bleiziffer S, et al. Standardized imaging for aortic annular sizing: implications for transcatheter valve selection. *JACC Cardiovasc Imaging*. 2013;6(2):249–62.
14. Piazza N, de Jaegere P, Schultz C, Becker AE, Serruys PW, Anderson RH. Anatomy of the aortic valvar complex and its implications for transcatheter implantation of the aortic valve. *Circ Cardiovasc Interv*. 2008;1:74–81.
15. Kodali SK, Williams MR, Smith CR, et al.; PARTNER Trial Investigators. Two-year outcomes after transcatheter or surgical aortic-valve replacement. *N Engl J Med*. 2012;366(18):1686–95.
16. Athappan G, Patvardhan E, Tuzcu EM, et al. Incidence, predictors, and outcomes of aortic regurgitation after transcatheter aortic valve replacement: meta-analysis and systematic review of literature. *J Am Coll Cardiol*. 2013;61(15):1585–95.
17. Sinning JM, Hammerstingl C, Vasa-Nicotera M, et al. Aortic regurgitation index defines severity of peri-prosthetic regurgitation and predicts outcome in patients after transcatheter aortic valve implantation. *J Am Coll Cardiol*. 2012;59(13):1134–41.
18. Young Lee M, Chilakamarri Yeshwant S, Chava S, et al. Mechanisms of heart block after transcatheter aortic valve replacement - cardiac anatomy, clinical predictors and mechanical factors that contribute to permanent pacemaker implantation. *Arrhythm Electrophysiol Rev*. 2015;4(2):81–5.
19. Abdel-Wahab M, Mehilli J, Frerker C, et al.; CHOICE Investigators. Comparison of balloon-expandable vs self-expandable valves in patients undergoing

transcatheter aortic valve replacement: the CHOICE randomized clinical trial. *JAMA*. 2014;311(15):1503–14.
20. Steinberg BA, Harrison JK, Frazier-Mills C, Hughes GC, Piccini JP. Cardiac conduction system disease after transcatheter aortic valve replacement. *Am Heart J*. 2012;164(5):664–71.
21. Erdoes G, Basciani R, Huber C, et al. Transcranial doppler-detected cerebral embolic load during transcatheter aortic valve implantation. *Eur J Cardiothorac Surg*. 2012;41:778–783; discussion783–4.
22. Kahlert P, Knipp SC, Schlamann M, et al. Silent and apparent cerebral ischemia after percutaneous transfemoral aortic valve implantation: a diffusion-weighted magnetic resonance imaging study. *Circulation*. 2010;121:870–878.
23. Lansky AJ, Schofer J, Tchetche D, et al. A prospective randomized evaluation of the TriGuard™ HDH embolic DEFLECTion device during transcatheter aortic valve implantation: results from the DEFLECT III trial. *Eur Heart J*. 2015;36(31):2070–2078.
24. Amat-Santos IJ, Rodés-Cabau J, Urena M, et al. Incidence, predictive factors, and prognostic value of new-onset atrial fibrillation following transcatheter aortic valve implantation. *J Am Coll Cardiol*. 2012;59(2):178–88.
25. Kappetein AP, Head SJ, Généreux P, et al.; Valve Academic Research Consortium-2. Updated standardized endpoint definitions for transcatheter aortic valve implantation: the Valve Academic Research Consortium-2 consensus document. *J Thorac Cardiovasc Surg*. 2013;145(1):6–23.
26. Généreux P, Webb JG, Svensson LG, et al.; PARTNER Trial Investigators. Vascular complications after transcatheter aortic valve replacement: insights from the PARTNER (Placement of AoRTic TraNscathetER Valve) trial. *J Am Coll Cardiol*. 2012;60(12):1043–52.
27. Chiam PT, Koh AS, Ewe SH, et al. Iliofemoral anatomy among Asians: implications for transcatheter aortic valve implantation. *Int J Cardiol*. 2013;167(4):1373–9.
28. Makkar RR, Fontana G, Jilaihawi H, et al. Possible subclinical leaflet thrombosis in bioprosthetic aortic valves. *N Engl J Med*. 2015;373(21):2015–24.
29. Kapadia SR, Leon MB, Makkar RR, et al. 5-year outcomes of transcatheter aortic valve replacement compared with standard treatment for patients with inoperable aortic stenosis (PARTNER 1): a randomised controlled trial. *Lancet*. 2015;385(9986):2485.
30. Mack MJ, Leon MB, Smith CR, et al.; PARTNER 1 Trial Investigators. 5-year outcomes of transcatheter aortic valve replacement or surgical aortic valve replacement for high surgical risk patients with aortic stenosis (PARTNER1): a randomised controlled trial. *Lancet*. 2015;385(9986):2477–84.
31. Adams DH, Popma JJ, Reardon MJ, et al.; U.S. CoreValve Clinical Investigators. Transcatheter aortic-valve replacement with a self-expanding prosthesis. *N Engl J Med*. 2014;370(19):1790–8.
32. Reardon MJ, Adams DH, Kleiman NS, et al. 2-year outcomes in patients undergoing surgical or self-expanding transcatheter aortic valve replacement. *J Am Coll Cardiol*. 2015;66(2):113–21.
33. Deeb GM, Reardon MJ, Chetcuti S, et al.; CoreValve US Clinical Investigators. Three-year outcomes in high-risk patients who underwent surgical or transcatheter aortic valve replacement. *J Am Coll Cardiol*. 2016;67(22):2565–74.
34. Frerker C, Schewel J, Schewel D, et al. Expansion of the indication of transcatheter aortic valve implantation--feasibility and outcome in "off-label" patients compared with "on-label" patients. *J Invasive Cardiol*. 2015;27(5):229–36.
35. Dvir D, Webb J, Brecker S, et al. Transcatheter aortic valve replacement for degenerative bioprosthetic surgical valves: results from the global valve-in-valve registry. *Circulation*. 2012;126(19):2335–2344.
36. Linke A, Woitek F, Merx MW, et al. Valve-in-valve implantation of Medtronic CoreValve prosthesis in patients with failing bioprosthetic aortic valves. *Circ Cardiovasc Interv*. 2012;5(5):689–697.

37. Eggebrecht H, Schafer U, Treede H, et al. Valve-in-valve transcatheter aortic valve implantation for degenerated bioprosthetic heart valves. *JACC Cardiovasc Intv.* 2011;4(11):1218–1227.
38. Seiffert M, Diemert P, Koschyk D, et al. Transapical implantation of a second-generation transcatheter heart valve in patients with noncalcified aortic regurgitation. *JACC Cardiovasc Intv.* 2013;6(6):590–597.
39. Mack MJ, Leon MB, Thourani VH, et al.; PARTNER 3 Investigators. Transcatheter aortic-valve replacement with a balloon-expandable valve in low-risk patients. *N Engl J Med.* 2019;380(18):1695–1705.

TRANSCATHETER AORTIC VALVE IMPLANTATION (TAVI)
Alternative Approaches for Transcatheter Aortic Valve Implantation

FAIZUS SAZZAD AND THEO KOFIDIS

INTRODUCTION

At the moment, the most common practice for aortic valve implantation (for selective group of patients) requiring aortic valve implantation is transfemoral transcatheter aortic valve implantation (TF-TAVI). In cases of difficult anatomical approach, the next most common method is the transapical transcatheter aortic valve implantation (TA-TAVI) technique. Besides these approaches, there are a number of ways to perform transcatheter aortic valve implantation (TAVI) safely. These other methods have their own pros and cons, but are mostly less frequently practiced and require more precise wire skills (Figure 8.3.1).

The feasibility of alternative approaches is dependent on the factors that hinder the possibility of carrying out the aforementioned, most common approaches. In other words, these alternative approaches should only be a last resort when all other more common options have been exhausted [1,2].

Although there is no direct comparison available between the common and alternative routes of TAVI, there is no valid reason for either technique to be favored over the other. However, the availability of alternative vascular accesses for TAVI should not affect the principle for which this procedure was conceived. Therefore, the choice of vascular access should remain patient-centered rather than driven by the preferences of the operating surgeon.

ALTERNATIVE APPROACHES

A. Subclavian transcatheter aortic valve replacement (SC-TAVI)
B. Transaxillary transcatheter aortic valve replacement (TAX-TAVI)
C. Direct aortic transcatheter aortic valve replacement (DA-TAVI)
D. Transcarotid transcatheter aortic valve replacement (TC-TAVI)
E. Transcaval transcatheter aortic valve replacement (TCA-TAVI)

HOW TO DO IT/STEP BY STEP

SUBCLAVIAN TRANSCATHETER AORTIC VALVE REPLACEMENT (SC-TAVI)

The subclavian approach is currently approved as an alternative to the transfemoral approach for TAVI. The learning curve for an SC-TAVI is relatively shorter in terms of procedural duration, use of different balloon-dilatable TAVI valves and vascular complications [1]. Importantly, the trans-subclavian access does not require the use of general anesthesia and allows for an early patient shift. The current standard is local anesthesia with mild sedation, which is a major advantage of the subclavian over the transapical and transaortic accesses in elderly patients with multiple concurrent sicknesses (Figure 8.3.2 and Figure 8.3.3).

TECHNIQUE

The cardiac/vascular surgeon usually isolates and prepares the subclavian artery. The insertion of the sheath is usually done by using standard surgical techniques with local anesthetic agents, in combination with a mild sedative/analgesic. General anesthesia is avoided. Some surgeons prefer performing an arteriotomy or placing a graft conduit, followed by the introduction of a standard 18 Fr sheath, which is then advanced over a stiff guide wire through the subclavian artery into the aortic arch and ascending aorta, stopping just below the origin of the brachiocephalic artery.

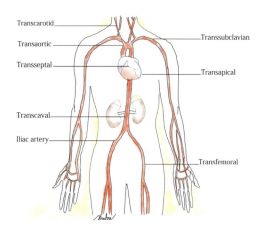

FIGURE 8.3.1 Alternative approaches for TAVI. (Courtesy: Shaghayegh Shahrigharahkoshan, 2019.)

FIGURE 8.3.2 TAVI: the Trans-subclavian route.

FIGURE 8.3.3 Subclavian access for TAVI.

The rest of the procedure is the same as the standard transfemoral approach. At the end of the procedure, hemostasis is achieved by simply tightening the purse-string sutures, and the skin layers are closed in the usual fashion. A drainage tube is rarely required (Figure 8.3.4).

PROS AND CONS

- ∞ The subclavian artery is more fragile than the common femoral artery.
- ∞ Due to its anatomy and location deep within the body, it is unfavorable for a vessel rupture of the subclavian artery to be repaired.
- ∞ The subclavian artery is quite tortuous in very elderly patients.
- ∞ Sometimes SC-TAVI can cause focal stenosis, and there is often calcification or narrowing at the origin of the subclavian artery.
- ∞ SC-TAVI in the presence of a patent left internal mammary artery (LIMA) graft to the left anterior descending coronary artery may cause myocardial ischemia.
- ∞ The contralateral subclavian access is a feasible alternative in patients with a permanent pacemaker implanted in the ipsilateral pectoral region.

TRANSAXILLARY TRANSCATHETER AORTIC VALVE REPLACEMENT (TAX-TAVI)

According to BIBA (BIBA Med Tec, UK) in 2017, TAVI via the transaxillary route was usable in only 3% of cases as a significant number of patients suffer from peripheral vascular disease [3]. The anatomical advantage of the axillary artery makes it superior to the subclavian artery in terms of vascular access during complications (Figure 8.3.5).

TECHNIQUE

The axillary artery can be prepared by surgical isolation or by direct percutaneous puncture with a predefined closure technique. The subclavian artery runs above the first rib and subsequently becomes the axillary artery, which then courses posterior to the pectoralis minor muscle and becomes the brachial artery at the inferior border of the teres minor muscle.

To determine if a TAX-TAVI can be performed, it is necessary for the following selection criteria to be fulfilled:

- ∞ Diameter of the axillary ≥6 mm.
- ∞ Absence of heavy calcification in the artery.
- ∞ Severe stenosis of the access vessel, which cannot be treated with balloon angioplasty.
- ∞ In patients with a patent left internal mammary artery (LIMA) coronary bypass graft, a minimal vessel diameter of 7–8 mm and no significant atherosclerotic disease proximal to or at the ostium of the LIMA is necessary in order to prevent myocardial ischemia.

The ideal access site of the axillary artery is in its first segment between the lateral border of the first rib and the medial border of the pectoralis minor muscle due to the absence of major side branches. The left axillary artery is preferred, because it allows for coaxial orientation of the valve prosthesis within the aortic annulus. To adequately evaluate the transaxillary access route, a multi-slice computed tomography scan should be performed prior to

TAX-TAVI. Vasculography or duplex study of the axillary will provide additional useful information.

Most surgeons prefer a surgical cut-down of the axillary artery with purse-string suture securing. Some surgeons prefer to attach a short conduit to gain access to the axillary artery. The rest of the procedure is similar to the SC-TAVI.

PROS AND CONS

- In contrast to SC-TAVI, pacemakers implanted ipsilateral to the access site are not a contraindication for TAX-TAVI.
- The transaxillary access is less invasive than SC-TAVI.
- Truly percutaneous delivery is possible.

DIRECT AORTIC TRANSCATHETER AORTIC VALVE REPLACEMENT (DA-TAVI)

DA-TAVI is a minimally invasive approach mostly preferred in patients with inherently small arteries and/or severe peripheral vascular disease [4,5] (Figure 8.3.6 and Figure 8.3.7). A transaortic approach is preferred over a transapical approach in patients who have compromised transfemoral access in the following clinical settings:

- Diseases of the descending and abdominal aorta, including:
  - Severe calcification/atheroma of the aortic arch
- History of aortic occlusion, aortic aneurysm or aortic dissection
- Left ventricular functional or anatomical abnormalities, including:
  - Severe systolic or diastolic dysfunction
  - Small ventricular cavity, with severely hypertrophic myocardium
  - Thin left ventricular wall, or severe dilated cardiomyopathy
  - Extremely frail myocardial tissues

Relative contraindications for a DA-TAVI include calcified or atheromatous ascending aorta, vein grafts with very high origins and cardiac anatomic variations, including:

- Grafts close to the sternum, placing patient at risk for sternotomy
- Variations preventing a good coaxial prosthesis deployment (e.g., pectus excavatum)

TECHNIQUE

1. Identify the puncture site: A favorable puncture site is one found on the greater curve of the aorta, typically on the right lateral side (at the surgeon's 1 to 3 o'clock when standing at the head of the bed), and 2 to 3 cm proximal to the innominate artery.

2. Surgical access to puncture site:

- Upper J mini sternotomy
- Right anterior mini thoracotomy
- Suprasternal approach (Figure 8.3.8)

FIGURE 8.3.4 Live case: TAVI through subclavian.

FIGURE 8.3.5 Right axillary TAVR, CTS.net.

PROS AND CONS

- ∞ Mostly requires surgical access.
- ∞ Wire exchange is challenging.
- ∞ Favorable in arch and descending thoracic aortic disease scenarios.
- ∞ Opens the way for extra-sternal and extra-thoracic approaches for TAVI (Figure 8.3.9).

TRANSCAROTID TRANSCATHETER AORTIC VALVE REPLACEMENT (TC-TAVI)

Transcarotid access is only reserved for a specific group of patients who require TAVI. Patient groups with advanced age and multiple comorbidities mostly undergo TF-TAVI [6]. However, for a selective group of patients, where the peripheral vessels are diseased and SC-TAVI and DA-TAVI options are unavailable, TC-TAVI is a favorable alternative surgical technique for treatment, especially for those with severe calcified ascending aorta (Figure 8.3.10 and Figure 8.3.11).

TECHNIQUE

1. Pre-operative multi-slice CT scan to confirm suitable supra-aortic anatomy. The carotid artery minimal diameter should be ≥6 mm without significant stenosis (≥50%).
2. Under general anesthesia, perform a surgical cut-down and exposure of the common carotid artery to at least 3–4 cm. Secure the vessel with proximal and distal control.
3. Transcranial Doppler and cerebral oximetry are needed to monitor cerebral blood flow.
4. Before insertion of the 14 Fr sheath, clamp the distal common carotid artery and ensure that there is no change on the neurological monitor. Keep the artery clamped during delivery to prevent embolism.
5. Extend the arteriotomy over the wire transversely to allow sheath entry without injuring the vessel.
6. After delivery of the valve and removal of the sheath, flush the artery proximally and distally in a similar fashion to any carotid repair.

PROS AND CONS

The presence of atherosclerotic plaque at the carotid artery means there is a high risk for embolization.

Anatomic variants: The absence of subclavian, vertebral and contralateral carotid stenosis or occlusion, or congenital variants of the aortic arch is a relative contraindication for TC-TAVI.

Compression of the recurrent laryngeal nerve could cause dysphonia, and insufficient hemoptysis could lead to compressive hemoptysis and subsequent asphyxia.

It has recently been reported to have similar outcomes to transfemoral access in terms of mortality and morbidity.

Arguably, left carotid access for TAVI should be favored to the right because it provides superior coaxial alignment.

FIGURE 8.3.6 Direct aortic TAVI delivery route.

FIGURE 8.3.7 Direct aortic TAVI, MMCTS.

FIGURE 8.3.8 Suprasternal direct aortic approach TAVI.

FIGURE 8.3.10 Transcarotid approach for TAVI.

FIGURE 8.3.9 Balancing risks and benefits of subclavian, direct aortic and transapical approaches.

FIGURE 8.3.11 Transcarotid TAVI: an optimal alternative.

TRANSCAVAL TRANSCATHETER AORTIC VALVE REPLACEMENT (TCA-TAVI)

A new, innovative approach to bypass the issues in suboptimal access vessels is the transcaval access method (Figure 8.3.12). This involves the use of femoral vein access, followed by a small puncture made in the aorta above the problematic regions with the wire continuing toward the heart [7]. The catheter crosses over in the retroperitoneal space between the vena cava and the aorta. The rest of the procedure continues as a standard TAVI procedure (Figure 8.3.13 and Figure 8.3.14).

TECHNIQUE

1. CT-guided identification of the crossover point from IVC to aorta.
2. Angiography alone is used to guide access and closure.
3. A transcatheter electrosurgery ablation system is used to create the hole in the walls of the vessels.

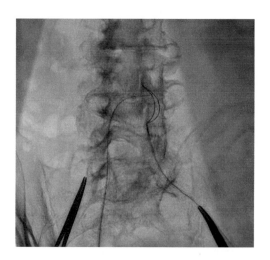

FIGURE 8.3.12 Transcaval TAVI procedure, showing a guide wire in the vena cava and a snare located in the aorta to pull the guide wire through. (After Adam B. Greenbaum, How to Perform Transcaval TAVR Access, Diagnostic and Interventional Cardiology, accessed from www.wainscotmedia.com, © 2018 Wainscot Media LLC, with permission.)

4. Escalating wire sizes are then used across the opening from the IVC to gradually enlarge the opening.

FIGURE 8.3.13 Transcaval access in TAVI procedures.

FIGURE 8.3.15 Transcaval TAVR, discussion.

PROS AND CONS

Gaining access to the caval vessel and cross-over to the descending thoracic aorta is the main concern.

It is important to determine if the vascular access routes can accommodate the large diameters of TAVI devices.

FIGURE 8.3.14 Transcaval TAVI, Oklahoma Heart Institute.

5. Vessel closure is performed using a deflectable catheter.

This alternative approach can be used when heavy calcification or large lesions are present in the femoral artery, or popcorn-type calcifications are present in the aorta (Figure 8.3.15).

DEVICES

Boston Scientific's Lotus Valve System is a controlled mechanical expansion TAVI valve that allows for full control over the release, repositioning, retrieval and redeployment of the valve, with an Adaptive Seal™ technology that reduces the risk of paravalvular leak (Figure 8.3.16).

The ACURATE neo Transfemoral and ACURATE neo Transapical Aortic Valve Systems are self-expanding supra-annular valves deployed in a top-down fashion that allows for better hemodynamic stability (Figure 8.3.17).

The Edwards Lifesciences' SAPIEN XT Valve and SAPIEN 3 Valves are

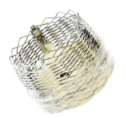 

FIGURE 8.3.16 LOTUS *Edge*™ Aortic Valve System. ©2020 Boston Scientific Corporation or its affiliates. All rights reserved.

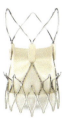

FIGURE 8.3.17 A. ACURATE neo Valve system. ©2020 Boston Scientific Corporation or its affiliates. All rights reserved.

FIGURE 8.3.17   B. ACURATE neo Valve System by Boston Scientific.

FIGURE 8.3.19   D. Medtronic's TAVI valves

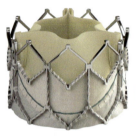
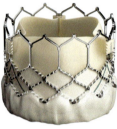

FIGURE 8.3.20   C. Portico TAVI solution.

FIGURE 8.3.18   A. Edwards SAPIEN XT™. B. Edwards SAPIEN 3™ Transcatheter Heart Valve. Reproduced with permission of Edwards Lifesciences LLC, Irvine, CA.

Medtronic's Evolut Pro+, Evolut Pro and Evolut R are self-expanding, recapturable TAVR valves with nitinol frames that adjust according to the shape of the stenotic valve, thereby reducing paravalvular regurgitation (Figure 8.3.19).

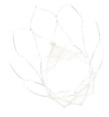
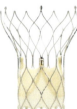

FIGURE 8.3.18   C. SAPIEN 3™ valve by Edwards.

FIGURE 8.3.20   A. Portico™ Valve (from top). B. Portico™ Valve (lateral view). Reproduced with permission of Abbott, © 2020.

balloon-expandable valves designed to minimize the risk of paravalvular leak (Figure 8.3.18).

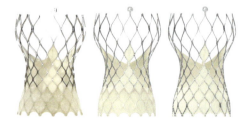

FIGURE 8.3.19   A. Evolut™ Pro+ B. Evolut™ Pro and C. Evolut™ R. Reproduced with permission of Medtronic, Inc.

Abbott Vascular's Portico Valve features a self-expanding nitinol frame that accommodates the structure of the calcified aortic valve and reduces paravalvular leak (Figure 8.3.20).

PERI-PROCEDURAL CONSIDERATIONS

FIGURE 8.3.21   Anatomy for TAVI, PCR online.

FIGURE 8.3.22   Imaging for TAVI, PCR online.

1. For a better understanding of the anatomy of the aortic valvar complex, a virtual atlas providing detailed descriptions is available at the following link (Figure 8.3.21).
2. To gain a better understanding of TAVI imaging, the following link (Figure 8.3.22) provides examples of pre-procedural and peri-procedural TAVI imaging. The section titled "pre-procedural imaging" includes the categories "patient selection", "prosthesis size" and "procedure access", which will provide greater detail on using TAVI imaging for evaluating the degree of aortic stenosis and the anatomy of the aortic valve, the various advantages and disadvantages of the different techniques used to measure the size of the aortic annulus and determining which method of access is suitable for the patient. In "peri-procedural imaging", a better look at TAVI imaging for direct visualization during the procedure can be found under the sections "valve implantation" and "post-implantation assessment".

FIGURE 8.3.23   The heart valve team.

3. The heart valve team case study, accessible in the following link (Figure 8.3.23), provides more information on the dynamics of a heart valve team, with the various roles of each member described in detail.

WHERE AND HOW TO LEARN

The links in the images below provides greater detail on the challenges and complications that one is likely to meet when performing TAVI:

Chapter 8.3 – Transcatheter Aortic Valve Implantation (TAVI)   179

- ∞ Figure 8.3.24 TAVI: What to expect.
- ∞ Figure 8.3.25 is a lecture comparing the SAPIEN and CoreValve TAVR valves.
- ∞ For a more in-depth explanation of patient characteristics that indicate patient suitability for a TAVI procedure, the following link is available for access from Figure 8.3.26.
- ∞ An animation on the use of Sentinel to minimize the risk of brain embolism and peri-procedural stroke during a TAVI procedure can be found in Figure 8.3.27.

TAVI FELLOWSHIP

For information on applying for a TAVI fellowship, please access the link in Figure 8.3.28.

FIGURE 8.3.24   TAVR: What to expect?

FIGURE 8.3.25   Choice of prosthesis for TAVI.

FIGURE 8.3.26   TAVI: Who should be evaluated?

FIGURE 8.3.27 Sentinel during a TAVI procedure.

FIGURE 8.3.28 TAVI Fellowship, Emory University.

REFERENCES

1. T. Dahle, N. Castro, B. Stegman, et al. Supraclavicular subclavian access for SAPIEN transcatheter aortic valve replacement—a novel approach. *J Cardiothorac Surg*, 13 (2018), p. 16.
2. Prakash A. Patel Peter J. Neuburger. Ongoing obstacles for universal use of sedation for transfemoral transcatheter aortic valve replacement. *J Cardiothorac Vasc Anesth*, 2019; 33(1), pp. 36–38.
3. U. Schäfer, F. Deuschla, N. Schofera, et al. Safety and efficacy of the percutaneous transaxillary access for transcatheter aortic valve implantation using various transcatheter heart valves in 100 consecutive patients. *Int J Cardiol*, 232 (2017), pp. 247–254. doi: 10.1016/j.ijcard.2017.01.0100167-5273.
4. U. Schafer, Y. Ho, C. Frerker, et al. Direct percutaneous access technique for transaxillary transcatheter aortic valve implantation. *J Am Coll Cardiol Intv*, 5 (2012), pp. 477–486.
5. Eduardo Alegría-Barreroa, Pak Hei Chana, Carlo Di Marioa, Neil E. Moatb. Direct aortic transcatheter aortic valve implantation: a feasible approach for patients with severe peripheral vascular disease. *Cardiovasc Revascul Med*, 13 (2012), pp. 201.e5–201.e7. doi: 10.1016/j.carrev.2011.12.004.
6. D. Mylotte, A. Sudre, E. Teiger, et al. Transcarotid transcatheter aortic valve replacement: feasibility and safety. *J Am Coll Cardiol Intv*, 9 (2016), pp. 472–480.
7. A. Greenbaum, V. Babaliaros, M. Chen, et al. Transcaval access and closure for transcatheter aortic valve replacement—a prospective investigation. *J Am Coll Cardiol*, 69 (2017), pp. 511–521.

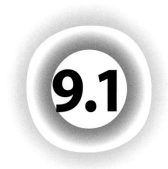

THE MITRAL VALVE
Minimally Invasive Mitral Valve Surgery

HUGO VANERMEN

HISTORY AND INTRODUCTION

Minimally invasive mitral valve surgery (MIMVS) is 20 years old!

The first question: what is it?

In a century in which lifestyle has changed considerably, where awareness is ubiquitous, where, for a lot of elderly, quality of life is likely to be more important than longevity, where patients are very active in making their own choices, less invasive procedures are a need and percutaneous interventions have become pure frenzy. Let's make the point that all surgery is percutaneous as well! Interventional cardiologists are surgeons, who operate through a puncture hole on a beating heart, whereas surgeons do interventions through every sort of approach. That is more than a puncture hole on a beating or an arrested heart. Basically, in this book chapter, we are going to elaborate on the typical approach as it is pursued on an arrested, empty heart with visual control of the action of the interventional person on the object they're operating on. The first aim of minimally invasive surgery is to minimize the lesions of the bony structure of the thorax, in the first place by not making them at all. The purpose is to work through the smallest possible "true ports" in the intercostal spaces without causing any lesions to the ribs, cartilages, intercostal nerves and vessels.

FIGURE 9.1.1 MIMVS incision by CMHVI.

What we do NOT consider MIMVS: the old-fashioned approach from the side that was done in the late 1970s and 1980s in redo situations through what we commonly call a lateral thoracotomy. The purpose was to avoid a mid-sternotomy in redo cases or to avoid a big scar in the middle of the thorax for esthetic reasons. The second aim of minimally invasive surgery is to minimize the deleterious effects of the extracorporeal circulation (ECC).

The general purpose is obtaining the best possible of the three "Cs":

- Better *comfort*: less or virtually no pain
- Better *cosmesis*: almost no visible scars
- Shortest fast-track to *complete* rehabilitation

MIMVS becomes "totally endosopic" when it is totally impossible for the surgeon to directly "look" through the working port, that they created for their instruments in order to reach the mitral valve, let alone a working port, that is big enough to bring hands or head through. As a result, a lot of "classical" aspects of the surgery DO change considerably: the visualization becomes "assisted", two-pronged instruments become shafted, the cannulation for the ECC, the clamping, the myocardial preservation and the monitoring of hemodynamics are different.

The approach remains the lateral side, a "mini-thoracotomy" skin incision, peri-areolar for men and in the submammary groove for ladies, but certainly without any form of rib-cutting or cartilage removing and avoiding at all times a sternal saw except for bailing out situations. Nevertheless, let's keep in mind that the overall strategy of all interventions is changing. The new paradigm is one where, in the future, cardiac surgery, interventional cardiology and imaging techniques are going to merge and where the "ideal" heart team knows and respects each other's methodology and armamentarium, goes for early treatment, stepwise and sometimes combined strategies and has one question in mind: what is the best option for the patient, that is presented to our team (Figure 9.1.1)?

HOW TO DO IT/STEP BY STEP

POSITION THE PATIENT

Patient is placed supine on the operating table with an inflatable cushion (Shoulder-Float™) under the chest to elevate the right hemi-thorax and to open up the intercostal spaces (ICS). The right arm is slightly flexed. The anesthesiologist places a central venous line, a right radial arterial line, a double-lumen endotracheal tube and a TEE probe (Figure 9.1.2, Figure 9.1.3 and Figure 9.1.4).

INSTALLING EXTRACORPOREAL CIRCULATION

Every extracorporeal circulation (ECC) requires the safe introduction of both an arterial return cannula and a venous drainage cannula. In the setting of "tru-port" surgery, this is much less obvious than in a sternotomy setting, where the ascending aorta and the caval veins are very easily reachable.

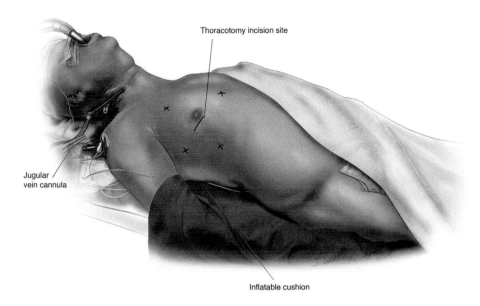

FIGURE 9.1.2 Patient positioning and skin marking for MiMVR. (Reprinted from *Oper Tech Thorac Cardiovasc Surg*, 16(4), Vanermen A, Van Praet F, Degrieck I et al. Endoscopic Mitral Valve Repair, 278-292, © 2011, with permission from Elsevier.)

In addition to that, possible candidates should have an MRI study of the peripheral vessels. Severe peripheral vessel disease, a very dilated ascending aorta (>41 mm) and known pleural adhesions should be excluded.

The sternotomy setting has certain advantages but also drawbacks. Venous drainage is not assisted and allows white cells to be sequestrated in the lungs, which may be a serious threat as lysis may lead to the release of pretty vaso-active substances. There is a significant blood–air interface with remnants of blood in the pericardium, where hemolysis takes place and thrombocytes are activated. Fatty cells from the bone marrow may be aspirated in the system as well. None of all this occurs in the percutaneous ECC. Active drainage will lead to empty lungs; there are no fatty cells and there is virtually no blood–air interface. In the setting of femoral arterial access, retrograde flow may have disadvantages, although there is no firm evidence for that in the literature. Ninety-five percent of mitral valve degenerative patients have normal peripheral arteries, and as a result, femoral artery access for arterial return is legitimate.

All "rules" about femoral cannulation from the past have to be forgotten. The rules should be: never tape the artery, and do not clamp or incise it, as this may lead to the introduction of a false lumen with disastrous consequences as a result! The "Seldinger" technique is imperative. It can be done through a 2.5-cm cutdown but also completely percutaneously in thin patients with the aid of an appropriate "closure" device. Prostar or ProGlide can be used safely up to 21 French cannulas.

The final access to the true lumen of the vessel is then obtained by the puncture-guidewire-dilation-introduction technique, obviously only under very accurate TOE-guidance. To avoid any misunderstanding, the surgeon should have their own echo-image-screen to make sure the images on the screen correlate perfectly well with the movements of the pigtailed guidewire.

FIGURE 9.1.3　Operating room setup.

FIGURE 9.1.5　MiMVr with Gore-Tex loops by Joseph Lamelas.

FIGURE 9.1.4　Double lumen endotracheal tube insertion.

FIGURE 9.1.6　Subclavian artery cannulation.

The general rule is that guidewires should advance as if they were pushed through olive oil! The slightest resistance should be an alarm as the dislodging of an intimal flap may be disastrous, as the purpose – unlike a "cath lab" procedure – is to install high retrograde flow in a fully heparinized body. In case of peripheral vascular disease, the subclavian artery is a very valid alternative. It has the advantage of antegrade flow, but a slightly bigger cutdown in a less convenient area is the drawback. Longitudinal transmural "U" stitches with 5/0 or 4/0 Gore-Tex, that are 4 mm in length, do give the advantage that their puncture holes don't produce any drops of blood in the small operative field, ensure an immediate dry closure on removal of the cannula and refrain from causing restrictions of the artery in diameter (Figure 9.1.5 and Figure 9.1.6).

Venous cannulation should be done the same way but with extreme caution to avoid perforation of the iliac or hepatic veins. Avoid the premature pulling down of the dome of the diaphragm as it may create a different angle between the inferior vena cava (IVC) and the hepatic vein. The visualization (and recognition by two observers) of the presence of the guidewire in the upper caval vein is therefore utterly important. Two-stage cannulas do produce enough drainage, when vacuum- or centrifugal pump-assisted. Be aware that the more the approach to the atrial groove is medial, the more left atrial retraction will be required. This action may cause the cannula to be "kinked" or pulled out of the superior vena cava (SVC) with massive and very disturbing pulmonary return as a result.

An additional jugular vein cannula is necessary for tricuspid valve surgery and, then, snaring of the caval veins allows for bloodless access of the right atrium. It is advisable to have your anesthesiologist put in a jugular vein cannula (17, 19 or 21 French) every now and then to allow them to practice their skills as it will be absolutely necessary in some cases. It is possible to proceed without double cannulation when your perfusionist is very experienced and perfectly able to monitor the blood levels in a "open" right atrium.

MYOCARDIAL PRESERVATION

More than in conventional surgery, myocardial protection is crucial in MIMVS, as cross clamp times will have the tendency to be longer, certainly in the beginning of a surgeon's experience.

As it will be impossible to apply a conventional cross clamp, there are actually three possibilities left:

1. No clamping, which means ventricular fibrillation.
2. An "adapted" clamp, either transthoracic ("Chitwood" clamp), flexible or detachable.
3. An endoclamp, an intravascular balloon, that, when inflated will provide adequate clamping, a root-pressure line, a venting and a cardioplegia line.

There are definite advantages and drawbacks for every form of clamping and according myocardial preservation.

1. Ventricular fibrillation is to be discouraged as it will lead to subendocardial ischemia and invariably give way to leaking of blood through the aortic valve during left atrial retraction. This is going to be very disturbing during complex valvular repairs with intracardiac gestures. It should be considered only in very easy annuloplasty repairs or in bailout situations like redos with open grafts.
2. Other chapters will discuss largely on all sorts of clamps adapted to mini-approaches.
3. Therefore, in this chapter, the endoclamp is going to be looked at extensively.

The *endoclamp* (Intraclude, Edwards Lifesciences) is a device that is brought in through a side-arm of the arterial return cannula, and placed in the femoral artery or subclavian artery. It can be inserted independently through a specific straight 21 French introducer as well (Figure 9.1.7).

The Intraclude (Edwards Lifesciences, USA) has three lumina: one for balloon inflation and balloon-pressure monitoring, one for root-pressure monitoring and one for venting and cardioplegia administration; the latter is equipped with a guidewire that is designed to be advanced in first under echo-guidance and have the endoclamp safely slide over (Figure 9.1.8).

Needless to say, in a particular groups of patients (with peripheral vascular disease) the condition of the peripheral vessels has to be checked first (MRI) to ensure safe placement of the endoclamp. In some individuals (young smoking females with very tortuous iliac arteries) the advancement of the endoclamp has to be carried out with extreme caution to avoid vascular injury. Under the echo-guidance of an expert, with great experience or with the coaching of an experienced wire-skilled surgeon, vascular injury should never be the case anymore (Figure 9.1.9).

FIGURE 9.1.7 Femoral cannulation by Joseph Lamelas.

FIGURE 9.1.8 ThruPort IntraClude from Edwards.

FIGURE 9.1.9 Aortic endoclamping for MiMVR.

Expert echo-guidance, basic wire-skills and intense communication between surgeon, anesthesiologist and perfusionist are needed to have the guidewire reach the aortic root safely, that is to say to avoid subclavian and/or carotid artery entry and migration. Once the endoclamp is positioned in the ascending aorta, just above the sino-tubular junction, the ECC can be initiated (Figure 9.1.10).

It has to be mentioned that this should always be done very slowly to prevent the iliac arteries from becoming spastic on the endoclamp-catheter. Arterial line-pressures in excess of 300 mm mercury should be avoided. Vasodilating drugs may help in finding the necessary balance between flow and acceptable pressures. If not, an additional arterial cannulation is to be considered in another artery, most often the contralateral femoral artery: the smallest possible cannula (size 17Fr) will invariably provide enough pressure drop on the arterial line.

Once acceptable flows are obtained and the interatrial groove sufficiently exposed, the balloon can be positioned and inflated. Inflation can only be initiated when all parties are agreed that the endoclamp is in the right position. Once it is about to fill the aortic lumen, the heart should be stopped. Cardiac arrest can be obtained by injecting adenosine or potassium in the aortic root through the cardioplegia line or – even better as it will provide a longer arrest – by rapid pacing or with a fibrillator pad behind the left ventricle. This will make the balloon act like a kite in the flow to stretch its catheter and take all slack out of it. This is important to avoid the balloon from migrating any further into the root during the procedure.

Once it is correctly positioned under echo-guidance, and paying attention to balanced pressures in both radial arteries, it can be inflated to secure complete clamping and fixed to the arterial cannula with a "locking" device. Adequate clamping can be obtained whilst observing balloon pressures going up to over 350–400 mm mercury depending on the size of the ascending aorta. Diameters of the ascending aorta in excess of 40 mm should certainly be avoided in unexperienced hands.

A single dose of cardioplegia (Bretschneider Custodiol) is preferable as most repairs and/or replacements will be done with one dose of cardioplegia and as the exposure of the mitral valve with the left atrial retractor may lead to less efficient subsequent cardioplegia delivery. After administration of the appropriate dose, the position and the adequate clamping of the balloon have be checked again on echo. All this may look complicated, but it will, in experienced hands, lead to a very reliable and long-lasting myocardial protection. Balloon migration and vascular lesions can be excluded completely.

EXPOSURE

The saying "Surgery is exposure" is even much more "ad rem" than in open conventional surgery. The smaller the access ports, the more their position and their angle towards the valve are important to have a good enough visualization of the mitral valve.

All this basically depends on

a. The Right Port-Placement

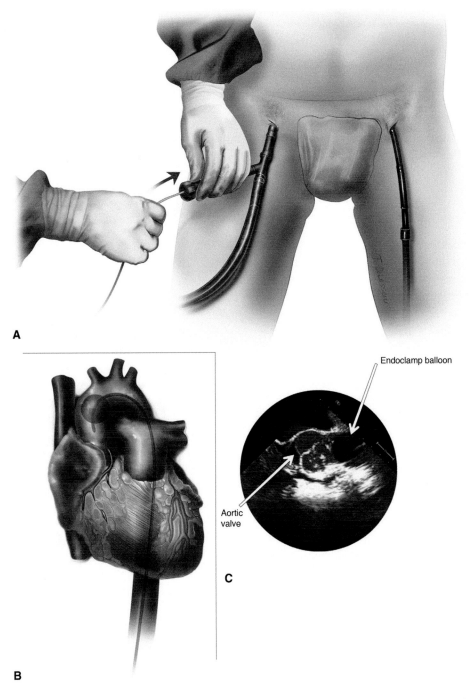

FIGURE 9.1.10 Echo-guided endoclamp placement. (Reprinted from *Oper Tech Thorac Cardiovasc Surg*, 16(4), Vanermen A, Van Praet F, Degrieck I et al. Endoscopic Mitral Valve Repair, 278-292, © 2011, with permission from Elsevier.)

TABLE 9.1.1 Comparison of external and internal clamping

External	Advantages:	Close to conventional clamping, less worrying about efficiency
		No additional learning curve
	Disadvantages:	Injury to left atrial appendix
		Necessity of cannulation and purse-strings on ascending aorta and hazardous closing at the end of surgery
		More time-consuming
		May be very hazardous in redo-situations
Internal	Advantages:	Very fast and reliable in experienced hands
		Very useful in redo-cases, applicable on grafts and/or repaired aortas
	Disadvantages:	Long learning curve
		Concerns about efficacy of myocardial preservation in unexperienced teams

The "working port" is the opening we create in an intercostal space, that we are going to bring all working, shafted instruments through. As a result, it should be at the mid-atrial level. In the vast majority of the patients this is going to be the fourth intercostal space. In a male patient, the skin incision can be purely peri-areolar or with a little extension laterally: the advantage is that in 99% of the cases the fourth interspace will be directly underneath. In a female patient though, in order to avoid an incision in breast tissue and have an invisible scar at the end, the incision should be in the infra-mammary groove. Whilst preparing the thorax (both in men and women) one should pay particular attention to make sure the right hemothorax is lifted at the level of the nipple to free the axillary area and in a female patient with a large breast, one should retract the right breast tissue towards the left shoulder with an adhesive drape. This maneuver will allow the infra-mammary groove to get in front of the fourth interspace. The more lateral the working port, the farther from the mitral, and the more medial, the closer, but sometimes with an awkward angle to overcome. It is about taking the best option with the size of the thorax in mind.

It is advisable to test the interspace after introducing a finger in the pleural space. Is it much narrower than the upper one? Is the dome of the diaphragm way above or way beneath? That's the moment when we can still change our decision about the right interspace to go through. In a minority it may become the fifth space. From that particular digital access in the pleural space, we can then make a 5-mm trocar port at middle finger's length all the way down in the seventh or eighth space. (Allied Medical™ provides two disposable 5.5-mm ports with an interesting inflatable balloon in one package). That will be the port for the venting cannula and the CO_2 influx (2.5 L/min). Only when CO_2 is flooding the right hemi-thorax, should the right lung be deflated. One may assume that only CO_2 (and no nitrogen) will fill the space and will make later de-airing almost unnecessary.

After enlarging the incision in the fourth space, a soft tissue retractor (Perivue™, Edwards Lifesciences) will make it a truly great space to work through (Figure 9.1.11).

FIGURE 9.1.11 Edwards ThruPort Systems Soft Tissue Retractor.

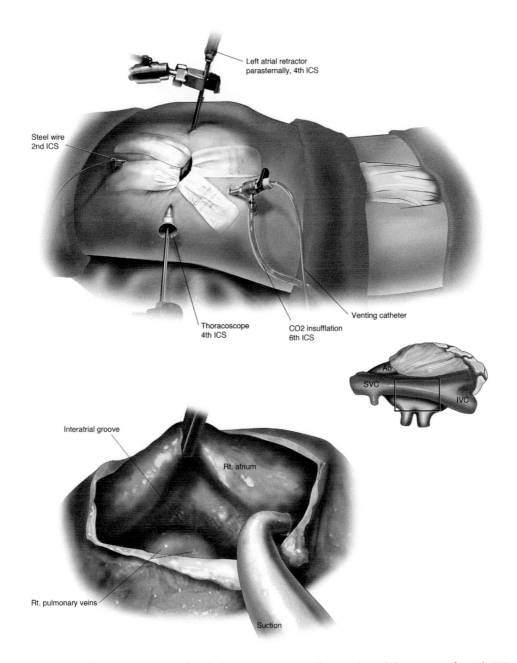

FIGURE 9.1.12 Thoracotomy, use of soft-tissue retractor and steps in gaining access for MiMVR. (Reprinted from *Oper Tech Thorac Cardiovasc Surg*, 16(4), Vanermen A, Van Praet F, Degrieck I et al. Endoscopic Mitral Valve Repair, 278-292, © 2011, with permission from Elsevier.)

Keep in mind that a rigid rib retractor will be much more of an obstacle for the movements of your shafted instruments! The next 5.5-mm port is made towards the axilla, in the same interspace somewhere at the front axillary line (Figure 9.1.12). It is the camera-port. The introduction of a 5-mm 30° endoscope will give a great view of the pericardium. If the diaphragm is still an obstacle for a nice view, one can

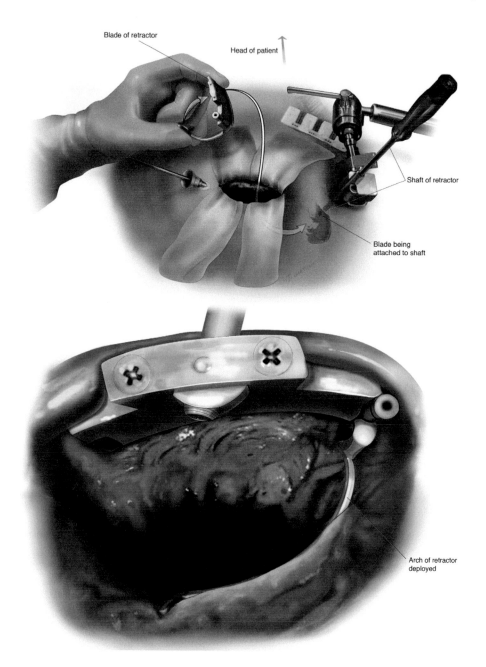

FIGURE 9.1.13 The "Vanermen" maneuver. (Reprinted from *Oper Tech Thorac Cardiovasc Surg*, 16(4), Vanermen A, Van Praet F, Degrieck I et al. Endoscopic Mitral Valve Repair, 278-292, © 2011, with permission from Elsevier.)

bring it down with a very superficial, preferably pledgeted monofilament U-stitch in the fibrous center, that is pulled down and exteriorly with a hook (Endoclose™) in the seventh or eighth space (Figure 9.1.13). One should avoid doing this maneuver prior to the cannulation of the right atrium to avoid a considerable alteration of the angle of the hepatic veins and the IVC. The last move is the introduction of a steel wire through

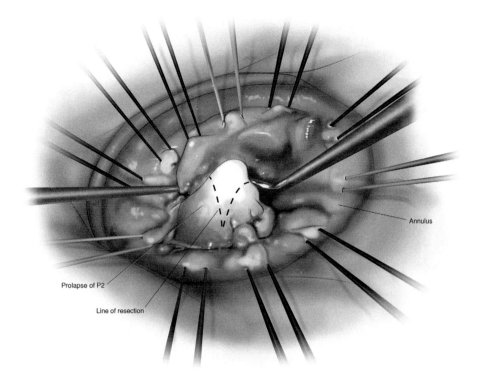

FIGURE 9.1.14 Exposure of mitral valve for prolapsed P2 repair. (Reprinted from *Oper Tech Thorac Cardiovasc Surg,* 16(4), Vanermen A, Van Praet F, Degrieck I et al. Endoscopic Mitral Valve Repair, 278-292, © 2011, with permission from Elsevier.)

the second space above the working port. Make sure venflon is protected when passed through the space and gliding over the upper edge of the third rib to avoid any damage to the intercostal artery.

Once on CPB the pericardial sac can be opened 3–4 cm above the phrenic nerve, and both edges over the interatrial groove can be suspended: the upper edge-stitch tied to the soft tissue retractor and two bottom edge-stitches brought exteriorly with a hook dorsal to the camera-port.

b. The Left Atrial Retraction

MITRAL VALVE REPAIR TECHNIQUE

The endoscopic mitral valve surgeon should come up with simple, fast, reproducible and efficient techniques for a variety of pathologies of the leaflets (Figure 9.1.14).

Actually, there is no reason why the sternotomy surgeon shouldn't do exactly the same. Complex and cumbersome techniques add to the complexity of the armamentarium and are more difficult to adopt for younger, inexperienced surgeons.

The ultimate goal of every repair is a reliable long-term result, and the requirements are the same:

1. *A high surface of coaptation* between the free edges of anterior and posterior leaflet (AL and PL) all the way from antero-lateral commissure to posteromedial commissure.
2. The closure line should occur *early in systole.*
3. And be located *in the inflow of the left ventricle.*

FIGURE 9.1.15 Mitral quadrangular repair in wet lab.

FIGURE 9.1.17 Extracorporeal cannula, Medtronic.

FIGURE 9.1.16 MiMVR – the Mohr technique.

FIGURE 9.1.18 ThruPort IntraClude, Edwards.

The repair history all started with the quadrangular resection as P2 prolapse is responsible for more than 60% of the degenerative lesions: a rectangle of the prolapsing leaflet tissue is resected and in doing so a gap is created [1] (Figure 9.1.15). Plicating sutures in the posterior annulus will allow the approximation of the edges of the leaflet tissue, and the gap is then closed with separate or running sutures. It often gave way to a situation, where now more rigid area in the PL, that (after the push-up of the annulus by the plication and the restriction of the anterior-posterior diameter with the remodeling annular ring) protrudes in the mitral orifice and impairs the full excursion of the AL: this situation will inevitably create the most dramatic complication of mitral valve repair: anterior leaflet motion, or SAM.

Alain Carpentier and Patrick Perier came up with the idea of the sliding plasty. It is all about reducing the height of the PL, avoiding the plicating stitch and in doing so avoiding the phenomenon of SAM. The result is a reduction of height of the posterior leaflet, and no more protruding or SAM, but the technique is cumbersome and time-consuming because of the long suturing time, and the final result is a smaller surface of coaptation.

In order to nearly exclude the possibility of SAM, to enhance the surface of coaptation and to simplify the repair techniques, the simplest "toolbox" should be advocated.

1. The most up-to-date techniques favor a ***triangular resection*** of a prolapse of the posterior leaflet scallops: the highest point is taken away and – as most P2s have the tendency to sort of flare out – the indentations remain intact; the scallop is lowered by the closing of the gap and there's no reason to fear SAM.
2. ***Gore-Tex sutures***: in some cases, though, even after a triangular resection with a very high P2 and P3, the portion may still be rigid and may give way to SAM. What is the solution? Well, it is to lower the new P2-scallop by pulling it down with a Gore-Tex! Gore-Tex sutures should originate from both papillary muscles to allow

for a nice symmetrical result and guarantee a high surface of coaptation and a durable repair. Needless to say that even in a full-blown Barlow, two small triangular resections together with two Gore-Tex sutures may generate a very good result in terms of both simplicity and durability.

Finally, if we want tissue to create a surface of coaptation and we want to avoid the opening of indentations, why would we resect in the first place? The concept of *"Respect"* was born. This is the idea: when there is excess tissue, we don't resect and we pull down the big P2 with two Gore-Tex sutures. Make sure they do not cross the midline and pull down symmetrically. This is very important. The length is to be fixed *after* the ring is in place and determined in accordance with a normal scallop. The same technique is used for anterior leaflet prolapse.

3. ***Papillary muscle repositioning (PMR)***: a very efficacious way to cure posteromedial commissural prolapse is the repositioning of the intermediate head of the papillary muscle. It is the head that all the "fan" chords originate from; it is usually very individual or can easily be individualized and pulled into the ventricle with a double reinforced Gore-Tex stitch towards the posterior head, that is invariably some 8–9 mm deeper. The PMR is very effective as it pulls down part of A3 and P3 together with the commissure. The free edges move down together and create a high surface of coaptation (Figure 9.1.16).

The aim of the simplified toolbox is to be faster, more effective and avoid SAM at all times. It came up as a spontaneous evolution of the P2 treatment; it is not the result of an intention to make endoscopic maneuvers more facile!

TOOLS/INSTRUMENTS AND DEVICES

MEDTRONIC EXTRACORPOREAL CANNULA

Medtronic Venous Cannulae are flexible and offers a wide range of insertion and drainage techniques. Medtronic Venous Cannulae are available with or without wire winding in single, double and triple stage designs in a variety of tip configurations to accommodate both bi-caval and caval-atrial cannulation. Medtronic Bio-Medicus NextGen is designed for femoral, arterial or jugular venous access (Figure 9.1.17).

THRUPORT INTRACLUDE FROM EDWARDS LIFESCIENCES

ThruPort is designed to eliminate an external cross clamp in minimal incision valve surgery (MIVS) cases. The device is delivered via the femoral artery approach and occludes the ascending aorta between 2.0 cm to 4.0 cm in width by an inflatable balloon. A case of MiMVR has been demonstrated in the linked video ((Figure 9.1.18 and Figure 9.1.19).

FIGURE 9.1.19 Port Access (Thru-Port System) video-assisted mitral valve surgery.

PERIOPERATIVE CONSIDERATIONS

The decision to start an MIMVS program is not an overnight decision. It is utterly important to assess whether the right team members and the right skills are available (Figure 9.1.20). Therefore, certain questions have to be asked.

Mitral valve repair surgery should be a discipline that is done on a very regular basis, as only in centers with enough volume, will the rates of repair and the long-term outcomes be good enough. This applies even more so for MIMVS. The lowest acceptable minimum of MIMVS case frequency should be once every week.

MIMVS certainly requires the right team approach. Hence, the decision to start a program has to be taken not only by the surgeon, but as a group after a multidisciplinary meeting with the anesthesiologists, the perfusionists, the scrub nurses, the referring cardiologists and intensive care specialists.

There are more burning questions to be asked:

∞ Do we have the right equipment?
3D TEE-equipment, adhesive defibrillation pads, double lumen tracheal tube, multiple pressure domes with appropriate monitoring, inflatable cushion or pad, high-definition camera-tower with multiple screens, an arm or "endoboy" to stabilize the endoscope during surgery, an appropriate left atrial retractor with stabilizing arm (Figure 9.1.21), shafted instruments, knot-pusher or Cor-Knot, shafted clip appliers.

FIGURE 9.1.20 How to start a minimal access mitral valve program.

∞ Do we have the right skill-sets?

Is *the anesthesiologist* an expert in TOE or is the expert-cardiologist present at the critical moments? Purpose: follow the guide-wires during cannulation, positioning the endoclamp when used, evaluate the quality of the mitral surgery (repair or replacement) (Figure 9.1.22).

Did *the surgeon* practice with shafted instruments; is he/she a seasoned endoscopic surgeon? Did *the perfusionist and the scrub nurse* have a theoretical and a practical teaching session? Is *the intensivist* aware of the novel strategies in terms of rapid awakening and rehabilitation?

CAVEATS AND CONTROVERSIES

Endoscopic mitral valve surgery has resulted in reduced intensive care unit and hospital stays, accelerated recovery times, less discomfort, reduced rehabilitation requirements and improved cosmesis. Some studies indicate lower rates of infection, use of foreign blood and postoperative arrhythmias. Postoperatively, patients are monitored overnight in the intensive care unit. Chest tubes can be removed after 36 hours. Results, in terms of mortality and repair quality, are comparable to sternotomy approaches. Practicing endoscopy and shafted instruments skills are mandatory, and as a result enough case load is necessary (Figure 9.1.23).

FIGURE 9.1.21 Medtronic ThoraTrak retractor.

FIGURE 9.1.23 Pros and cons discussions – MiMVR.

FIGURE 9.1.22 ProPlege device, Edwards.

Totally endoscopic surgery is a great asset for the surgeons in times where transcatheter techniques become widely adopted and are often the first choice for the patient of the 21st century. The non-rib-spreading technique limits scarring, discomfort and physiologic responses to the intervention, ensures a 2-week rehab period. Theses comes very close to puncture hole, no pain, no rehabilitation requirements, but with a long-term repair-for-life result in a very good number of cases (Figure 9.1.24).

RESEARCH, TRENDS AND INNOVATION

Minimally invasive mitral valve surgery has been adopted by many heart surgery centers throughout the globe. In a meta-analysis Cao et al compared clinical outcomes of repair for patients with degenerative mitral disease. They found no significant differences between the two surgical techniques [2]. Further multiple centered randomized trials are need to further valid the benefits and risks of minimally invasive mitral valve surgeries (Figure 9.1.25).

WHERE AND HOW TO LEARN

FOCUS VALVE WORKSHOPS

FOCUS Valve is a 4-day training course including live surgeries transmitted in 3D from our OR, lectures, how-to-do-it presentations, workshops, MICS wet labs and valve interventions in a beating heart model (Figure 9.1.26).

NUHCS SINGAPORE MINIMALLY INVASIVE MITRAL VALVE PROGRAMME

There are structured training programs for minimally invasive surgery throughout the year. NUHCS offers clinical fellowships and advanced clinical fellowships in minimally invasive cardiac surgery (Figure 9.1.27).

CLEVELAND CLINIC MINIMALLY INVASIVE MITRAL REPAIR

Cleveland offers an accredited fellowship program in minimally invasive cardiac and robotic-assisted surgery (Figure 9.1.28).

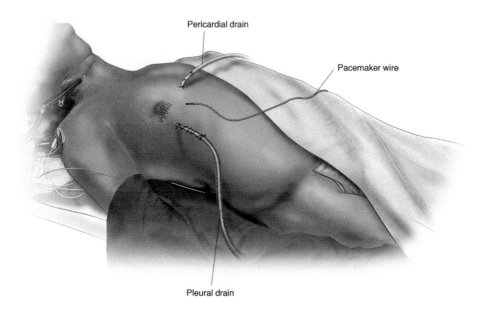

FIGURE 9.1.24 Post-MiMVR scar and chest drains in situ. (Reprinted from *Oper Tech Thorac Cardiovasc Surg,* 16(4), Vanermen A, Van Praet F, Degrieck I et al. Endoscopic Mitral Valve Repair, 278-292, © 2011, with permission.)

FIGURE 9.1.25 MiMVR: a systematic review.

FIGURE 9.1.27 NUHCS MICS programme.

FIGURE 9.1.26 FOCUS valve workshops.

FIGURE 9.1.28 Cleveland clinic training program.

REFERENCES

1. Anthony Vanermen, Frank Van Praet, Ivan Degrieck, et al. Endoscopic mitral valve repair. *Operative Techniques in Thoracic and Cardiovascular Surgery.* 2011;16(4):278–292. doi: 10.1053/j.optechstcvs.2011.11.002.

2. Cao C, Gupta S, Chandrakumar D, et al. A meta-analysis of minimally invasive versus conventional mitral valve repair for patients with degenerative mitral disease. *Ann Cardiothorac Surg.* 2013;2(6):693-703. doi:10.3978/j.issn.2225-319X.2013.11.08.

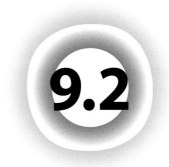

THE MITRAL VALVE
Alternative Approaches to Minimally Invasive Mitral Valve Surgery

CHANG GUOHAO AND THEO KOFIDIS

HISTORY OR INTRODUCTION

Andreas Vesalius suggested the term "mitral" to describe the left atrioventricular valve owing to its resemblance to a plane view of a bishop's miter. Perloff emphasized that the mitral valve requires all its components – the valve leaflets, the annulus, the subvalvular apparatus – together with the adjacent atrial and ventricular musculature working in concert to ensure the valve functions at its optimal capacity. This valve can be affected in many pathological conditions.

The first successful valve surgery of any kind was performed on the mitral valve before the introduction of pump oxygenators and open heart surgery. The surgeon works on the mitral valve blindly, purely relying on the sense of touch. It was performed in the then Peter Bent Brigham Hospital in 1923, now known as Brigham and Women's Hospital, by Dr Elliott C. Cutler, one of the trainees of Dr Harvey W. Cushing, and cardiologist Samuel A. Levine. The patient was a young girl with rheumatic mitral stenosis which was complicated by low cardiac output. Cutler performed a blind mitral commissurotomy with a knife through the apex of the left ventricle [1]. This was the first-in-the-world mitral valve repair and was reported in the Boston Medical and Surgical Journal, now known as the New England Journal of Medicine. The patient was discharged from the hospital a few days later. Less than

2 months later, Cutler developed a device to relieve mitral stenosis. He named it the cardiovalvulotome [2]. It is passed through the ventricular wall retrogradely through the mitral valve into the left atrium. The device removes a piece of the mitral valve so as to reduce the obstruction in mitral stenosis. The cardiovalvulotome was unfortunately difficult to use and conferred high complication rates of severe mitral regurgitation and high mortality rates. All of Cutler's patients died, and he discontinued mitral valve repair in 1929.

Yet another attempt was made in 1925, 2 years after Cutler's successful blind mitral commissurotomy, in the London hospital. Henry S. Souttar operated on a 19-year-old girl with mitral stenosis. This time, the mitral valve was approached from above – the left atrium – and the stenotic mitral valve was dilated with Souttar's finger (Figure 9.2.1).

Over the years, many techniques have been developed to repair or replace the mitral valve. Surgical procedures on the mitral valve, especially repairs, demand precise anatomical assessment of the valvular pathology in order to guide decisions regarding repair, reconstruction or replacement with preservation of the subvalvular apparatus. With the increasing sophistication of cardiovascular surgeries and reoperations, together with the growing popularity (among patients and surgeons) of minimally invasive surgery, alternative techniques and technologies have become a necessary armamentarium (Figure 9.2.2).

In this chapter, we will not be describing specific operative procedures on the mitral valve; instead we will focus on the various minimally invasive technologies for mitral valve repair or replacement in the operating room.

HOW TO DO IT/STEP BY STEP

In this day and age, mitral valve operations can be performed through incisions smaller than the conventional median sternotomy. Some use traditional cannulation techniques and conventional instruments to work on the mitral valve, but through smaller incisions, e.g. ministernotomy, right paramedian approach or an upper sternotomy. Others employ port-access mitral valve surgery, using catheter-based techniques for both cardiopulmonary bypass and cardioplegia and specially designed instruments to work on the mitral valve through a small port, e.g. right or left thoracotomy.

RIGHT PARAMEDIAN APPROACH

An incision is made over the third and fourth costal cartilages and the two cartilages are transected and folded laterally. The internal mammary vessels are usually

FIGURE 9.2.1 Evolution of the concept and practice of mitral valve repair.

FIGURE 9.2.2 Mitral heart valve surgery – Hugo Vanermen and Harriett Seager.

FIGURE 9.2.3 Video-atlas on MiMVS – the David Adams technique.

FIGURE 9.2.4 Upper ministernotomy for MiMVR.

preserved. If exposure of the aorta is limited, the femoral artery and vein can be used for cannulation for cardiopulmonary bypass, following which, a trans-septal approach, superior septal or traditional left atriotomy approach can be used to access the mitral valve (Figure 9.2.3).

UPPER STERNOTOMY APPROACH

The upper sternotomy is performed with an oscillating saw from the sternal notch extending caudally to the fourth or fifth interspace. A J-shaped sternotomy is created by sawing through the right hemisternum, with preservation of the right internal mammary vessels. Cardiopulmonary bypass can be instituted via ascending aorta and right atrium cannulation. In this approach, there is a smaller operating space; hence vacuum-assisted drainage will enable the usage of smaller than usual cannulas. Left atriotomy via this approach will be challenging. A trans-septal or superior septal approach will be more feasible (Figure 9.2.4).

RIGHT THORACOTOMY APPROACH

This approach utilizes the port access technique through a limited lateral right fourth intercostal space thoracotomy. Cardiopulmonary bypass, venting of the heart and cardioplegia are achieved through peripheral catheters in the femoral vessels. Aortic occlusion and cardioplegia are done through the thoracotomy incision. The mitral valve can be accessed easily through the Sondegaard's groove.

TOOLS/INSTRUMENTS AND DEVICES

In order to facilitate the above non-conventional accesses for the mitral valve, advancements in medical technology have been made. A myriad of new products have surfaced, and are key enablers for innovations in various approaches to the mitral valve.

MitraClip™

The MitraClip™ is a novel percutaneous method of treatment suitable for interventional treatment of mitral valve regurgitation. It is approved by the FDA as an alternative to surgical treatment of mitral valve regurgitation [3]. It is made of cobalt and covered in polyester, which promotes tissue growth. The implantation of MitraClip reproduces the surgical method of edge-to-edge valve repair, but does not involve open heart surgery (Figure 9.2.5).

This procedure is done under general anesthesia as a catheter-based technique via the femoral vein with the aid of fluoroscopy and echocardiography. It involves passage of the catheter across the atrial septum

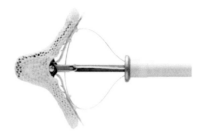

FIGURE 9.2.5 MitraClip™. Reproduced with permission of Abbott, © 2020.

FIGURE 9.2.6 Mitraclip™ procedure.

to reach the left atrium and under precise localization under echocardiographic and fluoroscopic guidance; the clip is fastened to the anterior and posterior mitral valve leaflets to reduce regurgitant flow (Figure 9.2.6). Usage of the EchoNavigator software can merge the images from echocardiography and fluoroscopy. In addition to the aforementioned device for transcutaneous mitral valve repair, TransCardiac Therapeutics patented MitraFlex, a novel method for mitral valve repair via a direct thoracoscopic approach through the apex on a beating heart. It involves implantation of an artificial chordae tendineae that controls the movement of the valve leaflets and reduces the annulus, hence reducing or eliminating mitral valve regurgitation. The MitraFlex mitral repair system provides an option for the minimally invasive repair of mitral regurgitation due to annular dilatation or chordal rupture without conventional sternotomy and cardiopulmonary bypass. This is still in its developmental stage and is not for human use.

TIARA VALVE

Neovasc's Tiara valve [4] is a self-expanding mitral prosthesis designed to treat mitral valve regurgitation by replacing the diseased valve. It is made of bovine pericardium and is delivered in a minimally invasive transapical transcatheter approach using a 32 French sheathless system under rapid pacing to replace the diseased native mitral valve without the need for open heart surgery or use of cardiopulmonary bypass. It has a fabric-covered skirt to prevent paravalvular leak and deploys two tabs to help engage the native valve for anchoring. The Tiara valve is the first transcatheter mitral valve to receive an FDA conditional investigational device exemption approval to initiate the U.S. arm of its Tiara-I Early Feasibility Trial.

As of December 12, 2016, a total of 22 patients have been treated with the Tiara valve in Canada, the U.S. and Europe. The technical success rate was 86%. Paravalvular leak levels were mild, trace or absent in 100% of these patients. The longest patient follow up available is nearing 3 years post-implant, where the Tiara valve remains fully functional and there have been no reported adverse events related to the valve performance. The Tiara valve has demonstrated the ability to treat patients with different anatomies, including patients with pre-existing prosthetic aortic valves (both mechanical and biological) and those with prior mitral repair surgery including mitral rings, which may be contraindications for other devices (Figure 9.2.7 and Figure 9.2.8).

ACCUFIT VALVE

The AccuFit mitral valve device is a novel transcatheter mitral valve developed by SINOMED as a pericardial valve

FIGURE 9.2.7 Results of the trans-apical Tiara bioprosthesis.

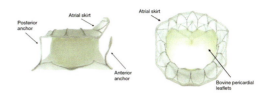

FIGURE 9.2.8 The Tiara™ transcatheter mitral valve. (Reprinted from Cheung A. Early experience of TIARA transcatheter mitral valve replacement system. *Ann Cardiothorac Surg.* 2018;7(6):787-791, © 2018, with permission from AME Publishing Company.)

mounted on a super elastic nitinol frame. It is designed to address the challenges faced by minimally invasive mitral valve replacement, specifically with a patented circumferential-coapt leaflet design which eliminates both central leakage and paravalvular leakage if the valve frame is deformed after implantation.

This is a self-expanding, self-centering valve made from three bovine pericardial leaflets secured within an atrial flange. Other components include a ventricular flange (of maximum height 14 mm) and an annulus support. The annulus support consists of a ring of anchors in a radial arrangement. There is an annular clipping space between the atrial flange and the ring of anchors. This "levelled" anchoring feature design minimizes paravalvular leakages and systolic anterior motion and provides improved valve stability. For controlled deployment, there is a set of tails extending from the ventricular aspect. The bovine pericardial leaflets are arranged uniquely in a reverse fashion with a central attachment and a circumferential coaptation (Figure 9.2.9, Figure 9.2.10).

Abdelghani et al. [5] described the transapical delivery fashion which utilizes a 0.035" or a 0.038" guidewire. This system is sheathless and made of polyvinylidene fluoride (PVDF) and polytetrafluoroethylene (PTFE) to reduce friction during deployment, during passage through the apex and through the mitral

FIGURE 9.2.9 AccuFit TMVR device by SINOMED.

valve complex. For this construct, sizing is based on echocardiographic mitral valve orifice average dimension (i.e. [mediolateral dimension + anteroposterior dimension]/2), and the manufacturer recommends to oversize by 3 mm.

TENDYNE™ VALVE

The Tendyne™ Bioprosthetic Mitral Valve System, by Abbott Laboratories, has been successfully implanted in patients using an off-pump transpical approach. It is fully retrievable, and fully repositionable. The Tendyne™ valve is made up of apically tethered tri-leaflet porcine pericardial valve sewn onto a nitinol frame and is able to address complex mitral valve anatomy of functional, degenerative and mixed etiology mitral regurgitation (Figure 9.2.11, Figure 9.2.12 and Figure 9.2.13).

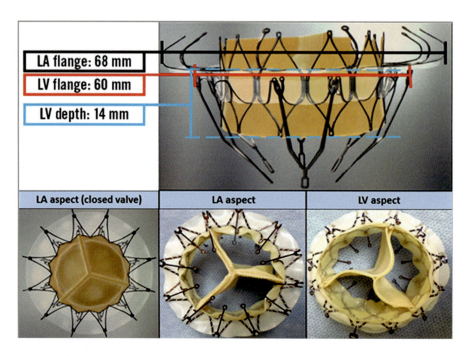

FIGURE 9.2.10 The Accufit TMVR prosthesis. The atrial aspect (left, lower) and the ventricular aspect (right, lower) displaying the reverse leaflet design [5]. (Republished with permission of Europa Group from EuroIntervention on behalf of the EuroPCR and EAPCI, Abdelghani M, Onuma Y, Zeng Y, et al. The Sino Medical AccuFit transcatheter mitral valve implantation system, 11, Suppl W:W84-W8, © 2015.)

CARDIAQ VALVE

The CardiAQ Valve, developed by Edwards Lifesciences, is made of porcine pericardium, mounted on a self-expandable nitinol stent designed for trans-septal implantation. This is the first percutaneous valve implanted in the mitral position [6]. The first-in-human percutaneous mitral valve implantation was performed in Denmark on an 86-year-old man with severe MR with residual MR grade 1+ post-replacement. However, the patient succumbed to multi-organ failure 3 days later. Autopsy did not find any structural failure of the valve (Figure 9.2.14).

CORONARY SINUS-BASED PERCUTANEOUS MITRAL ANNULOPLASTY

The Carillon Mitral Contour System is a fixed-length, double-anchor nitinol device that is designed to be positioned within the coronary sinus to reduce functional mitral regurgitation (FMR).

It is one of the devices used for indirect annuloplasty. Three prospective, multi-center trials involving more than 100 patients have shown that this system is effective, efficient and flexible. There is improvement of at least one NYHA class and at least a 50% reduction in regurgitation volume as a result of reversal of annular dilation in 80% of patients [7] (Figure 9.2.15).

In addition, the AMADEUS study has shown improved clinical and echocardiographic parameters when used in patients with FMR, with an acceptable safety profile. However, there were problems of wire-form fractures seen next to the proximal anchor locking mechanism at high-strain locations on the device. Even though the wire-form fractures were clinically benign,

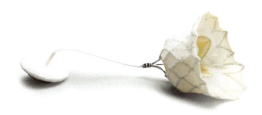

FIGURE 9.2.11 The Tendyne™ transcatheter mitral valve replacement (TMVR) system with Apical Pad. Reproduced with permission of Abbott, © 2020.

FIGURE 9.2.12 Transcatheter mitral valve implantation by Neil E. Moat.

the device was modified and named mXE2, which underwent the TITAN II study to further evaluate its safety and integrity [8]. Of 36 patients with congestive heart failure, reduced left ventricular function and at least moderate FMR who underwent implantation of the mXE2, there was one major adverse event within 30 days – non-device-related mortality – which occurred 17 days post-implantation. There was clinical improvement as evidenced by echocardiographic reductions in degree of FMR and better 6-min walk test results, as per the two previous studies. In addition, the previously seen device fractures were not seen in TITAN II. The next phase will be for the use of Carillon device in a blinded randomized trial of symptomatic patients with FMR in Europe and Australia (Figure 9.2.16 and Figure 9.2.17).

VALTECH CARDIOBAND

The Valtech Cardioband system reconstructs the mitral valve by direct annuloplasty which is delivered transfemorally with no need for open heart surgery. It is done under echocardiographic and fluoroscopic guidance and is anatomically fitted. The system easily conforms to each patient's specific annular geometry. It is composed of three elements: a standard polyester fabric sleeve, stainless-steel anchors and an adjustment mechanism which allows adjustment of each step to ensure safety and control throughout the implantation procedure. This implant is available in six sizes to cover the entire spectrum of functional mitral regurgitation. The sleeve has a unique design where the attaching anchors are kept safely within. The adjustment mechanism that is embedded inside the sleeve allows a homogeneous circumferential annular cinching after full deployment of the implant (Figure 9.2.18, Figure 9.2.19 and Figure 9.2.20).

A feasibility study was designed to evaluate the Cardioband implant (tranatrial) that enrolled five patients with mitral regurgitation in two centers in Europe. The primary endpoint was overall device-related safety at 30 days and technical feasibility. Endpoints included hemodynamic measures by echocardiography and mitral regurgitation reduction. There was a 30% average reduction in septo-lateral dimension of the mitral annulus. Another study to investigate the performance and safety of the Cardioband for mitral valve repair is currently ongoing and aims to be completed in 2018.

MITRALIGN

The Mitralign is the only direct transcatheter system that is designed to treat both mitral and tricuspid regurgitation. The Mitralign Percutaneous Annuloplasty

FIGURE 9.2.13 Animation of the implantation of the Tendyne™ valve.

System (MPAS) is intended for the treatment of symptomatic functional mitral regurgitation (MR 3+ or more) for annular reduction through tissue plication. It has an extremely small footprint, hence leaving a significant amount of native anatomy undisturbed. It is also possible to customize the location and plication distance on the mitral annulus. It uses a transfemoral retrograde approach to deliver pairs of pledgets connected with a suture. Each pledget pair is then cinched to achieve plications of the annulus at selected areas. More than two pairs of pledgets can be implanted along the posterior annulus (Figure 9.2.21 and Figure 9.2.22).

GDS ACCUCINCH

The GDS Accucinch is another novel transcatheter approach to mitral valve repair by direct annuloplasty. This was designed to reduce congestive cardiac failure in patients with mitral regurgitation who are not healthy enough for surgery. Access is via the femoral artery, to cinch the mitral annulus after measuring the size of the mitral opening. A series of anchor elements is implanted in the subvalvular space from trigone to trigone. These anchors are then connected by a cable to cinch the annulus and the basal portion of the left ventricle. This increases contact between the mitral valve leaflets to reduce regurgitant flow. The feasibility and the safety of the device have both been shown in ten patients, with no conversion to surgery and no 30-day major events. However, mitral regurgitation reduction was inconsistent, most probably due to the challenge of implantation of the anchors from trigone to trigone and at close proximity to the annulus [9] (Figure 9.2.23).

TRANSAPICAL OFF-PUMP NEOCHORD IMPLANTATION

Whilst not yet percutaneous, the NeoChord device and the Harpoon Medical device (Harpoon Medical, Inc., Baltimore, MD) both deliver expanded polytetrafluoroethylene artificial chords via an anterolateral minithoracotomy and transapical left ventricle puncture under echo guidance on a

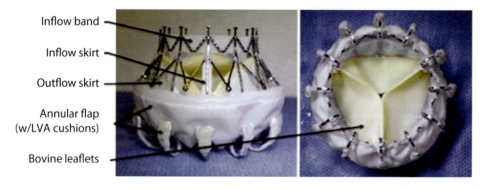

FIGURE 9.2.14 The CardiAQ™ transcatheter mitral valve implantation (TMVI) system. (Republished with permission of Europa Group from EuroIntervention on behalf of the EuroPCR and EAPCI, Sondergaard L, Ussia GP, Dumonteil N, Quadri A. The CardiAQ transcatheter mitral valve implantation system, 11 Suppl W:W76-W77© 2015.)

FIGURE 9.2.15 Animation of the implantation of a Carillon device.

FIGURE 9.2.16 Patient case demonstrating real-time implantation of Carillon device.

beating heart without need for cardiopulmonary bypass (transapical off-pump mitral valve repair with NeoChord implantation [TOP-MINI]). A successful TOP-MINI procedure was performed with five NeoChords implanted on the posterior mitral valve leaflet [10]. These devices allow for the adjustment of the prolapsed leaflet tethering chords and anchoring to the left ventricular epicardium using transesophageal echocardiographic guidance to optimize native leaflet coaptation (Figure 9.2.24).

VALTECH V-CHORDAL

The Valtech V-Chordal is an alternative solution for chordal shortening to reduce the degree of mitral regurgitation. It involves implantation of an artificial chorda to enable post-pump chordal length modification with echocardiography guidance (Figure 9.2.25).

MITRA-SPACER

The Mitra-Spacer is a reversible implantable device designed to be placed in the mitral valve via a trans-apical procedure aimed to improve mitral valve coaptation by providing a sealing surface for the mitral valve leaflets, hence reducing or eliminating mitral regurgitation (Figure 9.2.26). The first-in-human implantation of the Mitra-Spacer system was presented at PCR London Valves in Berlin, Germany, in 2015. This device is intended to treat or bridge heart failure patients whose perioperative mortality for conventional open heart surgery is deemed to be prohibitive (Figure 9.2.27).

The Mitra-Spacer, by Cardiosolutions Novel Technology, uses a tethered atraumatic inflatable and volume-adjustable balloon placed between the anterior and posterior mitral valve leaflets via a transapical approach on the beating heart (Figure 9.2.28). It does not repair anatomical abnormalities of the mitral valve, but serves to fill the defect between the native leaflets, hence reducing the mitral regurgitation. The first-in-human implantation was performed by Professor Olaf Wendler, Professor of Cardiac Surgery, in King's College Hospital London.

PERIOPERATIVE CONSIDERATION

Minimally invasive mitral valve surgery, as you would have already come to have a better understanding of from the previous chapters, is a highly subspecialized therapeutic approach for the treatment of mitral valve pathologies. The main principal consideration in undertaking a successful surgery is the patient selection and, subsequently, the assembly of an excellent, if not perfect, team. Patient selection has been alluded to in the previous chapters. The team is the key ingredient to achieving a

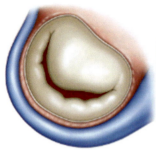
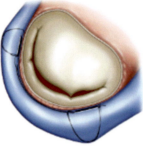
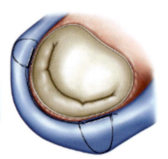

Mitral annulus dilation before implantation of Carillon device

Mitral annulus cinched with Carillon device

Mitral annulus remodeled with Carillon device

FIGURE 9.2.17 Carillon® Mitral Contour System: right-heart transcatheter mitral valve repair (TMVr) device. Reproduced with permission of Cardiac Dimensions Pty. Ltd. © 2020.

good patient outcome. This team, consisting of the minimally invasive mitral valve surgeon, his highly trained surgical and nursing assistants and the anesthesiologist who is well-versed in management of the changing physiology in the "on-and-off" ventilated lungs during the initial set up and final hemostatic phases of the surgery. All these have to work in tandem in order to achieve success (Figure 9.2.29).

ALTERNATIVE APPROACHES

TRANSCATHETER MITRAL VALVE REPLACEMENT

At the 2014 Transcatheter Cardiovascular Therapeutics (TCT) meeting, it was obvious that mitral valve technology will become the next major trend. At the 2015 Transcatheter Valve Therapies meeting, Juan Granda, M.D., executive director and chief scientific officer of the Cardiovascular Research Foundation's Skirball Center for Innovation spoke on the various transcatheter mitral valve therapies in development (Figure 9.2.30).

In addition, the same meeting saw an interview with Ted Feldman, M.D., FACC, MSCAI, FESC, cardiac lab director, Evanston Hospital, North Shore Health System and principal investigator for the Everest II MitraClip U.S. pivotal trial on the various technologies available for TMVR.

Besides minimally invasive surgical approaches to the mitral valve, this is an alternative for patients who are medically

FIGURE 9.2.18 Live procedure of mitral valve repair of Cardioband.

FIGURE 9.2.19 Cardioband procedure on a patient- Francesco Maisano.

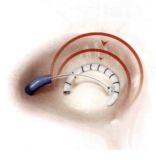

FIGURE 9.2.20 Cardioband™. Reproduced with permission of Edwards Lifesciences LLC, Irvine, CA.

FIGURE 9.2.21 Animation of the Mitralign procedure.

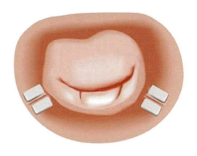

FIGURE 9.2.22 Mitralign™ Percutaneous Annuloplasty System (MPAS) for repair of functional mitral regurgitation. (After Gasior T, Gavazzoni M, Taramasso M, Zuber M, Maisano F. Direct Percutaneous Mitral Annuloplasty in Patients With Functional Mitral Regurgitation: When and How. *Front Cardiovasc Med*, 6:152, © 2019.)

FIGURE 9.2.23 Animation of the use of Accucinch.

not suitable for surgery. Transcatheter aortic valve replacement (TAVR) was originally intended for patients who could not undergo surgery, but it has now been established as an excellent alternative to surgical aortic valve replacement in patients at high or intermediate risk. The progress in developments of TAVR with well-designed devices of acceptable safety and efficacy has inspired manufacturers to push the boundaries of innovation to transcatheter mitral valve replacement (TMVR). TMVR is likely to follow a similar path to the one that TAVR has taken, starting with the sickest patients and a narrow indication, but likely attracting less sick patients who would rather have this minimally invasive procedure over surgery.

Surgical mitral valve repair and replacement is well established as a safe and effective procedure in patients with degenerative or functional mitral regurgitation. However, some patients have multiple comorbidities that place them at extreme risk, making less invasive surgery a better option – TMVR. With careful patient selection in highly experienced centers, the mortality with TMVR is low. TMVR can be performed either via a retrograde transapical approach or an antegrade trans-septal approach (Figure 9.2.31).

PERCUTANEOUS MITRAL VALVE REPAIR

In the 2012 European Society of Cardiology guidelines for the management of valvular diseases, mitral valve repair surgery, when feasible, is preferred over valve replacement as it is associated with lower rates of short- and long-term mortality and morbidity, better preservation and a greater likelihood

FIGURE 9.2.24 Transapical off-pump mitral valve repair with NeoChord implantation (TOP-MINI).

FIGURE 9.2.26 The Mitra-Spacer™ Cardiosolutions.

FIGURE 9.2.25 Cardioband: clinical reality for mitral and tricuspid valve repair.

FIGURE 9.2.27 Mitra-Spacer first-in-human news.

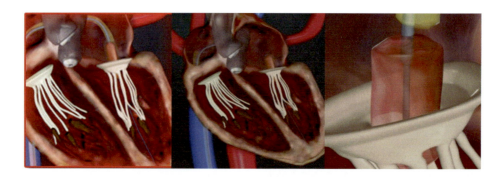

FIGURE 9.2.28 Percu-Pro Mitra-Spacer. (Reprinted from *JACC Cardiovasc Interv,* 4(1), Chiam PT, Ruiz CE. Percutaneous transcatheter mitral valve repair: a classification of the technology, 1-13, © 2011 American College of Cardiology Foundation, with permission from Elsevier.)

FIGURE 9.2.29 MiMVR by Ralph Damiano Jr.

FIGURE 9.2.30 Transcatheter mitral valve therapies in development, TCT.

FIGURE 9.2.31 Overview of transcatheter mitral valve repair technologies.

FIGURE 9.2.32 Percutaneous approach for the mitral valve – Anita Asgar.

FIGURE 9.2.33 Preclinical evaluation of the Tiara transapical mitral valve.

FIGURE 9.2.34 The current results of transcatheter mitral valve implantation.

of avoiding warfarinization and/or reoperation for structural valvular dysfunction. Percutaneous mitral valve repair (a possibility in the near future as an alternative and perhaps, some would argue, more attractive option) follows the same principles as conventional open mitral valve repair: NeoChord placement, leaflet plication, annuloplasty, papillary modification and left ventricular remodeling. Approaches include targeting coronary sinus implantation and transapical implantation of NeoChordae (not percutaneous at this stage) (Figure 9.2.32, Figure 9.2.33 and Figure 9.2.34).

WHERE AND HOW TO LEARN

We have just described a number of alternative approaches and techniques for the mitral valve in the minimally invasive era. Transcatheter mitral valve replacement in patients with regurgitant valves, failing mitral valve bioprosthesis and rings and calcified mitral annuli has been effectively conducted in patients with no surgical options due to prohibitive surgical risks. There are many products in the market, most of them undergoing large-scale prospective trials, and the long-term result is yet to seen. The development of various products in the arena of TMVR heralds the beginning of a new era.

REFERENCES

1. Cohn, L. H., Tchantchaleishvili, V., & Rajab, T. K. (2015). Evolution of the concept and practice of mitral valve repair. *Annals of Cardiothoracic Surgery*, 4(4), 315.
2. Weisse, A. B. (2002). *Heart to Heart: The Twentieth Century Battle against Cardiac Disease: An Oral History.* London U.K: Rutgers University Press.
3. Sündermann, S. H., Biaggi, P., Grünenfelder, J., Gessat, M., Felix, C., Bettex, D., et al. (2014). Safety and feasibility of novel technology fusing echocardiography and fluoroscopy images during MitraClip interventions. *EuroIntervention*, 9(10), 1210–6.
4. Cheung, A., Stub, D., Moss, R., Boone, R. H., Leipsic, J., Verheye, S., et al. (2014). Transcatheter mitral valve implantation with Tiara bioprosthesis. *EuroIntervention: Journal of EuroPCR in collaboration with the Working Group on Interventional Cardiology of the European Society of Cardiology*, 10, U115–9.
5. Abdelghani, M, Onuma, Y, Zeng, Y, Osama I.I. Soliman, Jim Ma, Yong Huo, Andrea Guidotti, Fabian Nietlispach, Francesco Maisano, Patrick W. Serruys. (2015). The sino medical AccuFit transcatheter mitral valve implantation system. *Eurointervention 11*, W84–W85. doi: 10.4244/EIJV11SWA26.
6. Sondergaard L, Ussia GP, Dumonteil N, Quadri A. The CardiAQ transcatheter mitral valve implantation system. *EuroIntervention*. 2015;11 Suppl W:W76–W77. doi:10.4244/EIJV11SWA22
7. Siminiak, T., Wu, J. C., Haude, M., Hoppe, U. C., Sadowski, J., Lipiecki, J., et al. (2012). Treatment of functional mitral regurgitation by percutaneous annuloplasty: results of the TITAN trial. *European Journal of Heart Failure*, 14(8), 931–938.
8. Lipiecki J, Kaye DM, Witte KK, et al. Long-Term Survival Following Transcatheter Mitral Valve Repair: Pooled Analysis of Prospective Trials with the Carillon Device. *Cardiovasc Revasc Med.* 2020;21(6):712-716. doi:10.1016/j.carrev.2020.02.012
9. Kleber, F; Reddy, V; Neuzil P. (2012). *GDS Accucinch Program Update, TCT Meeting*, Miami. Online content: https://www.tctmd.com/slide/accucinch-guided-delivery-systems-program-update
10. Colli A, Besola L, Gerosa G. Transapical Off-pump neochord implantation for mitral regurgitation recurrence. *Rev Esp Cardiol (Engl Ed)*. 2016 May;69(5):515. English, Spanish. doi: 10.1016/j.rec.2015.09.020. Epub 2015 Dec 28. PMID: 26739826.

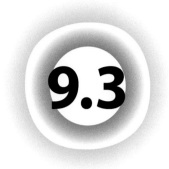

THE MITRAL VALVE
Robotic Mitral Valve Surgery

NIRAV C PATEL, MEGHAN K TORRES AND JONATHAN M HEMLI

HISTORY AND INTRODUCTION

A robotic-assisted approach to mitral valve surgery is the next logical step in the natural evolution of operating on the mitral valve through minimal-access techniques. Although excellent clinical outcomes have certainly been reported utilizing a mini-thoracotomy approach alone, with or without port-assist, addition of the robotic technology to the procedure facilitates better surgical exposure, greater dexterity for the surgeon and the ability to replicate the excellent quality of valve repair (or replacement) that would otherwise be traditionally achieved via sternotomy.

Any patient who requires mitral valve surgery, possibly combined with an anti-atrial fibrillation procedure and/or a tricuspid valve operation, is a potential candidate for a robotic-assisted approach, including those patients who have had prior cardiac or thoracic surgery. There is certainly, however, a definite learning curve to the procedure, and some patients may still prove to be better served by a more traditional surgical approach, particularly if they require more complex surgery in less experienced centers.

With this in mind, the rapid and relentless continued improvements in robotic technology will only serve to reduce the complexity of the operation, ease the learning curve and make the procedure more attractive to a larger number of surgeons. Patients demand excellent results using minimally invasive techniques, and there remains little doubt that robotic-assisted technology is ideally suited to fill this niche with respect to operating on the mitral valve.

The first robotic-assisted mitral valve repair using an early prototype of the da Vinci system (Intuitive Surgical, Sunnyvale, CA)

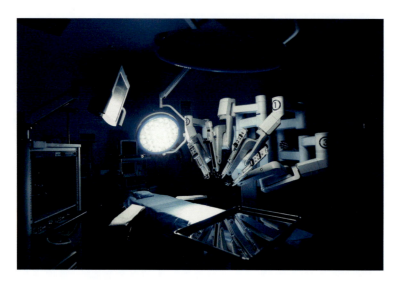

FIGURE 9.3.1   Robotic operating room, general outline.

was performed by Carpentier and associates in 1998 [1], followed immediately thereafter by Mohr and colleagues [2]. The feasibility and safety of performing cardiac surgery via a minimally invasive approach, using long-shafted instruments, with or without the assistance of two-dimensional videoscopes, had already been well established [3–9].

Chitwood's group performed the first complete robotic-assisted mitral valve repair in the United States under an FDA safety and efficacy trial in 2000 [10]. In 2002, after a multi-center phase II trial, the commercial da Vinci system was approved for mitral valve surgery by the FDA [11]. The progressive evolution of robotic-assisted mitral valve surgery has been relentless ever since, with iterative advancements in technology resulting in enhanced three-dimensional (3D) stereoscopic visual systems, improved ergonomic instruments

FIGURE 9.3.2   Robot-assisted MiMVr – Mayo Clinic.

with greater flexibility, dexterity and multiple degrees of freedom of movement, programmable instrument carts with integrated energy sources and the capability for the surgeon to continually hone their skills on a training simulator. In addition, the current da Vinci system is able to seamlessly integrate more than one video console, aptly facilitating the training of the next generation of robotic valve surgeons (Figure 9.3.1 and Figure 9.3.2).

HOW TO DO IT/STEP BY STEP

PATIENT SELECTION

Theoretically, any patient requiring isolated mitral valve surgery is a candidate for a robotic-assisted, minimally invasive approach, and the indications for intervention are the same as those outlined in the

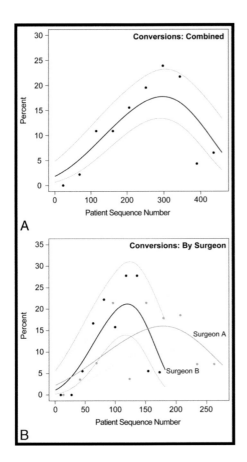

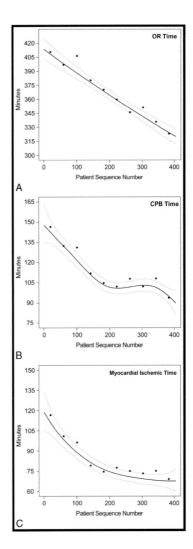

FIGURE 9.3.3A Learning curves for operative success in terms of conversion from robotic to conventional surgical approaches. A, combined for both surgeons. B, individual surgeons. (After Goodman A, Koprivanac M, Kelava M, et al. Robotic Mitral Valve Repair: The Learning Curve. *Innovations (Phila)*, 12(6):390-397. 2017 by the International Society for Minimally Invasive Cardiothoracic Surgery. Reprinted by Permission of SAGE Publications, Inc.)

AHA/ACC and European guidelines for the management of patients with valvular heart disease [12,13].

Robotic mitral repair techniques can be applied to both degenerative and functional valve pathology, and robotic-assisted valve replacement can be undertaken for those patients not deemed candidates for repair, irrespective of disease etiology. Patients with a history of atrial fibrillation requiring

FIGURE 9.3.3B Learning curves for technical performance in terms of operative efficiency. Solid lines depict estimate of the mean response based on the nonparametric function, enclosed within 95% confidence intervals. Closed circles depict average of the observed data for deciles of patient sequence number. A, operating room time continuously declined. B, cardiopulmonary bypass time plateaued after 200 cases. C, myocardial ischemic time plateaued after approximately 200 cases. CPB, cardiopulmonary bypass; OR, operating room. (After Goodman A, Koprivanac M, Kelava M, et al. Robotic Mitral Valve Repair: The Learning Curve. *Innovations (Phila)*, 12(6):390-397. c 2017 by the International Society for Minimally Invasive Cardiothoracic Surgery. Reprinted by Permission of SAGE Publications, Inc.)

a concomitant ablation or maze procedure are good candidates for a robotic-assisted approach, as are those who need concurrent intervention on the tricuspid valve.

Patients with poor left ventricular function, a heavily calcified mitral annulus, severe pulmonary hypertension, poor pulmonary function, aortic insufficiency, peripheral arterial disease and moderate to severe pectus excavatum tend not to be ideal candidates for a robotic approach. Although these are not necessarily all absolute contraindications to the use of the robot, we suggest that caution be exercised when assessing these patients for a minimal-access strategy, especially by a surgeon who is still in the earlier stage of their learning curve for robotic-assisted techniques [14]. These patients may indeed be better served by a sternotomy.

Any patients with medical co-morbidities (such as advanced liver or renal dysfunction, or a systemic bleeding diathesis) that place them at higher inherent risk for perioperative complications may also be more suitable for a sternotomy approach, given the longer cardiopulmonary bypass and cross-clamp times that tend to be associated with robotic-assisted techniques. Patients who require concomitant coronary artery bypass grafting or aortic valve and/or ascending aortic surgery cannot be adequately treated via minimal-access robotic surgery and should be managed through a median sternotomy (Figure 9.3.3A,B).

PREPARATION

Right-lung isolation is typically facilitated through the use of a double-lumen endotracheal tube, although a bronchial blocker could potentially be utilized instead. We find that the former option provides more reliable and consistent lung deflation. After endotracheal intubation, a 17-Fr cannula is percutaneously inserted via the right

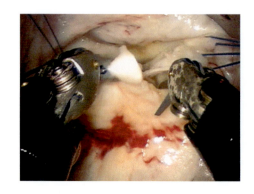

FIGURE 9.3.4 Valve repair. Prolapsing segment resection using micro-scissors and valve forceps. (Republished with permission of Elsevier Science & Technology Journals, from Robotic mitral valve repair: trapezoidal resection and prosthetic annuloplasty with the da vinci surgical system, Chitwood WR Jr, Nifong LW, Elbeery JE, et al. *J Thorac Cardiovasc Surg*. 120(6):1171-1172, © 2000 The American Association for Thoracic Surgery; permission conveyed through Copyright Clearance Center, Inc.)

internal jugular vein into the superior vena cava (SVC), using a standard Seldinger technique, the position of the cannula being confirmed by transesophageal echocardiography. Although not necessarily always mandatory for minimal-access mitral valve surgery, we find the SVC cannula to be invaluable in ensuring adequate venous drainage for cardiopulmonary bypass. This is particularly so, given that our preferred method of attaining cardiac arrest is through the use of a trans-thoracic aortic cross-clamp. We have found that, without an SVC cannula in place, a long aortic cross-clamp, coupled with superior retraction of the roof of the left atrium, can potentially "kink" the SVC, partially obstructing venous return from the cerebrum and upper body, resulting in inadequate venous drainage (Figure 9.3.4 and Figure 9.3.5).

External defibrillator pads are attached to the patient's chest, and a padded support is placed underneath the right scapula in order to achieve a 30-degree elevation of

FIGURE 9.3.5 Robotic approach to mitral valve repair: Mayo Clinic experience.

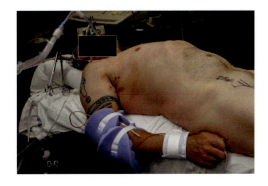

FIGURE 9.3.6 The patient is appropriately positioned for the procedure. Note the venous cannula that has been percutaneously inserted into the superior vena cava via the right internal jugular vein.

this side. The patient's right arm hangs by the side of the table, such that the posterior axillary line is exposed. Special attention needs to be given to the positioning of the right arm in order to avoid undue strain on the brachial plexus and prevent a neurapraxic or traction injury to the ulnar nerve. The whole operating table is tilted approximately five to seven degrees to the patient's left, further elevating the right chest, making it more accessible to the surgeon (Figure 9.3.6).

At this point, a thorough and complete interrogation of the mitral valve utilizing three-dimensional TEE is absolutely imperative in order to generate a model of the valve and engender a detailed plan for the operation. Any unexpected findings should be noted, and, if the surgeon is not comfortable proceeding, there should be no hesitation in electively converting the surgical strategy to a sternotomy approach, even at this early stage. The tricuspid valve should also be examined, with detailed measurements of its annular dimensions, in order to determine whether a concomitant tricuspid procedure should be undertaken as well.

SURGICAL EXPOSURE AND ACCESS

After the right lung is deflated, a 3- to 4-cm slightly curvilinear incision is made in the right inframammary crease, lateral to the nipple, and the pleural cavity is entered through the fourth intercostal space (ICS) (Figure 9.3.7).

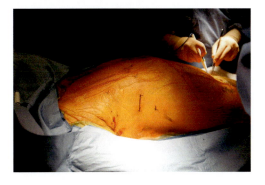

FIGURE 9.3.7 The patient is prepped and draped and ready for surgery. The positions of the "working incision" and the robotic port sites are marked out on the chest wall. Note that preparation of the left femoral vessels for cannulation has already commenced.

This "working incision" serves as the primary means of access into the chest for the bedside surgical assistant. The robotic camera can also be directly inserted into the pleural space at the medial aspect of this incision, or alternatively, the camera trocar can be passed through a separate entry point in the chest wall, more towards the sternum. An Alexis soft-tissue wound retractor (Applied Medical, Rancho Santa Margarita, CA) is used to provide circumferential atraumatic retraction and improve

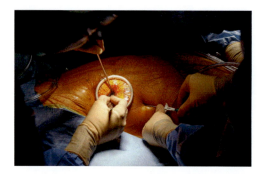

FIGURE 9.3.8 The soft-tissue retractor aids surgical exposure and prevents the need for rib-spreading, reducing postoperative pain.

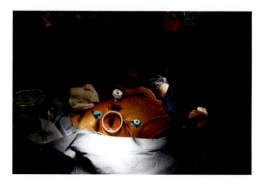

FIGURE 9.3.9 The trocars for the robotic instruments have been inserted into the right pleural space.

exposure. A rib-spreading retractor is usually not required (Figure 9.3.8). Avoidance of rib-spreading significantly reduces postoperative pain.

It is often helpful to displace the diaphragm caudally, utilizing a retraction suture placed in the right diaphragmatic dome, anchored outside the chest wall, the suture tails being externalized using the Endo Close™ traction device (Medtronic, Minneapolis, MN).

Trocars for the left- and right-arm robotic instruments are inserted through the third and fifth interspaces, respectively, just anterior to the mid-axillary line. An additional trocar is passed through the fifth ICS more medially, just lateral to the mid-clavicular line, for insertion of the left atrial retractor. All trocars are introduced under direct vision.

The camera is placed into the chest first and then directly visualizes the insertion of each trocar through the chest wall from within the right pleural cavity, ensuring safe entry and making sure that there is no undue bleeding (Figure 9.3.9). The robot can then be docked to the operating field (Figure 9.3.10A, B). Carbon dioxide is insufflated into the right pleural space at a rate of 6 L/minute through the left arm trocar. Alternately, a separate catheter can be inserted through the chest wall for this purpose.

We currently use the four-arm da Vinci Xi surgical system. The da Vinci robot cart is typically rolled into the bedside at a 0–30° angle to accommodate for the natural position of the mitral valve in the chest (dependent on individual patient anatomy) (Figure 9.3.11).

A sample layout of the entire operating suite, demonstrating relative positions of the patient, da Vinci robot system, robot control console, anesthesiologist and heart-lung machine, is depicted in Figure 9.3.12.

CARDIOPULMONARY BYPASS AND MYOCARDIAL PROTECTION

The patient is heparinized (dose adjusted for weight), and a long venous cannula is inserted percutaneously, using a Seldinger technique, via the right common femoral vein, its position in the right atrium being confirmed with TEE. We typically use a 23-Fr distal/25-Fr proximal LivaNova femoral venous cannula for this purpose (LivaNova, London, UK). Concurrently, an incision is made in the left groin, and the common femoral artery is exposed and controlled. This vessel is cannulated directly, utilizing an appropriately

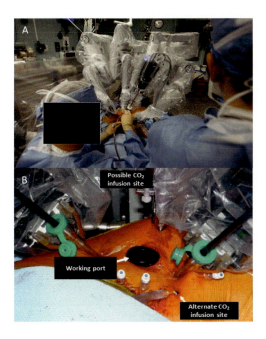

FIGURE 9.3.10 A. The robot is docked at the operating table. B. Close-up of robot arms docked within the ports. CO_2 infusion sites are demonstrated. Reproduced with permission of Intuitive Surgical, © 2020.

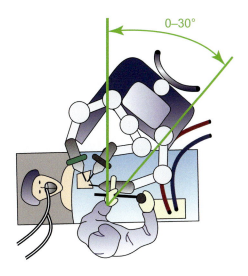

FIGURE 9.3.11 The robot is rolled in at a 0–30° angle to better accommodate for the variable natural position of the mitral valve in the chest. Reproduced with permission of Intuitive Surgical, © 2020.

sized OptiSite arterial cannula (Edwards Lifesciences, Irvine, CA) passed over a guidewire. We prefer not to place the arterial and venous cannulas on the same side, such that both the inflow and outflow of the one lower extremity are not synchronously obstructed. Nevertheless, in smaller patients, we occasionally do use a cut-down approach in the right groin only, in order to insert both the arterial and venous cannulas directly on this side.

After cardiopulmonary bypass has been established, the patient is cooled to a systemic temperature of between 28 and 32 degrees centigrade, depending on the anticipated complexity and duration of the operation. The pericardium is opened using the robotic instruments, 3 to 4 cm anterior to the right phrenic nerve (Figure 9.3.13). It is critical to positively and definitively identify the phrenic nerve and ensure that it is kept well away from the operative field. The pericardium is secured to the chest wall using retraction sutures (Figure 9.3.14), once again externalized using the Endo Close™ instrument (Figure 9.3.15). A long MiAR™ aortic root cannula (Medtronic, Minneapolis, MN) is directly inserted into the proximal ascending aorta through the working incision in order to facilitate antegrade delivery of cardioplegia, as well as venting of the root (Figure 9.3.16).

Our preferred method for attaining cardiac arrest is through the use of a long trans-thoracic Chitwood Debakey aortic cross-clamp (Scanlan International, Saint Paul, MN), passed through a separate stab incision in the chest wall, typically through the second or third ICS, as posteriorly and cephalad as possible, so as to avoid conflict with the left robotic-arm trocar. It is important to visualize the cross-clamp traversing the entirety of the ascending aorta, without causing injury to the pulmonary artery

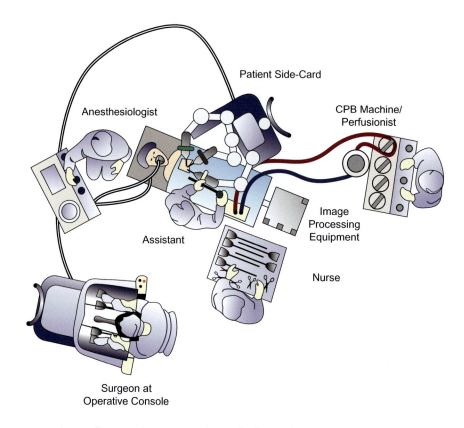

FIGURE 9.3.12 A sample operating room suite ready for a robotic-assisted mitral valve procedure, depicting relative positions of all key components and personnel. Reproduced with permission of Intuitive Surgical, © 2020.

FIGURE 9.3.13 The pericardium is opened anterior to the right phrenic nerve.

FIGURE 9.3.14 Pericardial retraction sutures are placed.

(Figure 9.3.17). Once the cross-clamp has been applied, cardioplegia is administered via the aortic root cannula. We prefer to use Custodiol HTK (Essential Pharmaceuticals, Durham, NC) as our cardioplegia of choice, and we have indeed described our experience with this previously [15], although there is no specific reason that each surgeon cannot administer their own particular cardioplegia solution of preference.

OPERATING ON THE MITRAL VALVE

Once the heart has been adequately arrested, the robotic instruments are used to dissect out the inter-atrial groove and

FIGURE 9.3.15 Retraction sutures are externalized utilizing the "Endo Close" device.

FIGURE 9.3.17 A long clamp is introduced into the surgical field through a separate incision in the chest wall and the aorta is cross-clamped.

FIGURE 9.3.16 Insertion of a long, flexible aortic root cannula.

FIGURE 9.3.18 The left atrium is opened and the mitral valve is exposed.

open the left atrium. The left atrial retractor is inserted through its separate trocar, and the mitral valve is exposed (Figure 9.3.18).

The actual specifics of the valve repair (or replacement) procedure should proceed in an identical fashion as if the surgeon were accomplishing this through a sternotomy. The magnification, flexibility and excellent exposure afforded by the robotic system should facilitate all types of mitral valve repair, irrespective of complexity, whether it incorporates triangular/quadrangular resection of the posterior leaflet with/without sliding plasty, folding valvuloplasty, chordal transfer/translocation, Gore-Tex NeoChord implantation (Figure 9.3.19) or patch augmentation of the valve, as examples. All knots on the valve and the NeoChords themselves are either tied totally intra-corporeally, using the robotic arms, or are exteriorized and tied by the bedside assistant with the aid of a knot-pushing device. The sutures of an annuloplasty device (or those of a valve prosthesis, in the setting of a valve replacement) are secured with the Cor-Knot® device (LSI Solutions, Victor, NY) (Figure 9.3.20).

Once the valve procedure has been completed, the competency of the valve is tested by pressurizing the left ventricle using the StrykeFlow II laparoscopic suction/irrigation system (Stryker, Kalamazoo, MI). If an endocardial ablation or maze procedure needs to be undertaken to treat concurrent atrial fibrillation, this can be done at any time while the left atrium is open. Similarly, the orifice of the left atrial appendage can be closed with either a running suture or with multiple interrupted sutures, using the robotic instruments. The left atrium is closed using a running Gore-Tex suture (WL Gore & Associates, Flagstaff, AZ) as the patient is systemically rewarmed (Figure 9.3.21).

CONCLUDING THE OPERATION

A temporary epicardial placing wire is placed on the diaphragmatic aspect of the right ventricle prior to removal of the aortic

FIGURE 9.3.19 A Gore-Tex NeoChord is sutured into one of the papillary muscles in the process of repairing a flail posterior mitral leaflet.

FIGURE 9.3.20 An annuloplasty device is implanted around the mitral annulus utilizing braided sutures secured with the "Cor-Knot" device.

FIGURE 9.3.21 The left atriotomy is closed.

FIGURE 9.3.22 A temporary epicardial pacing wire is secured to the inferior aspect of the right ventricle prior to removal of the aortic cross-clamp.

cross-clamp (Figure 9.3.22), which is then itself removed only after meticulous de-airing of all cardiac chambers, as confirmed by real-time TEE.

After cardiopulmonary bypass has been weaned and the integrity of the valve repair has been confirmed using TEE, the long root cannula is removed, and its purse-string suture is secured using the Cor-Knot device, a technique that has also been reported by others [16]. After protamine has been administered, all robotic trocars are individually removed whilst being visualized using the camera from within the chest, so as to ensure that there is no residual chest wall bleeding that needs to be attended to.

The purse-string suture placed around the femoral venous cannula is primarily tied down and secured after decannulation at the conclusion of the operation, irrespective of whether the cannula was inserted percutaneously, or whether it had been directly advanced into the common femoral vein via a cut-down approach. We never, however, replicate this technique for the arterial access site, irrespective of the size of the vessel, the size of the cannula used or the side chosen for cannulation. We always re-fashion the arterial cannulation site into a transverse arteriotomy, and we then repair the femoral artery primarily.

Some surgeons have also described inserting a perfusion catheter distal to the arterial cannulation site, in order to maintain perfusion of the lower extremity for the duration of the procedure [17]. This has not been our approach, however, and it would also have to be removed at this juncture had it been utilized. To date, in over 400 minimal-access mitral valve procedures incorporating femoral arterial cannulation, we have yet to encounter an issue with a perioperative ischemic limb.

TOOLS/INSTRUMENTS AND DEVICES

DA VINCI XI SYSTEM

The da Vinci system is precise, flexible and well controlled to perform many cardiac procedures; it offers real-time feedback to operate easily (Figure 9.3.23).

ALEXIS WOUND PROTECTOR

Alexis wound atraumatic protectors protect and provide retraction 360° circumferentially. They can maintain moisture at the incision site and reduce superficial surgical site infections (Figure 9.3.24).

ENDO CLOSE™ TROCAR SITE CLOSURE DEVICE

This device has a potential application in robotic cardiac procedures and is used for tissue approximation and percutaneous suturing for closing of the incision site. It has a spring-loaded blunt stylet mechanism that can retract the needle and automatically advanced in the tissue has been penetrated (Figure 9.3.25).

LIVANOVA VENOUS RETURN CANNULAS

The LivaNova venous return cannula, with wire-reinforced tubing and with or without connector, features a third point of drainage for optimal flow performance. The distal tip is softer, yet it adds rigidity to prevent collapse during vacuum assistance procedures (Figure 9.3.26).

OPTISITE ARTERIAL CANNULAS

The Optisite arterial cannula from Edwards Lifescience has a blunt tip that allows safe insertion for additional arterial access sites such as the aorta, axillary and subclavian artery. It has a lock feature which reduces push-back of the introducer during insertion. As of all cannulas it also has dept

FIGURE 9.3.23 The Da Vinci Xi system from Intuitive Surgical.

FIGURE 9.3.25 Endo Close™ trocar site closure device, Medtronic.

FIGURE 9.3.24 Alexis wound protector.

FIGURE 9.3.26 LivaNova venous return cannulas.

Chapter 9.3 – The Mitral Valve   225

FIGURE 9.3.27 Optisite arterial cannulas, Edwards.

FIGURE 9.3.29 Chitwood Debakey aortic cross-clamp.

FIGURE 9.3.28 MiAR™ cardioplegia cannula, Medtronic.

FIGURE 9.3.30 StrykeFlow II suction irrigation pump.

marking; the sizes include 16, 18, 20 and 22 (Figure 9.3.27).

MIAR™ CARDIOPLEGIA CANNULA

This is a minimally invasive aortic root (MiAR) cardioplegia delivery cannula which allows access into the chest MICS. The long length of this cannula allows positioning of the luer connection to the cardioplegia line out of the surgeon's view. Additionally, the MiAR CP cannula includes the Flow-Guard™ feature to maintain hemostasis during removal of the needle from the cannula (Figure 9.3.28).

CHITWOOD DEBAKEY AORTIC CROSS-CLAMP

This instrument had been developed in collaboration with W Randolph Chitwood Jr, MD. It is mainly used for safe and atraumatic aortic clamping in minimally invasive cardiac procedures. They are suitable for all kinds of patients and anatomies (Figure 9.3.29).

STRYKEFLOW II SUCTION IRRIGATION PUMP

The StrykeFlow II suction irrigation pump is used for suction irrigation of the surgical field. It features a disposable battery-powered suction irrigator that spikes directly into the bag (Figure 9.3.30).

PERIOPERATIVE CONSIDERATION

PREOPERATIVE ASSESSMENT

Patients being screened for a robotic-assisted mitral valve procedure require the same preoperative investigations as any patient about to undergo mitral surgery, irrespective of surgical approach, although there are a number of unique caveats worth considering. The importance of a high-quality trans-thoracic and/or transesophageal echocardiogram (TEE) to accurately define the nature of the mitral valve pathology to be addressed cannot be overstated, especially if the surgeon is planning to embark upon a complex valve repair strategy.

Given that a robotic mitral valve procedure requires peripheral cannulation for cardiopulmonary bypass, patients should be assessed for the presence of aorto-iliofemoral atherosclerotic disease. Significant peripheral arterial disease may preclude femoral arterial cannulation. A CT angiogram of the chest/abdomen/pelvis is usually our investigation of choice in this regard, although a preoperative TEE can also provide valuable information as to the burden and nature of any atheroma and plaque that may be present in the aortic arch and descending aorta.

If the concern regarding retrograde arterial flow via the femoral artery is too great, with respect to the associated elevated risk of perioperative stroke, the surgeon is faced with a number of viable options:

1. Elect to pursue a robotic-assisted approach, but utilize the right axillary artery for perfusion, rather than the femoral artery, reducing the risk of an adverse neurological outcome [18].
2. Complete the operation via a minimal-access right thoracotomy (without using the robot) and cannulate the right axillary artery or indeed the ascending aorta directly.
3. Choose to undertake a median sternotomy.

A preoperative coronary angiogram is usually required to assess for the presence of coronary artery stenoses, although in the younger population, particularly in those with degenerative valve pathology, and in those who have a low pretest probability of having significant atherosclerotic disease, a CT coronary angiogram may, in fact, suffice [19].

As adequate right-lung isolation is critical for adequate exposure during robotic mitral valve surgery, chronic heavy smokers and patients with history of lung pathology such as chronic obstructive pulmonary disease (COPD) or restrictive lung disease warrant preoperative pulmonary evaluation with pulmonary function testing [20].

PREVIOUS CARDIAC SURGERY

Patients who have had prior cardiac surgery can derive great benefit from a minimal-access right chest approach. Peripheral cannulation, avoiding a re-sternotomy and attaining surgical exposure from the right side all serve to minimize the need for extensive dissection around the heart, reducing the risks of injury to the heart or to any patent bypass grafts, should they be present, while concomitantly reducing the incidence and extent of perioperative bleeding.

CLINICAL OUTCOMES

There is no doubt as to the benefits of a robotic-assisted approach in mitral valve surgery. Numerous reports confirm low perioperative complication rates, reduced transfusion requirements, shorter ventilation times, reduced intensive care unit and overall lengths of stay, diminished postoperative pain, faster return to normal activities and greater overall patient satisfaction [21–23]. In a systematic review of the literature, Seco and associates summarized the results of 27 studies that assessed the perioperative outcomes of robotic mitral valve surgery [24]. The investigators concluded that, although cardiopulmonary bypass and cross-clamp times tend to be on the longer side, the overall short-term mortality and morbidity are

FIGURE 9.3.31 Robotically assisted MVr – Cleveland Clinic.

FIGURE 9.3.32 Prop-matched analysis of robotic, mini-invasive and conventional MVR.

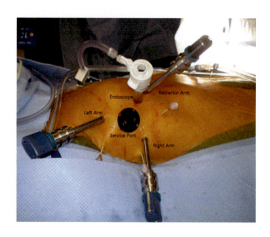

FIGURE 9.3.33 Port placement for lateral endoscopic approach using robotics (LEAR) surgery. (Reprinted from *Ann Thorac Surg*, 100(5), Murphy DA, Moss E, Binongo J, et al. The Expanding Role of Endoscopic Robotics in Mitral Valve Surgery: 1,257 Consecutive Procedures, © 2015 by The Society of Thoracic Surgeons, with permission from Elsevier.)

low, and that the increased cost of the procedure accrued by the use of the robot is more than offset by the patients' more expeditious return to work and by the rapid improvements in their quality of life. A meta-analysis of six studies comparing robotic and conventional mitral valve surgery by Cao and colleagues demonstrated that robotic mitral surgery is safe, with low perioperative complication rates, despite longer bypass and cross-clamp times, particularly if performed by experienced surgeons in designated centers of excellence [25]. re-iterating the concept that surgeons should undertake focused specialized training if they wish to truly become facile with the procedure.

Gillinov and co-workers recently analyzed the results of the first 1000 cases of robotically assisted mitral surgery performed at the Cleveland Clinic [26]. They found that, of the 992 patients who underwent valve repair for mitral regurgitation, 99.7% left the operating room with either no or mild residual regurgitation, and that 97.9% of patients had less than mild regurgitation by the time of hospital discharge.

Mortality was low (0.1%), perioperative stroke was infrequent (1.4%), and, importantly, the authors once again demonstrated a definite learning curve to the procedure, confirming that, over the longitudinal course of the review, bypass and cross-clamp times decreased, stroke rates diminished, transfusion rates improved and intensive care and hospital lengths of stay shortened. It is important to note that these excellent results were achieved in a patient population that was highly selected, and that tended to consist of younger, healthier, lower-risk subjects (Figure 9.3.31).

In an analysis of the Society of Thoracic Surgeons Adult Cardiac Surgery Database, Wang and associates reported the results of 503 patients over the age of 65 years who underwent robotic mitral valve repair and who were propensity-matched with 503 patients who had valve repair via a median sternotomy [27]. The investigators found that the robotic approach was associated with less postoperative atrial fibrillation, reduced rates of transfusion and shorter

FIGURE 9.3.34 Robotic MVr using the LEAR technique.

FIGURE 9.3.35 3D mini-mitral surgery: Why would you need a robot?

intensive care unit and hospital lengths of stay, with equivalent mortality at 3 years, and with no significant differences in the need for valve re-intervention in the midterm. Once again, however, bypass and cross-clamp times were indeed shown to be longer in the robotic group than in the sternotomy cohort. Chitwood reported his results of 944 cases performed between 2000 and 2014, including 38 reoperations [20]. For isolated primary mitral valve repair, he recounted a mortality rate of 0.15%, a perioperative stroke rate of 0.9% and a failure rate of the repair itself of 1.7% (Figure 9.3.32).

Disadvantages of robotic mitral surgery largely remain related to the longer bypass and myocardial ischemic times that are replicated in almost all studies. However, as demonstrated by the group at the Cleveland Clinic and by others [28], these do seem to improve over time as surgeons become defter with the procedure and advance along their learning curve. Moreover, the longer perfusion times do not seem to directly correlate with increased perioperative morbidity [29,30]. Other limitations of the robotic approach have included the lack of proprioception and the absence of tactile feedback provided by the robotic instruments; surgeons have had to learn to adopt an "ocular tactility" [31].

Future advances in robotic technology may address some of these limitations. Concerns regarding the potential for an increased risk of perioperative stroke associated with femoral arterial cannulation have largely been mitigated by appropriate preoperative screening for athero-occlusive disease, judicious patient selection and by the use of alternate cannulation sites where necessary.

The majority of the literature to date examining minimal-access mitral valve surgery in the reoperative setting describes those procedures performed via a right thoracotomy without robotic assistance [32]. However, more surgeons are now incorporating robotic techniques into these reoperations, so as to benefit from the improved visualization, exposure and dexterity afforded by the robotic apparatus [33]. Murphy and colleagues recently favorably reported on their experience in reoperating on 54 patients who had all previously undergone a robotic-assisted mitral valve operation, all of whom now required a second mitral procedure [34]. The reoperative mitral procedure was successfully completed robotically in 50 patients (92.6%), with no deaths or strokes reported in the series. The authors stated that four patients (7%) required a sternotomy for reoperation due to difficulties either with peripheral perfusion or with right chest access. Similarly, we have also found that the more significant hurdles in the reoperative patient do not usually tend to center around the mitral valve component of the operation itself, but rather relate to access issues through the right pleural space, which can be challenging, particularly if dense adhesions are present due to prior surgery.

ALTERNATIVE APPROACHES

LEAR TECHNIQUE

Carbon dioxide is infused through the endoscope port, and with the surgeon's finger blocking the service port, the pleural space is temporarily pressurized to 10 cm water to allow the safe insertion of additional robotic trocars and angiocatheters, which are used to exteriorize traction sutures (Figure 9.3.33 and Figure 9.3.34).

CARDIOPLEGIA

A long flexible Endoplege coronary sinus cannula (Edwards Lifesciences, Irvine, CA) can also be inserted percutaneously via the right internal jugular vein in order to administer retrograde cardioplegia. However, we have found this to be cumbersome and unnecessary in the current era of more effective cardioplegia solutions and thus no longer utilize this technique.

CROSS-CLAMP

Rather than utilize a cross-clamp, others have described employing an intra-aortic balloon approach in order to achieve endo-aortic occlusion and to deliver cardioplegia [35–37].

REOPERATIVE SURGERY

If the risk of introducing a long trans-thoracic aortic cross-clamp is thought to be prohibitive in a reoperative surgical field, hypothermic fibrillatory arrest represents an attractive alternative [38]. A patent internal mammary graft does not constitute a contraindication to this approach [39], although significant aortic insufficiency would need to be dealt with. An endo-aortic balloon occlusion technique could also be utilized in this situation.

CAVEATS AND CONTROVERSIES

If the surgeon does not feel that a minimal-access approach would facilitate a quality outcome, for whatever reason, based upon the pathology of the valve, or otherwise, then he/she should proceed with surgery via a sternotomy. The primary goal of the procedure remains the absolute correction of the patient's mitral valve pathology, safely, successfully and completely. Although we are confident that this can be accomplished using robotic-assisted methods in the majority of cases, we believe that it is not acceptable to compromise the integrity and durability of the intended valve operation merely for the sake of being able to utilize robotic techniques.

If a patient requiring mitral surgery is found to have isolated coronary disease that is deemed amenable to percutaneous intervention, then it may not be unreasonable to stent this lesion in some circumstances, and this can be followed by a robotic mitral valve procedure 4 to 6 weeks later, constituting a "hybrid strategy" [40]. More diffuse coronary disease that requires bypass grafting precludes a robotic-assisted operation and mandates a sternotomy. Right-lung isolation is critical for adequate exposure during robotic mitral valve surgery. Patients with poor pulmonary function who are unable to tolerate single-lung ventilation are therefore relatively poor candidates for this technique. Nevertheless, we have, to date, performed a number of robotic mitral valve procedures on patients with compromised lung function, although we have had to somewhat modify the conduct of the operation in order to ensure adequate gas exchange at all times and mitigate intraoperative hypoxemia.

RESEARCH, TRENDS AND INNOVATION

It seems clear that robotic mitral valve surgery will only continue to improve over time. Higher-resolution optics, smaller instruments with lower profiles allowing for finer motor control and coordination and the incorporation of some kind of "haptic" or tactile feedback system into the robotic arms will all combine to facilitate faster, smoother operations, with consistently reproducible results. Concomitant advances in imaging software may also allow the "fusion" of echocardiography, CT and computer modeling, such that the surgeon may be able to visualize a "blueprint" model of the desired final repaired mitral valve overlaid on the surgical field image at the console [41], providing a "roadmap" of the most efficacious way to complete the operation. To date, the surgeon operating at the console has always been physically co-located in the same operating suite as the patient and the bedside assistant, although the potential for remote tele-surgery utilizing robotic technology has long been speculated [42].

The rapidity with which some or all of these advances come to pass and the role that they will play in the current era of explosive growth of transcatheter mitral valve therapies still remain to be seen. We remain confident that the future for minimally invasive and robotic-assisted mitral valve surgery continues to be very bright. Nevertheless, the desire for less invasive therapy should not take precedence over the surgeon's primary goal, which is always to correct the patient's mitral valve pathology safely, completely, successfully, ideally and durably (Figure 9.3.35).

FIGURE 9.3.36 Video-atlas of robotically assisted MVS.

FIGURE 9.3.37 STS Workshop on Robotic Cardiac Surgery.

TABLE 9.3.1	Relative contraindications to robotic mitral valve surgery
Previous sternotomy	
• Moderate pulmonary dysfunction	
• Asymptomatic CAD (treated)	
• Coronary artery disease – requiring PCI	
• Limited peripheral vascular disease	
• Asymptomatic CVD	
• Poor left ventricular function (EF <30%)	
• Pulmonary hypertension (variable >60 torr)	
• Mild to moderate aortic stenosis or insufficiency	
• Moderate annular calcification	

Abbreviations: EF, ejection fraction; CAD, coronary artery disease; PCI, percutaneous coronary intervention; CVD, cerebrovascular disease.
Source: After Chitwood WR Jr. Robotic mitral valve surgery: overview, methodology, results, and perspective. *Ann Cardiothorac Surg.* 2016;5(6):544-555. © 2020, with permission from AME Publishing Company.

WHERE AND HOW TO LEARN

ANNALS OF CARDIOTHORACIC SURGERY (ACS) VIDEO ATLAS

This video (Figure 9.3.36) article provides a detailed description of our current approach to performing complex mitral valve surgery using the da Vinci™ system.

STS WORKSHOP ON ROBOTIC CARDIAC SURGERY

The STS Workshop on Robotic Cardiac Surgery offers extensive hands-on procedural experience and complementary lectures to surgeons and their team members of all skill levels (Figure 9.3.37).

REFERENCES

1. Carpentier A, Loulmet D, Aupecle B, et al. Computer assisted open heart surgery. First case operated on with success. *C R Acad Sci III* 1998; 321: 437–42.
2. Mohr FW, Falk V, Diegeler A, Autschback R. Computer-enhanced coronary artery bypass surgery. *J Thorac Cardiovasc Surg* 1999; 117: 1212–4.
3. Fann JI, Pompili MF, Burdon TA, et al. Minimally invasive mitral valve surgery. *Semin Thorac Cardiovasc Surg* 1997; 9: 320–30.
4. Navia JL, Cosgrove DM 3rd. Minimally invasive mitral valve operations. *Ann Thorac Surg* 1996; 62: 1542–4.
5. Kaneko Y, Kohno T, Ohtsuka T, et al. Video-assisted observation in mitral valve surgery. *J Thorac Cardiovasc Surg* 1996; 111: 279–80.
6. Chitwood WR Jr, Wixon CL, Elbeery JR, et al. Video-assisted minimally invasive mitral valve surgery. *J Thorac Cardiovasc Surg* 1997; 114: 773–80.
7. Mohr FW, Onnasch JF, Falk V, et al. The evolution of minimally invasive valve surgery –2 year experience. *Eur J Cardiothorac Surg* 1999; 15: 233–8.
8. Vanermen H, Farhat F, Wellens F, et al. Minimally invasive video-assisted mitral valve surgery: from port-access towards a totally endoscopic procedure. *J Card Surg* 2000; 15: 51–60.
9. Felger JE, Chitwood WR Jr, Nifong LW, et al. Evolution of mitral valve surgery: toward a totally endoscopic approach. *Ann Thorac Surg* 2001; 72: 1203–8.
10. Chitwood WR Jr, Nifong LW, Elbeery JE, et al. Robotic mitral valve repair: trapezoidal resection and prosthetic annuloplasty with the da vinci surgical system. *J Thorac Cardiovasc Surg* 2000; 120: 1171–2.
11. Nifong LW, Chitwood WR, Pappas PS, et al. Robotic mitral valve surgery: a United States multicenter trial. *J Thorac Cardiovasc Surg* 2005; 129: 1395–404.
12. Nishimura RA, Otto CM, Bonow RO, et al. 2014 AHA/ACC guideline for the management of patients with valvular heart disease: executive summary: a report of the American College of Cardiology/American Heart Association Task Force on Practice Guidelines. *J Am Coll Cardiol* 2014; 63: 2438–88.
13. Baumgartner, H, Falk, V, Bax, JJ, et al. ESC/EACTS guidelines for the management of valvular heart disease. *Eur Heart J* 2017; 38(36): 2739–2791.
14. Goodman A, Koprivanac M, Kelava M, et al. Robotic mitral valve repair: the learning curve. *Innovations (Phila)* 2017; 12: 390–7.
15. Patel N, DeLaney E, Turi G, Stapleton T. Custodiol HTK cardioplegia use in robotic mitral valve. *J Extra Corpor Technol* 2013; 45: 139–42.
16. Hashim SW, Pang PY. Antegrade cardioplegia decannulation using the COR-KNOT system in minimally invasive mitral valve surgery. *Innovations (Phila)* 2017; 12: 150–1.
17. Bonaros N, Wiedemann D, Nagiller J, et al. Distal leg protection for peripheral cannulation in minimally invasive and totally endoscopic cardiac surgery. *Heart Surg Forum* 2009; 12: E158–62.

18. Bedeir K, Reardon M, Ramchandani M, Singh K, Ramlawi B. Elevated stroke risk associated with femoral artery cannulation during mitral valve surgery. *Semin Thorac Cardiovasc Surg* 2015; 27: 97–103.
19. Morris MF, Suri RM, Akhtar NJ, et al. Computed tomography as an alternative to catheter angiography prior to robotic mitral valve repair. *Ann Thorac Surg* 2013; 95: 1354–9.
20. Chitwood RW Jr. Robotic mitral valve surgery: overview, methodology, results, and perspective. *Ann Cardiothorac Surg* 2016; 5: 544–55.
21. Murphy DA, Moss E, Binongo J, et al. The expanding role of endoscopic robotics in mitral valve surgery: 1257 consecutive procedures. *Annals of Thoracic Surgery* 2015; 100: 1675–82.
22. Mihaljevic T, Jarrett CM, Gillinov AM, et al. Robotic repair of posterior mitral valve prolapse versus conventional approaches: potential realized. *J Thorac Cardiovasc Surg* 2011; 141: 72–80.
23. Ramzy D, Trento A, Cheng W, et al. Three hundred robotic-assisted mitral valve repairs: the Cedars-Sinai experience. *J Thorac Cardiovasc Surg* 2014; 147: 228–35.
24. Seco M, Cao C, Modi P, et al. Systematic review of robotic minimally invasive mitral valve surgery. *Ann Cardiothorac Surg* 2013; 2: 704–16.
25. Cao C, Wolfenden H, Liou K, et al. A meta-analysis of robotic *vs.* conventional mitral valve surgery. *Ann Cardiothorac Surg* 2015; 4: 305–14.
26. Gillinov AM, Mihaljevic T, Javadikasgari H, et al. Early results of robotically assisted mitral valve surgery: analysis of the first 1000 cases. *J Thorac Cardiovasc Surg* 2018; 155: 82–91.
27. Wang A, Brennan JM, Zhang S, et al. Robotic mitral valve repair in older individuals: an analysis of the Society of Thoracic Surgeons Database. *Ann Thorac Surg* 2018;106(5): 1388–1393. doi: 10.1016/j.athoracsur.2018.05.074.
28. Yaffee DW, Loulmet DF, Kelly LA, et al. Can the learning curve of totally endoscopic robotic mitral valve repair be short-circuited? *Innovations (Phila)* 2014; 9: 43–8.
29. Suri RM, Burkhart HM, Daly RC, et al. Robotic mitral valve repair for all prolapse subsets using techniques identical to open valvuloplasty: establishing the benchmark against which percutaneous interventions should be judged. *J Thorac Cardiovasc Surg* 2011; 142: 970–9.
30. Hawkins RB, Mehaffey JH, Mullen MM, et al. A propensity matched analysis of robotic, minimally invasive, and conventional mitral valve surgery. *Heart* 2018;104(23):1970–1975. doi: 10.1136/heartjnl-2018-313129.
31. Suri RM, Dearani JA, Mihaljevic T, et al. Mitral valve repair using robotic technology: safe, effective and durable. *J Thorac Cardiovasc Surg* 2016; 151: 1450–4.
32. Bolotin G, Kypson AP, Reade CC, et al. Should a video-assisted mini-thoracotomy be the approach of choice for reoperative mitral valve surgery? *J Heart Valve Dis* 2004; 13: 155–8.
33. Patel H, Lewis CTP, Stephens RL, Angelillo M, Sibley DH. Minimally invasive redo mitral valve replacement using a robotic-assisted approach. *Innovations (Phila)* 2017; 12: 375–7.
34. Murphy DA, Moss E, Miller J, Halkos ME. Repeat robotic endoscopic mitral valve operation: a safe and effective strategy. *Ann Thorac Surg* 2018; 105: 1704–9.
35. Breves SL, Hong I, McCarthy J, et al. Ascending aortic endoballoon occlusion feasible despite moderately enlarged aorta to facilitate robotic mitral valve surgery. *Innovations (Phila)* 2016; 11: 355–9.
36. Yaffee DW, Loulmet DF, Fakiha AG, Grossi EA. Fluorescence-guided placement of an endoaortic balloon occlusion device for totally endoscopic robotic mitral valve repair. *J Thorac Cardiovasc Surg* 2015; 149: 1456–8.
37. Ward AF, Loulmet DF, Neuburger PJ, Grossi EA. Outcomes of peripheral perfusion with balloon aortic clamping for totally endoscopic robotic mitral valve repair. *J Thorac Cardiovasc Surg* 2014; 148: 2769–72.
38. Hollatz A, Balkhy HH, Chaney MA, Neuburger PJ, Gerlach RM, Guy TS. Robotic mitral valve repair with right ventricular pacing-induced ventricular fibrillatory arrest. *J Cardiothorac Vasc Anesth* 2017; 31: 345–53.
39. Byrne JG, Aranki SF, Adams DH, Rizzo RJ, Couper GS, Cohn LH. Mitral valve surgery after previous CABG with functioning IMA grafts. *Ann Thorac Surg* 1999; 68: 2243–7.

40. Ford RB, Rodriguez E, Nifong LW, Chitwood RW Jr. Robotic mitral valve repair or replacement. In: KL Franco and VH Thourani (Eds), *Cardiothoracic surgery review* (pp. 410–4). Philadelphia, PA: Lippincott Williams & Wilkins, 2012.
41. Bush B, Nifong LW, Alwair H, Chitwood RW Jr. Robotic mitral valve surgery – current status and future directions. *Ann Cardiothorac Surg* 2013; 2: 814–7.
42. Menkis AH, Kodera K, Kiaii B, Swinamer SA, Rayman R, Boyd WD. Robotic surgery, the first 100 cases: where do we go from here? *Heart Surg Forum* 2004; 7: 1–4.

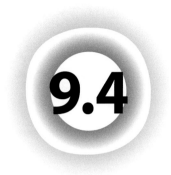

THE MITRAL VALVE
Percutaneous Mitral Valve Repair: MitraClip®

MOHAMMAD ABDULRAHMAN AL OTAIBY

HISTORY AND INTRODUCTION

PERCUTANEOUS MITRAL VALVE REPAIR USING THE MITRACLIP® SYSTEM

The MitraClip System (Abbot Vascular, Abbot Park, Illinois) mimics the surgical edge-to-edge stitch by implanting a clip via a transatrial transfemoral access under fluoroscopic and transesophageal echocardiographic guidance. This technique has emerged as the most used transcatheter approach to treat MR. Despite the high risk profile of treated patients, the MitraClip provides satisfactory results in terms of procedural safety and improvement of symptoms and quality of life. Current guidelines take into consideration transcatheter mitral valve repair via MitraClip System in case of symptomatic high-risk or inoperable patients with more than 1 year expected survival after Heart-Team discussion, both in functional and degenerative MR. A careful selection of the patients from an anatomical and clinical point of view is essential to achieve efficacy and avoid futility. See also Figure 9.4.1 to Figure 9.4.7.

FIGURE 9.4.1 The MitraClip story: First patient implanted with MitraClip.

FIGURE 9.4.3 TMVr with Mitraclip Therapy.

FIGURE 9.4.2 Summary of safety and effectiveness data.

FIGURE 9.4.4 MitraClip™ transcatheter mitral valve repair.

HOW TO DO IT/STEP BY STEP

A. STEPS

- ∞ Ideally, the MitraClip procedure is done in a hybrid OR, but it is possible to do in an ordinary cardiac catheterization laboratory, provided it is big enough to accommodate the necessary equipment, including an echocardiography machine, ventilator and MitraClip delivery system.
- ∞ It is mandatory for the procedure to be done under transesophageal echocardiography guidance with 3D capabilities.

FIGURE 9.4.5 Percutaneous approaches to valve repair for mitral regurgitation.

- ∞ It is done under general anesthesia.
- ∞ A new anesthetic approach of conscious sedation is being studied (Figure 9.4.8).
- ∞ The procedure must be performed in rooms following hygiene class 1B (after DIN 1946-4), with all hygienic measures followed (Figure 9.4.9).

B. SURGICAL APPROACH

MitraClip therapy is a completely percutaneous, minimally invasive intervention to treat mitral regurgitation. A short animation of how the procedure is done is depicted in the video embedded in this QR code (Figure 9.4.10).

The details of the procedure are as follows:

TRANSSEPTAL PUNCTURE

- ∞ An important and integral part of the procedure.
- ∞ Determines the success of the procedure.

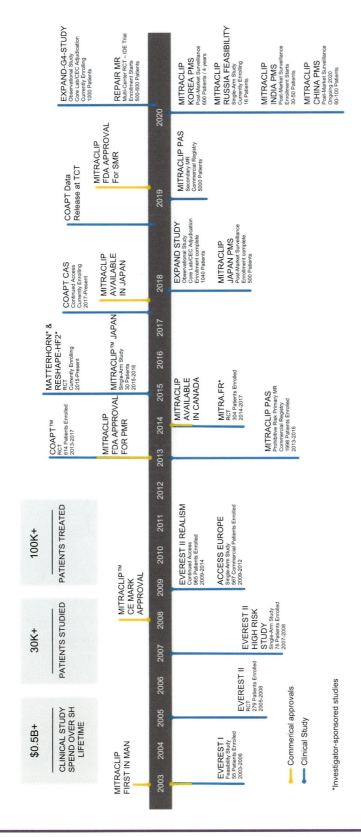

FIGURE 9.4.6   Brief history of the development of MitraClip. Reproduced with permission of Abbott, © 2020.

Chapter 9.4 – The Mitral Valve

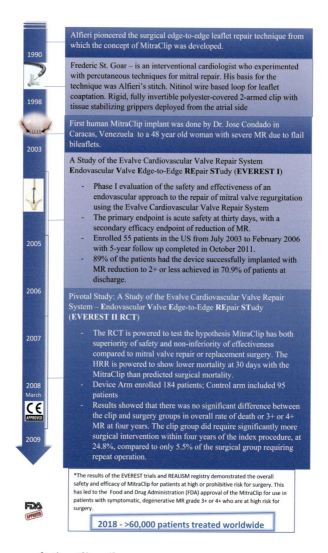

FIGURE 9.4.7 Summary of MitraClip milestones.

FIGURE 9.4.8 MitraClip placement under conscious sedation.

ANATOMY OF THE SEPTUM

For the purpose of the MitraClip procedure the transseptal puncture should be superior and posterior according to the etiology of the MR. The following measurements from the mitral coaptation line are recommended:

For primary MR: 4.0–5.0 cm
For functional MR: 3.5–4.0 cm

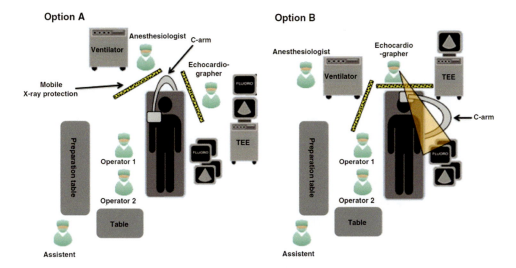

FIGURE 9.4.9 The figure shows two possible arrangements in the angiography suite. In A, the C-arm of the catheter display is cranial and the echocardiographer is positioned left lateral to the patient. The X-ray pictures are visible for the echocardiographer on a separate monitor (fluoro). The yellow lines represent mobile radiation protection walls. In B, the C-arm is positioned left lateral to the patient; the anesthetist and particularly the echocardiographer are found cranial to the patient and have better access to the head of the patient. The orange cone indicates the additional view angle onto the X-ray pictures on the angiography monitor arrangement. (Reprinted by permission from Springer Nature Customer Service Centre GmbH: Springer Nature, *Clin Res Cardiol*, 103(2):85-96. Percutaneous interventional mitral regurgitation treatment using the Mitra-Clip system, Boekstegers P, Hausleiter J, Baldus S, et al © 2014.)

FIGURE 9.4.10 MitraClip procedure animation.

Transseptal puncture should be done under direct guidance of transesophageal echocardiography to ensure the right puncture site and height. The usual multi-planar TEE views are the bi-caval, short axis and four-chamber views (Figure 9.4.11 to Figure 9.4.14).

However, special situations might require modifications to the above transseptal height. The following are examples:

∞ Flail leaflets: Distance from puncture to point of coaptation is 4 to 4.5 cm.
∞ Functional MR with very large left atrium: 4 to 4.5 cm.
∞ Medial jet MR.

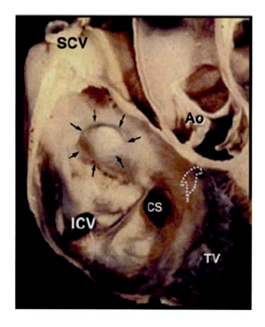

FIGURE 9.4.11 The intraarterial septum as seen from the right atrium. (After Ho SY, McCarthy KP, Faletra FF. Anatomy of the left atrium for interventional echocardiography. *Eur J Echocardiogr.* 2011;12(10):i11-i15. Reprinted by permission of Oxford University Press on behalf of the European Society of Cardiology.)

FIGURE 9.4.13   Echo measurements for MitraClip

FIGURE 9.4.14   Details of transseptal procedure.

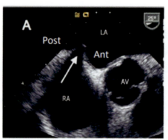
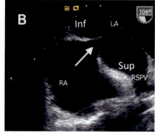
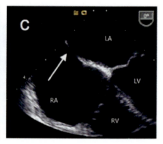

FIGURE 9.4.12   Multi-planar TEE views used in transseptal puncture: (A) short axis view at the base; (B) bi-caval view; (C) apical four-chamber view.

TOOLS/INSTRUMENTS AND DEVICES

Overview of the MitraClip® System: The MitraClip is a clip that attaches the leaflets of mitral valve designed to treat mitral regurgitation. It allows the mitral valve to coapt more completely and helps restore blood flow through left ventricle. It is a less invasive treatment option for MR which is a valid alternative to conventional mitral valve surgery for MR (Figure 9.4.15).

FIGURE 9.4.15 Percutaneous mitral valve repair with the edge-to-edge technique.

FIGURE 9.4.16 Live case MitraClip procedure XTR.

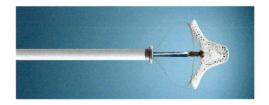

FIGURE 9.4.17 MitraClip™ XT Clip Delivery System. Reproduced with permission of Abbott, © 2020

FIGURE 9.4.18 New-generation MitraClip devices.

The device consists of:

∞ Steerable guiding catheter
∞ Clip delivery system
∞ Delivery catheter
∞ MitraClip device

Third generation of MitraClip:

MitraClip NTR: The improved clip delivery system (CDS) is designed to be more precise and predictable through new ease-of-use features.

MitraClip XTR: Longer clip arms for easier grasping on an improved CDS (Figure 9.4.16, Figure 9.4.17 and Figure 9.4.18).

PERIOPERATIVE CONSIDERATION

A. INDICATIONS FOR MICS PROCEDURE

1. *Symptomatic mitral regurgitation (MR) more than 3+ due to primary or degenerative MR in patients who have been determined to be at prohibitive risk for mitral valve surgery.* ACC/AHA recommendation for primary MR intervention: Transcatheter mitral valve repair may be considered for severely symptomatic patients (NYHA Class III to IV) with chronic severe primary MR (stage D) who have favorable anatomy for the repair procedure and a reasonable life expectancy but who have a prohibitive surgical risk because of severe comorbidities and remain severely symptomatic despite optimal GDMT for the heart failure (Class IIb) (Figure 9.4.19).

2. *Symptomatic severe secondary mitral regurgitation after failure of optimal medical treatment and no option for revascularization.* 2017 ESC/

TABLE 9.4.1 Indication for MitraClip therapy

Ideal treatment for MitraClip treatment	MitraClip to be considered	MitraClip not recommended or only in exceptional cases
Severe mitral regurgitation and Optimal valve morphology and SMR with LV-EF <30% and PMR (with operation-indication following guidelines) and A high operative risk or other risk constellation	Moderate to severe mitral regurgitation and Optimal valve morphology and SMR or PMR (with operation-indication following guidelines) and High operative risk, very high age or other risk constellations	Moderate to severe mitral regurgitation and Conditionally suitable valve morphology and Life expectancy <12 months or LV-EF <15% or cardiothoracic operation planned due to other indication and Previously operated mitral valve or As surgical/interventional hybrid procedure or At low operative risk

Source: With kind permission from Springer Science+Business Media, Springer Nature, *Clin Res Cardiol*, Percutaneous interventional mitral regurgitation treatment using the Mitra-Clip system, 103(2), 85–96, Boekstegers, P., Hausleiter, J., Baldus, S. et al. © 2014.

FIGURE 9.4.19 2017 AHA/ACC guidelines.

FIGURE 9.4.20 2017 ESC/EACTS guideline.

EACTS Guideline for the management of valvular heart disease; indication for mitral valve intervention in chronic secondary mitral regurgitation (Figure 9.4.20).

3. *MitraClip may be considered in the treatment of heart failure, after all other options are exhausted, to reduce hospitalization.*
4. *Other indications of MitraClip which require evidence-based studies.*
    1. MitraClip might be considered in patients with symptomatic severe mitral regurgitation in hypertrophic cardiomyopathy (HOCM) who are not surgical candidates (Figure 9.4.21).
    2. MitraClip as an emergency treatment for patients with cardiogenic shock due to acute ischemic papillary muscle rupture who are not surgical candidates (Figure 9.4.22).

Note: The other indications of MitraClip mentioned previously were only reported as case reports and/or case series and need to be studied further.

FIGURE 9.4.21 MitraClip in HOCM.

FIGURE 9.4.23 MitraClip by Boekstegers et al. 2014.

FIGURE 9.4.22 MitraClip as an emergency treatment.

B. PATIENT SELECTION

Risk determination: Prohibitive risk is determined by the clinical judgment of a heart team, including a cardiac surgeon experienced in mitral valve surgery and a cardiologist experienced in mitral valve disease, due to the presence of one or more of the following documented surgical risk factors:

- Thirty-day STS-predicted operative mortality risk score of
  - ≥8% for patients deemed likely to undergo mitral valve replacement or
  - ≥6% for patients deemed likely to undergo mitral valve repair
- Porcelain aorta or extensively calcified ascending aorta
- Frailty (assessed by in-person cardiac surgeon consultation)
- Hostile chest
- Severe liver disease/cirrhosis (MELD score >12)
- Severe pulmonary hypertension (systolic pulmonary artery pressure >2/3 systemic pressure)
- Unusual extenuating circumstance, such as right ventricular dysfunction with severe tricuspid regurgitation, chemotherapy for malignancy, major bleeding diathesis, immobility, AIDS, severe dementia, high risk of aspiration, high risk of injury to the internal mammary artery (IMA), etc.

Ideal Valve Morphology (Ref: Figure 9.4.23)

- Central pathology in segment 2
- No leaflet calcification
- Mitral valve opening area >4cm^2
- Mobile length of the posterior leaflet ≥10 mm
- Coaptation depth <11 mm
- Normal leaflet strength and mobility
- Flail width <15 mm
- Flail gap <10 mm

C. CONTRAINDICATIONS

The MitraClip® Delivery System is contraindicated in DMR patients with the following conditions.

ALTERNATIVE APPROACHES

A LOOK TO CURRENT AND SOON-TO-COME TRANSCATHETER MITRAL VALVE REPAIR OPTIONS

Transcatheter therapies for repair of MR are developing rapidly, and several devices are in development. There are distinct advantages and limitations offered by transcatheter devices, including improved procedural safety, better hemodynamics and often the avoidance of long-term anticoagulation and device dislodgement (Figure 9.4.24).

- ∞ *Pascal (Edwards Lifesciences)*: Transvenous transseptal edge-to-edge repair paddles with central spacer. Broad grasping zone and spacer reduce multiple device implant; single leaflet grasping.
- ∞ *NeoChord DS1000 (NeoChord, Inc.)*: Transapical artificial chordal repair (sutures at edge of leaflets). Precise placement and tensioning of ePTFE artificial chords under physiological conditions using TEE guidance.
- ∞ *Harpoon TSD-5 (Harpoon Medical, Inc.)*: Transapical artificial chordal repair (sutures can insert anywhere in leaflet). Precise placement and tensioning of ePTFE artificial chords under physiological conditions using TEE guidance; ability to place sutures anywhere in valve leaflet.
- ∞ *V-Chordal off-pump transseptal (Edwards Lifesciences)*: Transseptal adaptation of artificial chord off-pump tensioning system. Adaptation of surgical technique.
- ∞ *Carillon (Cardiac Dimensions, Inc.)*: Transvenous pre-shaped nitinol device placed in coronary sinus. Multiple anchor sizes and lengths available (37 combinations); treatment effect and complications (circumflex artery compression) can be evaluated before device release.
- ∞ *Arto (MVRx, Inc.)*: Suture-based tether between interatrial septum and coronary sinus. Simplified annuloplasty with brief learning curve; adjustable device tension titrated to effect.
- ∞ *Mitral Loop Cerclage (Tau-PNU Medical Co, Ltd.)*: Transvenous adjustable stainless-steel loop delivered via coronary sinus. Annuloplasty delivered to circumference of mitral annulus; adjustable device tension titrated to effect.
- ∞ *Mitralign (Mitralign, Inc.)*: Retrograde femoral arterial access and bident catheter-suture system direct annuloplasty. Customizable to patient anatomy with variable bident catheter size; asymmetrical or symmetrical annuloplasty can be performed (one or two pledget pairs).
- ∞ *Cardioband (Edwards Lifesciences)*: Transvenous transseptal direct posterior leaflet annuloplasty. Surgical-like direct annuloplasty from atrial surface; homogeneous circumferential annular cinching.

FIGURE 9.4.24 Update on transcatheter mitral valve repair.

FIGURE 9.4.25 MitraClip discussion.

FIGURE 9.4.26 IE after MitraClip implantation.

CAVEATS AND CONTROVERSIES

A. FROM THE CARDIOLOGIST'S POINT OF VIEW

TRANSCATHETER MITRAL VALVE REPAIR TODAY AND TOMORROW

MitraClip has evolved as a valuable catheter-based treatment option in patients with both primary and secondary (functional) MR (Figure 9.4.25).

EXPERIENCES SO FAR

Percutaneous edge-to-edge mitral valve repair with the MitraClip® has been shown to be a safe and feasible alternative compared to conventional surgical mitral valve repair. This section shows the real-world reported experiences on MitraClip therapy.

REAL-WORLD EXPERIENCE

B. BUTTERFLY IN THE HEART

Things can go wrong. MitraClip can get complicated with infected endocarditis (IE). Aslannif et al. (Figure 9.4.26) reported six cases of IE after MitraClip repair. The authors concluded that MitraClip implantation carries a very low risk for IE, and prompt diagnosis can be made easily by noninvasive echocardiography (Figure 9.4.26).

TABLE 9.4.2 Morphology for a MitraClip therapy		
Optimal valve morphology	**Conditionally suitable valve morphology**	**Unsuitable valve morphology**
Central pathology in segment 2	Pathology in segment 1 or 3	Perforated mitral valve leaflet or cleft
No leaflet calcification	Mild calcification outside of the grip-zone of the clip system; ring calcification, post-annuloplasty	Severe calcification in the grip-zone
Mitral valve opening area >4 cm^2	Mitral valve opening area >3 cm^2 with good residual mobility	Hemodynamically significant mitral stenosis (valve opening are <3 cm^2, MPG ≥5 mmHg)
Mobile length of the posterior leaflet ≥10 mm	Mobile length of the posterior leaflet 7–10 mm Coaptation depth ≥10 mm	Mobile length of the posterior leaflet <7 mm
Normal leaflet strength and mobility	Leaflet restriction in systole (Carpentier IIIB)	Rheumatic leaflet thickening and restriction in systole and diastole (Carpentier IIIA)
Flail width <15 mm flail Gap <10 mm	Flail-width >15 mm only with a large ring width and the option for multiple clips	Barlow's syndrome with multisegment flail leaflets

Source: With kind permission from Springer Science+Business Media, Springer Nature, *Clin Res Cardiol*, Percutaneous interventional mitral regurgitation treatment using the Mitra-Clip system, 103(2), 85–96, Boekstegers, P., Hausleiter, J. and Baldus, S. et al. © 2014.

TABLE 9.4.3 Contraindications of MitraClip®

Rheumatic mitral valve disease or mitral stenosis
- Mitral valve area <4 cm²
- Transmitral gradient >5 mmHg

Femoral venous, inferior vena cava or intracardiac thrombus

Active mitral valve endocarditis

Intolerance of procedural anticoagulation

Intolerance of postprocedural antiplatelet therapy

Life expectancy <1 year

Severe frailty or modified Rankin scale 5 (relative contraindication)

Source: After Vesely MR et al 2015, Surgical and Transcatheter Mitral Valve Repair for Severe Chronic Mitral Regurgitation: A Review of Clinical Indications and Patient Assessment. *J Am Heart Assoc.* 2015;4(12):e002424.

TABLE 9.4.4 Late-breaking data on the MitraClip System

	EVEREST II (30-day FU)	TRAMI (EuroSCORE $20%/EuroSCORE, 20%), data for in-hospital events	ACCESS-EU	Meta-analysis
Procedural death	0.0%	-	0.0%	0.1%
30-Day mortality	7.7%	4.3%/1.1% (in hospital)	3.4%	4.2%
All-cause mortality during FU	24.4%	13.4%/9.6% (mean FU of 72 days)	17.3% (12-month FU)	15.8% (mean FU of 310 days)
Vascular complications needing intervention	-	-	-	1.0%
Major bleeding requiring transfusion	17.9%	13.7%/8.7%	-	9.7%
Bleeding complications	-	-	3.9%	-
Tamponade or significant pericardial effusion	-	1.1%/1.6%	1.1%	0.7%
Emergent cardiac surgery	0.0%	-	0.4%	0.7%
Nonfatal myocardial infarction	2.6%	0.0%/0.2%	0.7%	0.4%
Chordal rupture	-	-	-	0.8%
Single leaflet clip detachment	-	-	4.8% (diagnosed within 6 months)	2.3%
Clip embolism	-	-	0.0%	0.04%
Hemorrhagic or ischemic stroke/TIA	2.6%	0.7%/0.0%	0.7%	1.3%
Acute renal failure	3.8%	1.8%/0.2% (dialysis at discharge)	4.8%	4.2%
Need for repeat MitraClip	0.0%	1.8%/1.6%	3.4%	1.6%

Abbreviations: EuroSCORE, European System for Cardiac Operative Risk Evaluation; FU, follow-up; TIA, transient ischemic attack.
Source: After Deuschl F et al, Critical evaluation of the MitraClip system in the management of mitral regurgitation. *Vascular Health and Risk Management* 2016:12 1—8. © 2020 Dove Medical Press.

FIGURE 9.4.27 Extended use of MitraClip beyond EVEREST.

C. BEYOND EVEREST

Guilherme et al. (Figure 9.4.27 and Figure 9.4.28) sought to compare high-risk patients (3+ to 4+ MR) with echocardiographic features different from endovascular valve edge-to-edge repair (EVEREST). They observed similar rates of safety and efficacy through 12-month follow-up.

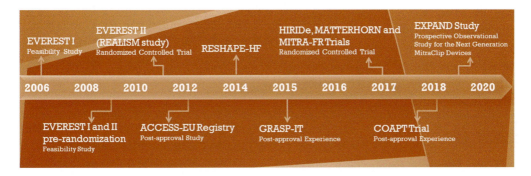

FIGURE 9.4.28 Clinical trials for MitraClip therapy.

RESEARCH, TRENDS AND INNOVATION

1. **Feasibility Study of a Percutaneous Mitral Valve Repair System (EVEREST I)**

Phase I evaluation of the safety and efficacy of an endovascular approach to the repair of mitral valve regurgitation using the Evalve Cardiovascular Valve Repair System. The study is a prospective, multicenter, Phase I study of the Evalve Cardiovascular Valve Repair System (CVRS) in the treatment of mitral valve regurgitation. A minimum of 20 patients will be enrolled (an additional maximum of 12 roll-in patients, a maximum of 2 per site, may be enrolled and analyzed separately). Patients will undergo 30-day, 6-month and 12-month clinical follow-up. The primary endpoint is acute safety at 30 days, with a secondary efficacy endpoint of reduction of MR.

2. **Pivotal Study of a Percutaneous Mitral Valve Repair System (EVEREST II RCT)**

This is a prospective, multicenter, randomized study of the safety and effectiveness of an endovascular approach to the treatment of mitral valve regurgitation using the Evalve Cardiovascular Valve Repair System (MitraClip® implant). A minimum of 279 evaluable patients randomized 2:1 to MitraClip or mitral valve surgery, respectively, are required to test the primary safety and effectiveness endpoints of the RCT. Enrollment in the RCT is now complete. Sixty roll-in patients were enrolled under EVEREST II RCT. Thirty-eight clinical sites throughout the US and Canada have participated in the RCT and HRR. Thirty-seven US sites are participating in

FIGURE 9.4.29 Percutaneous therapies for mitral regurgitation by Raviknath.

REALISM. The RCT is powered to test the hypothesis that MitraClip has both superiority of safety and non-inferiority of effectiveness compared to mitral valve repair or replacement surgery. The HRR is powered to show lower mortality at 30 days with the MitraClip than predicted surgical mortality (Figure 9.4.29).

3. Real-World Expanded Multicenter Study of the MitraClip® System (REALISM)

The EVEREST II REALISM study (REALISM study) is a continued-access registry designed for continued data collection on the use of Abbott's MitraClip System (MitraClip® Device) under more "real-world" conditions. After the completion of enrollment in the pivotal EVEREST II randomized controlled trial (RCT) NCT00209274 and EVEREST II High Risk Registry Study NCT01940120, continued access to the technology was warranted to collect additional data on the safety and efficacy of the MitraClip® Device. This continued-access study was approved by the FDA on November 21, 2008 (G030064). There are two arms (high risk and non-high risk) in the REALISM study. Patients who did not meet the REALISM high-risk or non-high-risk eligibility criteria were evaluated for consideration for either emergency use (EU) or compassionate use (CU). Enrollment in the non-high-risk arm of the study concluded on April 14, 2011, and enrollment in the high-risk arm concluded on December 19, 2013.

REALISM is a prospective, multicenter study of the safety and effectiveness of an endovascular approach to the treatment of mitral valve regurgitation using the Evalve Cardiovascular Valve Repair System (MitraClip® implant). Patients with moderate-to-severe (3+) or severe (4+) mitral regurgitation (MR), as determined by the site from a transthoracic echocardiogram (TTE), were considered for enrollment in this study. The TTE and a transesophageal echocardiogram (TEE) are used to assess eligibility criteria for MR severity, valve anatomy and left ventricular parameters.

4. EVEREST II Pivotal Study High Risk Registry (HRR)

Prospective, multicenter, single-arm registry. Clinical follow-up at discharge, 30 days, 6, 12, 18 and 24 months and 3, 4 and 5 years. The EVEREST II HRR is a single-arm prospective, multicenter clinical trial enrolling high-surgical-risk patients of the EVEREST II study (NCT00209274). Patients were considered to be of high surgical risk if either their Society of Thoracic Surgery (STS)-predicted operative mortality risk was ≥12%, or if the surgeon investigator determined the patient to be high risk (≥12% predicted operative mortality risk) due to the presence of, at bare minimum, one of the following pre-specified risk factors:

- ∞ Porcelain aorta or mobile ascending aortic atheroma
- ∞ Post-radiation mediastinum
- ∞ Previous mediastinitis
- ∞ Functional MR with ejection fraction (EF) <40%
- ∞ Over 75 years old with EF <40%
- ∞ Prior re-operation with patent grafts
- ∞ Two or more prior chest surgeries

- ∞ Hepatic cirrhosis
- ∞ Three or more of the following STS high-risk factors:
  - ∞ Creatinine >2.5 mg/dL
  - ∞ Prior chest surgery
  - ∞ Age over 75
  - ∞ EF <35%

Upon completion of enrollment in the HRR, a process was initiated to ensure patient consent to participate in a concurrent control (CC) group was in place. Patients were identified to determine survival through 12 months with current standard of care treatment. CC patients were derived from a cohort of patients who were screened for enrollment in the HRR, but did not enroll. All patients had moderate-to-severe (3+) or severe (4+) MR based on transthoracic echocardiography (TTE). To be considered eligible for inclusion in the CC group, the patient had to be classified as a high-surgical-risk patient using the same criteria used for the HRR. Upon follow-up with the clinical sites, it was determined that some of the initially identified patients with moderate-to-severe (3+) or severe (4+) MR met the criteria for high surgical risk. Of these patients, some were not included due to lack of institutional review board (IRB) approval at the site, lack of informed consent and some were non contactable, hence excluded. The remaining patients make up the CC group.

5. **A Randomized Study of the MitraClip® Device in Heart Failure Patients With Clinically Significant Functional Mitral Regurgitation (RESHAPE-HF)**

This trial is a randomized study of the MitraClip device in heart failure patients with clinically significant functional mitral regurgitation. A hierarchical composite of all-cause mortality and recurrent heart failure hospitalizations is hypothesized to occur at a lower rate with the use of the MitraClip device in addition to optimal standard medical therapy compared to optimal standard of care therapy alone. This study is a clinical evaluation of the safety and efficacy of the MitraClip System in the treatment of clinically significant functional mitral regurgitation in patients with chronic heart failure. The objective is to further study the safety and efficacy of the MitraClip System for the treatment of clinically significant functional mitral regurgitation in New York Heart Association Functional Class III or IV chronic heart failure patients.

6. **ACCESS-Europe A Two-Phase Observational Study of the MitraClip® System in Europe (ACCESS-EU)**

Phase I: The primary objective of ACCESS-EU Phase I is to gain information from countries in the European Union, regarding the use of the MitraClip System with respect to health economics and clinical care. Phase II: (HAS BEEN CLOSED BY SPONSOR). The primary objective of ACCESS-EU Phase II is to gather additional clinical data, specifically Echocardiography Core Laboratory measurements of MR severity and left ventricular volumes and diameters and other echocardiographic measures, on patients undergoing the MitraClip procedure in the European Union countries. Clinical data collected from both study phases are expected to contribute to decision making with regard to MitraClip therapy selection in patients with MR: (a) by establishing the value of the MitraClip therapy in the continuum of care; and (b) by providing practical information that will allow physicians to make therapeutic decisions, assist hospitals to make purchasing decisions and assist insurers in making coverage decisions.

Study design: ACCESS-Europe is a two-phase prospective, observational, multicenter

FIGURE 9.4.30 Patient selection for MitraClip – EACTS 2010.

FIGURE 9.4.31 Critical evaluation of the MitraClip System – Dovepress.

FIGURE 9.4.32 Critical evaluation of the MitraClip System – Dovepress.

FIGURE 9.4.33 Mitral valve disease – current management and future challenges by Nishimura et al.

post-approval study of the MitraClip System for the treatment of mitral regurgitation (MR) in the European Union countries. Patients will be evaluated per standard practice at baseline, discharge, 6 months and 12 months. Phase I of the study consists of patients who receive the MitraClip System for the treatment of MR and two concurrent comparator groups of (a) medically managed heart failure patients with MR and (b) patients who have undergone mitral valve surgery for MR. The two comparator groups will be followed and evaluated primarily from a health economic perspective. ACCESS EU Study Phase II will consist of only patients who receive the MitraClip System, with the objective of collecting additional clinical data, specifically Echocardiography Core Laboratory evaluation of MR severity and other echocardiographic measures. Enrollment of patients in each study phase is as follows (Figure 9.4.30).

ACCESS-EU PHASE I

- ∞ A minimum of 300 MitraClip therapy group patients
- ∞ A minimum of 100 patients in the mitral valve surgery comparator group
- ∞ As many patients as possible in the medical therapy comparator group

First patient enrollment projection: Q1, 2009. Last patient enrollment projection: Enrollment in the mitral valve surgery and medical therapy groups ceased on December 31, 2010. Enrollment in the MitraClip group will cease when Phase II of the study is initiated at each site.

ACCESS-EU PHASE II

A minimum of 300 MitraClip therapy subjects will be enrolled in Phase II. First patient enrollment projection: Q2, 2011. Last patient enrollment projection: Enrollment will cease when the sponsor has determined that an adequate number of patients have been enrolled.

7. Cardiovascular Outcomes Assessment of the MitraClip Percutaneous Therapy for Heart Failure Patients With Functional Mitral Regurgitation (The COAPT Trial)

Prospective, randomized, parallel-controlled, multicenter clinical evaluation of the MitraClip device for the treatment of clinically significant functional mitral regurgitation in symptomatic heart failure subjects who are treated per standard of care and who have been determined by the site's local heart team as not appropriate for mitral valve surgery. Eligible subjects will be randomized in a 1:1 ratio to the MitraClip device (device group) or to no MitraClip device (control group).

As part of the COAPT trial, a subset of patients (at least 50 up to 100 in total) will be registered in the CPX sub-study, which is designed as a prospective, randomized (1:1 ratio to the MitraClip or no MitraClip device), parallel-controlled, multicenter study registering approximately 50–100 subjects in up to 50 qualified US sites from the COAPT trial. Subjects registered and randomized in the CPX sub-study will contribute to the total enrollment of approximately 610 subjects in the COAPT trial. Roll-in subjects will not participate in the CPX sub-study.

The COAPT CAS study is designed as a prospective, multicenter, single-arm, continued-access registry study. A maximum of 800 subjects (anticipated) will be registered from up to 75 sites in the United States. The enrollment will end once pre-market approval (PMA) of the proposed expanded indication of the MitraClip System is obtained. Active follow-up of patients will be performed through 12 months with scheduled visits at 30 days and 12 months. The national Transcatheter Valve Therapy Registry (TVT Registry) will be used for data collection through 12 months. Annual follow-up data from 2 years through year 5 post-implant will be obtained by linkage to the Centers for Medicare and Medicaid Services (CMS) Claims database. COAPT CAS data may be used to support the PMA application of the labeling claims for the treatment of moderate-to-severe or severe FMR in symptomatic heart failure subjects. This single-arm registry will provide valuable new information regarding the use of the MitraClip® NT System under more "real-world" conditions.

8. The MitraClip® EXPAND Study

The MitraClip EXPAND study (a contemporary, prospective study evaluating real-world experience of performance and safety for the next generation of MitraClip devices) is designed to confirm the safety and performance of the MitraClip NTR System and MitraClip XTR System. The data collected in this study will be used to evaluate device outcomes and characterize trends in patient selection for MitraClip therapy in contemporary real-world use. Clinical outcomes and echocardiographic measures will be assessed in the context of historical data. Up to 1,000 subjects at a maximum of 60 sites in Europe and the US will be included in the MitraClip EXPAND study.

9. What is the future for MitraClip?

The conclusion is – first, transcatheter mitral valve treatment should be discussed by the heart team in symptomatic patients who are at high surgical risk or are inoperable. Secondly, more prospective, randomized controlled trials are needed to determine patients, potential adverse events, device durability and long-term follow-up, and lastly, MitraClip® should be used only in centers with high-quality surgical and interventional experience, and training.

10. Challenges in transcatheter mitral interventions

i) Efficacy and durability of MitraClip
ii) Feasibility and effectiveness of transcatheter mitral valve replacement
iii) Respective indications of repair and replacement
iv) Combination with tricuspid repair
v) Feasibility and effectiveness of combination of repair techniques

WHERE AND HOW TO LEARN

Referrals to Media:

FIGURE 9.4.34   Case presentation of a procedure by Randy Martin.

FIGURE 9.4.37   MitraClip patient success story.

Where to watch

FIGURE 9.4.35   Echocardiographic evaluation in MitraClip.

FIGURE 9.4.39   Treating MR with MitraClip therapy.

Where to train

FIGURE 9.4.38   Heart function, QoL improvements at 1 year – MitraClip Registry.

FIGURE 9.4.40   How do I get training?

FIGURE 9.4.36   Overview of transcatheter mitral valve repair technologies.

252   Minimally Invasive Cardiac Surgery

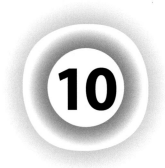

MINIMALLY INVASIVE TRICUSPID VALVE SURGERY

CHRISTOS ALEXIOU AND THEO KOFIDIS

HISTORY AND INTRODUCTION

Tricuspid valve surgery (TVS) may be needed for tricuspid regurgitation (TR), tricuspid stenosis (TS) or mixed tricuspid valve disease. Although median sternotomy (MS) has been, and probably remains, the most common surgical approach to TV, less invasive surgical techniques have emerged over time and are being increasingly used.

In this chapter we present the causes, natural history and indications for surgery for TR or TS and describe in detail the surgical technique for minimally invasive TVS through a right minithoracotomy.

TRICUSPID REGURGITATION

Most cases of TR are functional (around 80%), secondary to tricuspid annular dilation due to right ventricular (RV) enlargement. The pathological substrate in the majority of functional TR is a left-sided valvular heart pathology with ensuing pulmonary hypertension (PHT). The etiology in the remaining TR cases is organic, namely rheumatic, congenital, endocarditis, traumatic or iatrogenic, and myxomatous degeneration of TV. Rarely, isolated TR, secondary to a degenerative process causing severe annular and/or right atrial dilatation, is also seen [1]. TR was initially considered as a relatively benign condition; however, several studies have provided convincing evidence that untreated TR (isolated or concomitant with left-sided heart pathology) may deteriorate over time, adversely affecting the patient's symptoms, quality of life and survival [2–5].

Both American and European guidelines recommend surgical intervention (Class IIa indication) for isolated severe symptomatic TR, preferably before the onset of RV dysfunction [6–8]. However, a discrepancy is present in the suggestions of AHA/ACC and ESC/EACTS regarding the need and the optimal timing of TVS in patients with asymptomatic isolated severe TR. According to US guidelines, TVS could be considered in selected low-surgical-risk patients exhibiting progressive dilatation and reduction of RV function on serial ECHOs (Class IIb indication). The European guidelines [8] are more clear-cut, suggesting that TVS should be considered in asymptomatic or mildly symptomatic patients with severe isolated primary TR and progressive RV dilatation or deterioration of RV function (Class IIa indication).

TR AT THE TIME OF LEFT-SIDED HEART SURGERY

The threshold to operate on the TV during left-sided heart valve surgery is much lower compared to isolated TR cases for three reasons: (a) TR may not improve after successful treatment of left-sided valvular dysfunction particularly if the annulus is already dilated (40 mm), (b) TVS is not difficult to perform and it does not add significantly to the time and risk of the left-sided intervention and (c) re-operation for severe TR at a later stage would carry a significantly higher operative risk [6–11]. Currently, TV repair is recommended for severe TR (Class I indication) or mild-moderate functional TR at the time of left-sided valve surgery with either tricuspid annular dilatation or prior evidence of right heart failure (Class IIa indication). Furthermore, tricuspid valve repair should be considered (Class IIb indication) in patients with moderate functional TR and pulmonary hypertension at the time of left-sided valve surgery [6–8].

TRICUSPID STENOSIS

Most commonly, TS results from rheumatic heart disease. Other less common causes of TS include congenital abnormalities (Ebstein's anomaly or isolated tricuspid valve stenosis), metabolic or enzymatic abnormalities (Fabry's disease, Whipple's disease and carcinoid) and active infective endocarditis [12]. The 2014 AHA/ACC and ESC Valvular Heart Disease Guidelines recommend tricuspid valve surgery for (a) patients with severe TS at the time of operation for left-sided valve disease and (b) isolated, symptomatic severe TS (Class I recommendations). The guidelines further suggest percutaneous balloon commissurotomy in patients with isolated, symptomatic severe TS without accompanying TR and without calcified tricuspid valve [6–8].

HOW TO DO IT/STEP BY STEP

Historically, surgical access to the mitral valve was obtained via right thoracotomy (RT) incision [13], appreciating that this approach provides excellent visibility of both the right and left atrium. Subsequently, the advent of coronary artery bypass surgery led to the widespread adoption of median sternotomy as the universal approach for any type of cardiac surgery [14]. The realization of the risks associated with sternal re-entry in redo cases prompted many surgeons to resort again to an RT approach for right and left atrioventricular valve surgery [15–17]. The experience gained with the RT and advancements in surgical instrumentation and imaging technology helped in developing right port access mini thoracotomy techniques for mitral and tricuspid valve surgery in the last two decades of the previous century [18,19]. Minimally invasive cardiac surgery has rapidly expanded and has been increasingly adopted around the globe mainly for mitral valve and for tricuspid valve surgery. Currently, mini RT is employed in the setting of primary or redo isolated TVS or TVS at the time of mitral valve surgery. Many centers report significant benefits for the patient, which, in addition to improved cosmesis, include low morbidity and mortality, less tissue trauma, reduced bleeding and transfusion requirements for blood and blood products, shorter ventilation times, ITU and hospital stay, less pain, better chest stability, earlier mobilization and return to normal physical activities and work [20–37]. On the other hand, longer bypass and ischemic times (particularly during the surgeon's learning curve), the need for peripheral cannulation (careful patient selection essential to avoid vascular complications and stroke) and costs of the equipment are potential drawbacks for any type of MICS, all of which can be overcome with appropriate team preparation, planning and organization and proper patient selection [20–37].

In National University Hospital of Singapore, whenever feasible, a minimally invasive approach is preferred for mitral, aortic, tricuspid and CABG surgery [38]. In the following paragraphs we describe the standard technique utilized in our unit for mini TV surgery and alternative technical options employed in other minimally invasive cardiac surgery centers.

The right mini thoracotomy approach is indicated for patients undergoing primary or redo isolated TV or concomitant TV surgery during another left-sided heart procedure (Figure 10.1).

Prior to beginning surgery, in the operator theatre, it is good practice to carry out a briefing of the operating team where investigations, such as the coronary angiogram and contrast CT scan for evaluation of the status of the aorta, the iliac arteries and the femoral vessels, which will be used for peripheral arterial cannulation, are displayed (Figure 10.2).

The patient is placed in the supine position with the right chest slightly elevated using a shoulder pad and a lateral towel. In male patients, the right arm is positioned slightly off the side of the table. In female patients, the patient is rolled slightly to the left and the right arm is placed over the head.

The chest, abdomen and both groins are prepared and exposed. A double-lumen endotracheal tube is used for single-lung ventilation, to allow deflation of the right lung and facilitate exposure of the right chest cavity. An arterial line, central venous line and a pulmonary artery flotation catheter are also placed. A transesophageal (TOE) probe is inserted, prior to heparin administration, to guide correct placement

FIGURE 10.1 Double mini valve repair: Mitral and tricuspid.

FIGURE 10.2 Minimally invasive beating heart TV surgery in a redo case.

of venous drainage cannula and to evaluate the result of surgery.

Groin: The femoral vessels are exposed through a 3-cm oblique incision in the right groin. A 5/0 prolene purse-string suture is placed with a snugger in both the common femoral artery and vein (Figure 10.1, Figure 10.3 and Figure 10.4).

Chest: A 5–7-cm incision is made lateral to the nipple in males and in the mammary fold in females over the fourth or fifth intercostal space (ICS). The midpoint of the entire sternum is a useful external marker for the identification of the fourth space, which provides good exposure for both mitral and tricuspid valves. The right lung is deflated and the right chest entered in the fourth intercostal space (Figure 10.3 and Figure 10.5). In order to facilitate exposure of the chest cavity and to avoid rib fracture the parietal pleura is further incised 6 cm anteriorly and 6 cm posteriorly.

EXPOSURE OF THE HEART AND RIGHT ATRIUM

A soft tissue retractor Alexis® O ring (Applied Medical Resources Corporation, Rancho Santa Margarita, CA, USA) is inserted through the incision and unfolded. In addition, an MICS intercostal retractor system is optionally used to further aid exposure. A pledgeted 2-0 silk suture is placed on the diaphragm medially and is pulled through the chest wall laterally and inferiorly using a hock needle. This maneuver improves visibility of the lower aspect of the pericardium and the inferior vena cava (IVC) (Figure 10.5 and Figure 10.6).

The pericardium is opened where it looks easier and safer, 3 cm above the phrenic nerve, and a longitudinal incision is made from the superior vena cava (SVC) to the IVC, at which point the incision is ventralized towards the anterior chest wall to avoid local phrenic nerve injury (Figure 10.3). Two traction pericardial sutures are placed inferiorly and one or two anteriorly and pulled through the chest wall with a hook needle.

Before heparinization, a Chitwood clamp is inserted through the right second intercostal space at the mid-axillary line for subsequent aortic clamping. Likewise, a wide bore catheter is placed into the chest cavity through the fifth ICS at the

FIGURE 10.3 Minimal-access tricuspid valve surgery by Joseph Lamelas.

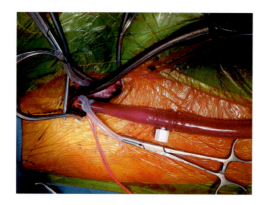

FIGURE 10.4 Cannulation of the right femoral artery and vein for cardiopulmonary bypass.

FIGURE 10.5 Tricuspid valve replacement on a beating heart via a right minithoracotomy.

mid-thoracotomy incision level for CO_2 insufflation.

CANNULATION AND CARDIOPULMONARY BYPASS

After full heparinization and under TEE guidance, the common femoral vessels are cannulated using Seldinger technique (Figure 10.2 and Figure 10.3).

Separate drainage of SVC and IVC. First, a long multistage cannula (Bio-Medicus® Multi-Stage Femoral Venous Cannula, Medtronic, Inc.) is inserted in the femoral vein and forwarded to just below the right atrium (RA). The SVC can be cannulated directly through the mini thoracotomy incision or (in order to avoid obstruction of the surgical view) via the chest wall, in which case a 12-mm trocar is used to introduce the SVC cannula through the sixth intercostal space. This site of trocar insertion is utilized for chest tube insertion at the end of the procedure (Figure 10.3). Alternatively, an appropriately sized cannula (12–14 mm) can be inserted through the neck into the right internal jugular vein and advanced into the SVC (Figure 10.2). Alternatively, effective SVC drainage with a pump sucker inserted in it is also possible (Figure 10.3 and Figure 10.8).

Single long two-staged cannula venous drainage. Alternatively, venous drainage can be accomplished using a single long two-staged venous cannula (Bio-Medicus® Multi-Stage Femoral Venous Cannula, Medtronic, Inc.) inserted with the Seldinger technique through the common femoral vein and advanced well into the SVC under TEE control. This technique obviates the need for double venous cannulation and provides good venous drainage. The femoral artery is then cannulated with an arterial cannula (Bio-Medicus® Femoral Arterial Cannulae, Medtronic, Inc.) using the Seldinger technique and secured to the leg. If atherosclerotic arterial disease precludes femoral cannulation, then the axillary artery or the ascending aorta can be utilized instead (Figure 10.3).

The sizes of the tubes selected for peripheral cannulation depend on the body surface area of the patient, and they tend to be smaller than those used for central cannulation (17–19 mm for femoral artery and 25–27 mm for femoral vein). After cannulation has been completed with the desired level of anticoagulation, CPB is commenced. If full-flow CPB with satisfactory emptying of the heart has not been obtained, vacuum assistance to the CPB circuit (negative pressure 35–65 mmHg) is applied as required. As mentioned above, in peripheral cannulation the tubes used are longer and smaller in size than those used for central cannulation. Vacuum-assisted venous drainage

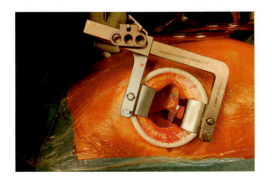

FIGURE 10.6 Retraction of the diaphragm.

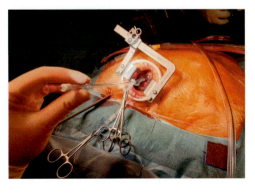

FIGURE 10.7 Chitwood clamp, CO_2 insufflation needle and antegrade cardioplegia placement.

greatly facilitates venous drainage in these circumstances and is commonly employed. Regardless of the selected cannulation strategy, upon establishment of CPB, both SVC and IVC are encircled with nylon tapes which are fed through tourniquets for subsequent bicaval occlusion. Rubber vessel loops for caval occlusion can also be used (Figure 10.1 and Figure 10.3).

AORTIC CLAMPING AND CARDIOPLEGIA DELIVERY

With the patient on CPB, a double pledgeted (optional) 5/0 or 4/0 prolene purse-string is placed in the ascending aorta, a dual catheter for cardioplegia delivery and aortic root venting is inserted through it, the CPB flow is reduced down to 1 L/min, the Chitwood clamp carefully applied with its concave surface pointing upwards so as to avoid injury to LA appendage and pulmonary artery (Figure 10.7 and Figure 10.9) and 1 L of modified Del Nido cardioplegia is administered, providing good protection for 90 min [39]. An additional 500-ml bolus is given if the duration of the aortic clamping exceeds 90 min or earlier if ventricular electrical activity becomes apparent. The temperature is allowed to drift to 32°C. The operative field is flooded with 3 L/min CO_2 for the entire procedure to displace air from the cardiac cavities, facilitating de-airing and preventing arterial air embolism [40].

MAIN OPERATION (TV REPAIR OR REPLACEMENT)

After completion of cardioplegia delivery, the IVC and SVC are snared, the RA opened longitudinally, stay sutures are placed in the atriotomy to expose the tricuspid valve and a separate suction placed in the coronary sinus to maintain a dry operative field. The TV is inspected and assessed, its pathology and lesions confirmed, and a decision is made to repair or replace the valve. Most repairs involve the placement of a TV annuloplasty incomplete ring (Figure 10.3), DeVega annuloplasty plus other repair techniques applied to the leaflets or subvalvular apparatus as appropriate. In cases of replacement (Figure 10.5), a bioprosthetic or mechanical valve is implanted, applying the same criteria as in a standard full sternotomy procedure. When placing annular sutures (for repair or replacement) great attention should be paid to keep clear from the triangle of Koch so as to avoid damage to the atrioventricular node and a possible heart block (Figure 10.3). Likewise, the repair and replacement techniques are the standard ones, the exception being the use (preferably) of long shafted endoscopic instruments and the knot pushers for knot tying (Figure 10.3). More recently, the Cor-Knot® (LSI solutions, Victor, NY, USA) device is increasingly used for convenience and shortening of cross-clamp and CPB times, particularly so in left-sided valve surgery.

FIGURE 10.8 Minimally invasive tricuspid valve repair technique (J Lamelas).

FIGURE 10.9 Chitwood clamp application (S Senai).

Upon completion of TV repair or replacement and de-airing, the right atrium is closed with a double layer of continuous 4/0 prolene (Figure 10.3), epicardial ventricular and atrial (when the patient is not in chronic atrial fibrillation) pacing wires secured, and the Chitwood clamp is removed.

COMPLETION OF THE PROCEDURE

The heart is allowed to recover and is weaned from CPB. Upon TEE confirmation of satisfactory TV repair or replacement and lack of intracardiac air, protamine is given, the cannulas removed and hemostasis at the cannula insertion points carefully secured. It should be noted that the aortic cardioplegia and vent cannula insertion site has been incriminated as a source of severe postoperative bleeding, morbidity and even mortality (personal communication). The sites of entry of ports and the Chitwood clamp in the chest wall may be used for the placement of one or two intercostal drains, of which a long and soft Blake drain (Ethicon, Sommerville, NJ, USA) is left within the intrapericardial space and a standard one in the right pleural space. It is important to remember to cut all pericardial traction sutures before asking the anesthesiologist to inflate the right lung, since forceful lung inflation against these sutures can cause major lung injury with disastrous consequences. After complete hemostasis has been ascertained, the diaphragmatic traction suture is also cut and the wounds closed in the usual fashion in layers.

REDO RIGHT MINI THORACOTOMY TV SURGERY (AFTER PREVIOUS PERICARDIOTOMY)

In redo TV surgery the techniques used are similar to first-time operations (Figure 10.1), bearing in mind the added difficulty posed by the intrapericardial adhesions, with the pericardium often being stuck onto the right atrium, the presence of grafts to the RCA or PDA and possible effects on cardiac anatomy, albeit subtle, caused by any previous valve surgery. We tend not to try to dissect out the adherent pericardium from the RA and include the adherent pericardium in the atriotomy incision. Also, we avoid encircling with tapes the IVC and SVC, which obviates the need for a potentially hazardous dissection. Although this may allow the entry of some amount of air into the venous drainage system, this is usually well tolerated and in our experience it does not seem to prevent effective venous drainage.

Concomitant mitral and tricuspid valve surgery. In cases of double valve surgery, the mitral valve is dealt with first (as described in the relevant chapters of this textbook) and the intervention to TV follows as described in this chapter, in the section titled, "How to do it".

TOOLS/INSTRUMENTS AND DEVICES

This is a list of specialized tools employed for the performance of minimally invasive tricuspid valve surgery:

1. **Soft tissue retractor Alexis® O ring** (Applied Medical Resources Corporation, Rancho Santa Margarita, CA, USA): The device retains moisture at the incision site, thus minimizing the risk of wound infections (Figure 10.10A,B).
2. **MICS intercostal retractor system**: This device features double swivel blades that are capable of adapting to different curvatures during the process of retraction in MICS (Figure 10.11A,B)

3. **Multistage cannula** (Bio-Medicus® Multi-Stage Femoral Venous Cannula, Medtronic, Inc.) or a single long two-staged venous cannula (Bio-Medicus® Multi-Stage Femoral Venous Cannula, Medtronic, Inc.) (Figure 10.12A,B).
4. **Bio-Medicus® Femoral Arterial Cannulae**, Medtronic, Inc.: A femoral arterial cannula for MICS surgery (Figure 10.13A,B).
5. **Chitwood aortic clamp**: The Chitwood aortic clamp is used for aortic cross-clamping during MICS (Figure 10.14A,B).
6. **Cor-Knot (LSI solutions, Victor, NY, USA) device**: This device is an automated suture fastener that eliminates the need for manual tying of suture knots (Figure 10.15A,B).

PERIOPERATIVE CONSIDERATION

Patients should have complete echocardiographic assessment with quantification of TR, pulmonary artery pressure (PAP), right ventricular (RV) size, left ventricular (LV) function and other valvular pathology. Coronary angiogram and 2D and 3D contrast CT scan to evaluate the status of the aorta, the iliac arteries and the femoral vessels, which will be used for peripheral arterial cannulation, are also recommended (Figure 10.2).

ALTERNATIVE APPROACHES

An attractive option in TV surgery (primary or redo) is to carry out the operation on a beating and perfused heart on full-flow CPB and normothermia (Figure 10.1). In this situation, it is important to ascertain with TOE that there is no interatrial communication. If there is, this should be closed straight after opening the RA so as to avoid air passing into left cardiac chambers. Large amounts of blood through the coronary sinus should be also expected and therefore extra suction in the RA (in addition to that placed within the coronary sinus itself) to assist in clearing the RA of excess blood and to aid visibility may be needed.

An innovative approach for establishing full CPB without having to undertake the risk of encircling both cavae is described by Misfeld Martin et al. After dual cannulation via femoral and internal jugular veins, two Fogarty catheters are inserted through the same venous cannulation sites and forwarded into the RA under TOE. Then, after pulling one cannula below the IVC and the upper cannula high in the SVC, the balloons of each of the two Fogarty catheters are inflated and pulled back so as to occlude the ostia of the SVC and IVC, allowing for the establishment of full CPB (Figure 10.2). The cannulation strategy and the management of CPB are otherwise similar to the primary right mini thoracotomy TV procedures.

CAVEATS AND CONTROVERSIES

Whilst patient outcomes are highly dependent on surgical techniques and the timing of surgery, it has been challenging to accurately determine the optimal time for which

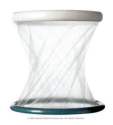

FIGURE 10.10A Alexis® soft tissue retractor. Reproduced with permission of Applied Medical, © 2020

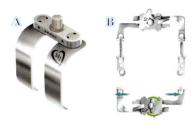

FIGURE 10.11A Joseph Lamelas Intercostal Retractor System. Reproduced with permission of LivaNova USA, Inc.

FIGURE 10.10B Alexis O Wound Protector – Retractor.

FIGURE 10.11B Joseph Lamelas Intercostal Retractor System – Double Swivel Blades

surgery should be performed, especially so in patients with isolated tricuspid valve disease. Evidently, a discrepancy is present in the suggestions of AHA/ACC and ESC/EACTS regarding the need and the optimal timing of TVS in patients with asymptomatic isolated severe TR. According to US guidelines, TVS could be considered in selected low-surgical-risk patients exhibiting progressive dilatation and reduction of RV function on serial ECHOs (Class IIb indication). The European guidelines [8] are more clear-cut, suggesting that TVS should be considered in asymptomatic or mildly symptomatic patients with severe isolated primary TR and progressive RV dilatation or deterioration of RV function (Class IIa indication).

RESEARCH, TRENDS AND INNOVATION

The global trend for mitral valve and for tricuspid valve surgery is towards minimally invasive access. Many centers report significant benefits for the patient, which, in addition to improved cosmesis, include low morbidity and mortality, less tissue trauma, reduced bleeding and transfusion requirements for blood and blood products, shorter ventilation times, ITU and hospital stay, less pain, better chest stability and earlier mobilization and return to normal physical activities and work [20–37]. On the other hand, longer bypass and ischemic times (particularly during the surgeon's learning curve), the need for peripheral cannulation (careful patient selection essential to avoid vascular complications and stroke) and the costs of the equipment are potential drawbacks for any type of MICS, all of which can be overcome with appropriate team preparation, planning and organization and proper patient selection [20–37].

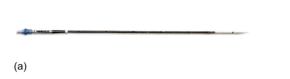

(a)

(b)

FIGURE 10.12A Bio-MedicusR Multi-Stage Femoral Venous Cannula. Reproduced with permission of Medtronic, Inc.

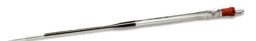

FIGURE 10.13 A. Bio-Medicus™ femoral arterial cannula. Reproduced with permission of Medtronic, Inc

FIGURE 10.13 B. Femoral arterial cannula, Medtronic

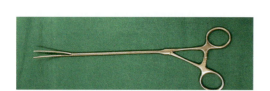

FIGURE 10.14 A. Chitwood aortic clamp.

FIGURE 10.14 B. Transthoracic aortic clamp by Chitwood

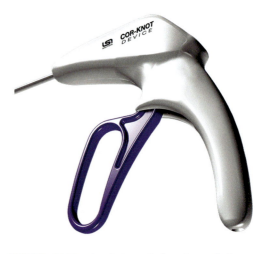

FIGURE 10.15 A. Automated suture fastener, Cor-Knot®. Reproduced with permission of LSI Solutions, Victor, NY, © 2020.

FIGURE 10.15 B. Cor-Knot® by LSI Solutions.

262   Minimally Invasive Cardiac Surgery

WHERE AND HOW TO LEARN

In the National University Hospital of Singapore (NUHS), whenever feasible, a minimally invasive approach is preferred for mitral, aortic, tricuspid and CABG surgery [38]. The "How to do it" section described step by step the techniques utilized in the NUHS and in Euromedica Kyanous Stavros Hospital, Thessaloniki, Greece, for mini TV surgery, and alternative technical options employed in other minimally invasive cardiac surgery centers.

REFERENCES

1. Topilsky Y, Khanna A, Le Tourneau T. Clinical context and mechanism of functional tricuspid regurgitation in patients with and without pulmonary hypertension. *Circ Cardiovasc Imaging* 2012;5(3):314–23.
2. Messika-Zeitoun D, Thomson H, Bellamy M. Medical and surgical outcome of tricuspid regurgitation caused by flail leaflets. *J Thorac Cardiovasc Surg* 2004;128(2):296–302.
3. Sagie A, Schwammenthal E, Newell JB. Significant tricuspid regurgitation is a marker for adverse outcome in patients undergoing percutaneous balloon mitral valvuloplasty. *J Am Coll Cardiol* 1994;24(3):696–702.
4. Nath J, Foster E, Heidenreich PA. Impact of tricuspid regurgitation on long-term survival. *J Am Coll Cardiol* 2004;43(3):405–9.
5. Topilsky Y, Nkomo VT, Vatury O. Clinical outcome of isolated tricuspid regurgitation. *JACC Cardiovasc Imaging* 2014;7(12):1185–94.
6. Nishimura RA, Otto CM, Bonow RO. 2014 AHA/ACC guideline for the management of patients with valvular heart disease: executive summary: a report of the American College of Cardiology/American Heart Association Task Force on Practice Guidelines. *J Am Coll Cardiol* 2014;63(22):2438–88.
7. Nishimura RA, Otto CM, Bonow RO. 2014 AHA/ACC guideline for the management of patients with valvular heart disease: a report of the American College of Cardiology/American Heart Association Task Force on Practice Guidelines. *Circulation* 2014;129(23):e521–643.
8. Vahanian A, Alfieri O, Andreotti F. Joint Task Force on the Management of Valvular Heart Disease of ESC and EACTS. Guidelines on the management of valvular heart disease (version 2012). *Eur Heart J* 2012;33(19):2451–96.
9. Dreyfus GD, Corbi PJ, Chan KM, Bahrami T. Secondary tricuspid regurgitation or dilatation: which should be the criteria for surgical repair? *Ann Thorac Surg* 2005;79(1):127–32.
10. Chopra HK, Nanda NC, Fan P. Can two-dimensional echocardiography and Doppler color flow mapping identify the need for tricuspid valve repair? *J Am Coll Cardiol* 1989;14(5):1266–74.
11. Fukuda S, Gillinov AM, McCarthy PM. Determinants of recurrent or residual functional tricuspid regurgitation after tricuspid annuloplasty. *Circulation* 2006;114(Suppl. 1):I582–587.
12. Waller BF, Howard J, Fess S. Pathology of tricuspid valve stenosis and pure tricuspid regurgitation—part I. *Clin Cardiol* 1995;18:167–74.
13. Dávila JC. The Birth of intracardiac surgery: A semicentennial tribute. *Ann Thorac Surg* 1998;65:1809–1820.
14. Julian OC, Lopez-Belio M, Dye WS, Javid H, Grove WJ. The medial sternal incision in intracardiac surgery with extracorporeal circulation: a general evaluation of its use in heart surgery. *Surgery* 1957;42:753–761.
15. Praeger PI, Pootey RW, Moggio A, Somberg ED, Sarabu MR, Reed GE. Simplified method for re-operation on the mitral valve. *Ann Thorac Surg* 1989;48:835–837.

16. Braxton JH, Higgins RS, Schwann TA, Sanchez JA, Dewar JL, Kopf GS, Hammond GL, Letsou GV, Elefteriades JA. Reoperative mitral valve surgery via right thoracotomy: decreased bloodloss and improved haemodynamics. *J Heart Valve Dis* 1996;5(2):169-173.
17. Adams DH, Filsifou F, Byrne JG, Karavas AN Aklog L. Mitral valve repair in redo cardiac surgery. *J Cardiovasc Surg* 2002;17:40–45.
18. Casselman FP, Van Slycke S, Dom H, Lambrechts DL, Vermeulen Y, Vanermen H. Endoscopic mitral valve repair: feasible, reproducible, and durable. *J Thorac Cardiovasc Surg* 2003;125:273–282.
19. Casselman FP, Van Slycke S, Wellens F, De Geest R, Degrieck I, Van Praet F, Vermeulen Y, Vanermen H. Mitral valve surgery can now routinely be performed endoscopically. *Circulation* 2003;108:II48–II54.
20. Ricci D, Boffini M, Barbero C, Qarra SE, Marchetto G, Rinaldi M. Minimally invasive tricuspid valve surgery in patients at high risk. *J Thorac Cardiovasc Surg* 2014;147:996–1001.
21. Pfannmüller B, Misfeld M, Borger M, Etz C, Funkat A, Mohr F. Isolated reoperative minimally invasive tricuspid valve operations. *Ann Thorac Surg* 2012;94:2005–10.
22. Peng R, Ba J, Wang C, Lai H, Hu K, Shi H. A new venous drainage technique in redo minimally invasive tricuspid valve surgery: vacuum-assist venous drainage via a single femoral venous cannula. *Heart Lung Circ* 2017;26(2):201–204.
23. Jeanmart H, Casselman F, Grieck Y, Bakir Y, Coddens J, Foubert L, Vaerenbergh G, Vermeulen Y, Vanermen H. Avoiding vascular complications during minimally invasive, totally endoscopic intracardiac surgery. *J Thorac Cardiovasc Surg* 2007;133:1066–70.
24. Peng R, Shi H, Ba J, Wang C. Single femoral venous drainage versus both vena cava drainage in isolated repeat tricuspid valve surgery. *Int Heart J* 2018;59:518–522.
25. Casselman F, La Meir M, Jeanmart H, Mazzarro E, Coddens J, Praet F, Wellens F, Vermeulen Y, Vanermen H. Endoscopic mitral and tricuspid valve surgery after previous cardiac surgery. *Circulation* 2007;116:I-270–I-275.
26. Färber G, Tkebuchava S, Dawson RS, Kirov H, Schlattmann P, Doenst T. Minimally invasive, isolated tricuspid valve redo surgery: a safety and outcome analysis. *Thorac Cardiovasc Surg* 2018;66(7):564-571. doi: 10.1055/s-0038-1627452.
27. Maimaiti A, Wei L, Yang Y, Liu H, Wang C. Benefits of a right anterolateral minithoracotomy rather than a median sternotomy in isolated tricuspid redo procedures. *J Thorac Dis* 2017;9(5):1281–1288.
28. Lamelas J, Williams R, Mawad M, LaPietra A. Complications associated with femoral cannulation during minimally invasive cardiac surgery. *Ann Thorac Surg* 2017;103:1927–32.
29. Mihos CG, Pineda AM, Santana O, Krishna RK, Lamelas J. Tricuspid valve repair with pericardial tube placement via a right minithoracotomy. *J Heart Valve Dis* 2015;24(3):338–41.
30. Mihos CG, Pineda AM, Davila H, Larrauri-Reyes MC, Santana O. Combined mitral and tricuspid valve surgery performed via a right minithoracotomy approach. *Innovations (Phila)* 2015;10(5):304–8.
31. Urbandt P, Santana O, Mihos CG, Pineda AM, Lamelas J. Minimally invasive approach for isolated tricuspid valve surgery. *J Heart Valve Dis* 2014;23(6):783–7.
32. Minol JP, Boeken U, Weinreich T, Heimann M, Akhyari P, Kamiya H, Lichtenberg A. Isolated tricuspid valve surgery: a single institutional experience with the technique of minimally invasive surgery via right minithoracotomy. *Thorac Cardiovasc Surg* 2017;65(8):606–611.
33. Pfannmüller B, Davierwala P, Hirnle G, Borger M, Misfeld M, Garbade J, Seeburger J, Mohr F. Concomitant tricuspid valve repair in patients with minimally invasive mitral valve surgery. *Ann Cardiothorac Surg* 2013;2(6):758–764.
34. Pfannmuller B, Moz M, Misfeld M, Borger M, Funkat A, Garbade J, Mohr F. Isolated tricuspid valve surgery in patients with previous cardiac surgery. *J Thorac Cardiovasc Surg* 2013;146:841–7.
35. Lee T, Desai B, Glower D. Results of 141 consecutive minimally invasive tricuspid valve operations: an 11-year experience. *Ann Thorac Surg* 2009;88:1845–5.
36. Kypson AP, Glower D. Minimally invasive tricuspid operation using port access. *Ann Thorac Surg* 2002;74:43–5.
37. Lamelas J. Minimal access tricuspid valve surgery. *Ann Cardiothorac Surg* 2017;6(3):283–286.

38. Kofidis T, Chang GH, Lee CN. Establishment of a minimally invasive cardiac surgery programme in Singapore. *Singapore Med J* 2017;58(10):576–579.
39. Ad N, Holmes SD, Massimiano PS, Rongione AJ, Fornaresio LM, Fitzgerald D. The use of del Nido cardioplegia in adult cardiac surgery: a prospective randomized trial. *J Thorac Cardiovasc Surg* 2018;155:1011–8.
40. Martens S, Dietrich M, Doss M. Optimal carbon dioxide application for organ protection in cardiac surgery. *J Thorac Cardiovasc Surg* 2002;124:387–91.

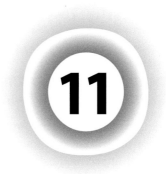

MINIMALLY INVASIVE COMBINED HEART VALVE SURGERY

FAIZUS SAZZAD AND THEO KOFIDIS

INTRODUCTION

Combined heart valve surgery and concomitant cardiac procedures comprise about one-third of all heart valve surgeries. However, the safety and benefits of combined procedure in a minimally invasive technique with one or more valve repairs or replacements have never been systematically analyzed. The reported evidence suggests that these procedures are effective. However, the fact remains that the technicality and challenge of completeness of the procedure through a small hole is the biggest challenge. For this reason, the chance of complications, and of converting the procedure to a full sternotomy approach as a result, is higher. Despite this, there are still many surgeons across the globe who have mastered these techniques [1].

The following procedures can be combined with each other:

∞ Minimally invasive mitral valve repair/replacement
∞ Minimally invasive aortic valve repair/replacement
∞ MICS tricuspid valve repair/replacement
∞ Secundum ASD closure
∞ Modified maze procedure
∞ Concomitant bypass surgery

HOW TO DO IT/STEP BY STEP

A. UPPER J STERNOTOMY APPROACH FOR DOUBLE VALVE REPAIR/REPLACEMENT (AVR+MVR)

A midline partial sternotomy with "J" extension to right third or fourth intercostal space. The upper mediastinum is exposed by using a single-blade chest spreader. The pericardium is usually retracted by using multiple stay sutures (Figure 11.1). The stay sutures are fashioned around the cut edge of the pericardium. Most of the stay sutures are used to create an exposed working area and separate the surrounding structures from the field of operation. Sometimes, an excess port is created to drag the sutures out (as described in famous "Miami" technique). The access port can be used as a drain tube site at the end of the procedure. Some of the stay sutures can be hitched to the skin.

If the anatomy is satisfactory, a groin-access femoro-femoral bypass is established. The femoral vessel cannula usually inserted using the Seldinger technique, within purse-string sutures and positioned under TEE guidance. Non-selective antegrade cardioplegia via the ascending aorta is used. A flexible cross clamp (i.e. Cygnet) is commonly carefully applied just at or above the level of the RPA.

After cardioplegic arrest, the standard oblique aortotomy is made on the ascending aorta with an extension towards the non-coronary sinus. The aortic valve is excised and the appropriate size of prosthesis is selected in the usual fashion.

The aorta is retracted anteriorly and leftwards with the help of the umbilical tape. This maneuver brings the superior surface of the left atrium closure to the surgical field and gives access to the LA roof. The LAtomy is made on the roof of left atrium. The mitral valve is then adequately exposed by inserting a USB-HV™ retractor. The rest of the mitral valve repair or replacement can be carried out using the standard MICS technique (refer to Chapter 9 for a more detailed discussion) (Figure 11.2).

After the completion of the mitral valve procedure LAtomy closure is preferred; it is difficult to suture the left atrial incision

FIGURE 11.2   DVR via J-type partial sternotomy – CTS.net.

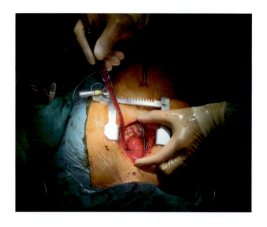

FIGURE 11.1   Upper J sternotomy for DVR.

FIGURE 11.3   Upper T mini sternotomy: DVR (AVR + MVR).

after aortic valve replacement. The AVR can be performed with supra-annular positioning of the valve with braided pledgeted sutures. The rest of the AVR follows standard AVR surgery techniques. An automated suture knotting device (i.e. Cor-Knot™) can be used to expedite the surgery. The pacing wires need to be attached to the intended locations before the release of the cross clamp. De-airing has always been a concern in the minimally invasive method. Routine use of CO_2 insufflations is useful. The process of de-airing should be monitored by TEE. After confirming complete de-airing and satisfactory prosthetic function on TEE, the rest of the procedure follows standard surgical steps for DVR.

B. UPPER T STERNOTOMY APPROACH

It is similar to the upper J sternotomy approach. An upper T sternotomy incision can provide a single surgical access site for a DVR. The prime consideration for an inverted "T" sternotomy is to preserve the internal mammary artery (Figure 11.3).

C. RIGHT MINI-THORACOTOMY APPROACH

1. Right mini thoracotomy (Kofidis technique) is a proven and trusted approach to minimally invasive mitral valve surgery. A combination of a number of concomitant surgeries can be carried out through the same incision. Along with the mitral valve repair or replacement surgery, tricuspid vale repair or replacement, right-sided coronary artery bypass, a modified atrial maze procedure, LA reductionplasty and left atrial appendage exclusion are the possible concomitant procedures. The closure of ASD is also done in combination with left or right heart minimally invasive surgery. Without appropriate caval isolation, ASD usually has a difficult access. The incision and exposure of the surgical field is similar to the standard MICS MVR technique. The strategical difference lies in the processes of cannulation and CPB establishment.

CAVAL ISOLATION

- ∞ Superior vena cava (SVC) cannulation: Wide-bore SVC cannulation from the right IJV commonly used. The linked video (Figure 11.4) shows the percutaneous cannulation of the SVC for extracorporeal circulation in minimally invasive cardiac surgery; a 17F Medtronic cannula is used.
- ∞ Inferior vena cava (IVC): Understanding of caval anatomy (Figure 11.5) is a crucial step to start an IVC cannulation and isolation. A wide-bore IVC cannula is commonly used. The cannulation technique is similar to the Seldinger technique used for usual SVC cannulation.
- ∞ Recently multistage caval cannula is used to cannulate both vena cavas together (Figure 11.6).

FIGURE 11.4   SVC cannulation for MICS.

FIGURE 11.5   Caval anatomy.

FIGURE 11.6 Multistage caval cannula, Medtronic.

- ∞ Percutaneous femoral vessel approach cannulation is a suitable option for peripheral cannulation [2] (Figure 11.7). The video link in Figure 11.8 demonstrates a percutaneous approach of femoral cannulation for MiMVR.

CAVAL OCCLUSION

- ∞ Caval isolation and occlusion can be particularly demanding in patients with enlarged and pressurized atria. The conventional way to isolate these vessels is to make a blunt dissection and use external snaring, where commonly umbilical tape snears are used.

2. Miami Method: However, the utility of a right anterior thoracotomy for aortic valve surgery is rising. The combination of an aortic valve procedure along with the mitral or tricuspid valve has been popularized as the "Miami Method" [3].

Preparation: Single lumen endotracheal tube, Swan Ganz catheter and transesophageal echocardiogram are prepared.

Exposition: The patient is placed in supine position, with a roll placed behind the scapula. The patient is then rolled to the left and the right arm placed over the head, with hips positioned as supine as possible.

Incision: The sternum is marked from the suprasternal notch to the lowest point of the xiphoid. Thereafter, the midpoint of the entire sternum is located. An imaginary line is drawn from this midpoint laterally. A 6-cm incision is then made lateral to, and starting at, the anterior axillary line. This will usually correspond to the

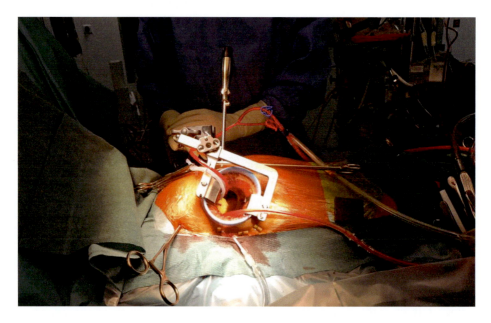

FIGURE 11.7 Operative setup for a right mini thoracotomy approach.

FIGURE 11.8 Percutaneous cannulation for minimally invasive surgery.

FIGURE 11.9 "Miami Method".

fourth intercostal space and provides excellent exposure to both the aortic and mitral valve. In female patients, the incision will be made in the inframammary crease laterally.

- ***Cardioplegia and cross clamp***: A retrograde cardioplegia cannula is inserted directly through the incision, with trans-incisional direct aortic cross clamping. One dose of antegrade cold blood cardioplegia is given, and thereafter, retrograde cold blood cardioplegia is delivered. Modified 4:1 blood to crystalloid Del Nido cardioplegia can also be used.
- ***Operation***: Usually a femoro-femoral bypass is performed; however, if severe peripheral vascular disease is present, the axillary artery in the axilla is cannulated instead. Venous drainage is augmented with vacuum assistance, which enables the application of negative pressures of between 35 and 65 mmHg as needed to decompress the right heart.

Complete circumferential aortotomy is made above the level of the sino-tubular junction. The aortic valve leaflets are removed and the annulus debrided. The LAtomy is carried out, and the MICS LA retractor is then utilized to retract the walls of the left atrium. Usually, repairs begin with the placement of the mitral annular sutures for better exposure. Carbon dioxide is infused into the operative field throughout the entire procedure. The LAtomy is then closed after mitral intervention.

Then with the aorta completely transected, three 3-0 prolene stay sutures are placed on the commissures. The aortic valve sutures are then placed through the annulus and, subsequently, the valve. The sutures are tied with a knot-setter. The circumferential aortotomy is closed with two running 5-0 prolene sutures.

Completion: The patient is returned to the Trendelenburg position once the cross clamp is removed. One Blake chest tube is left in the pleural cavity and another in the pericardial sac. A temporary ventricular pacer and the On-Q pain relief system (I-Flow, LLC, Irvine, CA, USA) are then passed through the chest tube incision.

The linked video in Figure 11.9 contains a clinical vignette, exposition, cardiopulmonary bypass and visualization, left atriotomy, mitral valve repair, aortic valve replacement and completion.

D. CONCOMITANT PROCEDURES

Heart valve surgery, along with CABG and other combinations, is also a valid option via different MICS approaches. Figure 11.10A depicts a concomitant procedure via upper J mini-sternotomy. A bypass conduit is seen to be used for the revascularization of the right coronary artery. In Figure 11.10B a unipolar maze is in progress during an MiMVr via right thoracotomy. Figure 11.10C showing right thoracotomy access for concomitant procedures with MICS CABG.

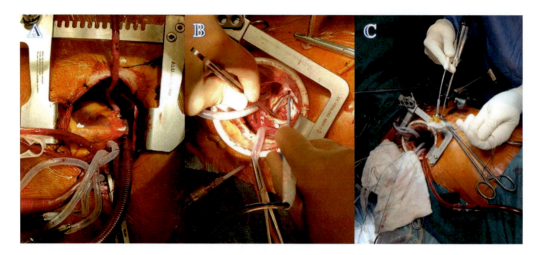

FIGURE 11.10 Concomitant MICS procedures: A. Upper J mini-sternotomy access for MiAVR + CABG (RCA). B. Right thoracotomy access for MiMVR + atrial ablation. C. Right thoracotomy access for MiMVR + CABG (RPDA).

TOOLS/INSTRUMENTS AND DEVICES

EXTERNAL DEFIBRILLATOR PADS

External defibrillator pads are placed on the patient prior to the operation. Whenever required, defibrillating shocks can be delivered to the patient during the procedure.

SOFT TISSUE RETRACTOR

Soft tissue retractors are a useful tool for good visualization through the keyhole (Figure 11.11).

ATRIAL LIFT SYSTEM AND VISOR

An atrial lift system can be used following the LAtomy or RAtomy in combined

FIGURE 11.12 Miami Instruments by LivaNova.

minimally invasive heart surgery, to achieve better exposure of the atria. The visor is used to hold open the valve orifice to make surgical intervention easier. The Atrial Lift System and Visor, Miami Instruments, Miami, FL, USA, is a useful commercially available retractor system (Figure 11.12).

ALTERNATIVES

CONVENTIONAL FULL STERNOTOMY APPROACH

The conventional full sternotomy approach is an alternative to minimally invasive combined heart surgery. Should severe complications develop during a minimally invasive combined heart surgery, the procedure can be converted to a full sternotomy approach.

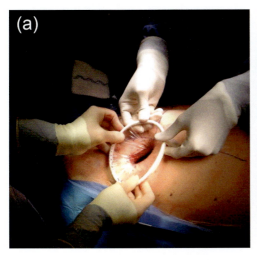 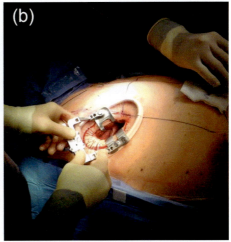

FIGURE 11.11 A. Use of soft tissue retractor at right thoracotomy. B. Thoracic rib retractors in situ.

CAVAL ISOLATION

An alternative technique to access the patient's IVC can be implemented via the left femoral vein (Figure 11.13). The route can be used to introduce a Coda balloon catheter (Cook Inc, Bloomington, IN), which can be placed at the junction of the IVC with the right atrium under transesophageal echocardiography guidance [4].

CAVEATS AND CONTROVERSIES

COMBINED PROCEDURES IN MINIMALLY INVASIVE VERSUS CONVENTIONAL APPROACHES

A study on the initial clinical outcomes of a combined mitral and aortic valve procedure via right mini-thoracotomy compared to a full median sternotomy is available in the link in Figure 11.14. The study observed that the minimally invasive approach produced slightly longer aortic cross clamp and cardiopulmonary bypass times as compared to the conventional, more invasive approach. **Conversion to sternotomy** Conversion to sternotomy is a primary bailout method for MICS, more often related to anatomical factors that creates difficulties [5]. Minoru Tabata et al has reported 2.6% conversion rate in their 9.5 years clinical experience [6].

RESEARCH, TRENDS AND INNOVATION

SOFT ROBOTICS IN MINIMALLY INVASIVE SURGERY

Robotic devices can be produced by using compliant and soft materials. The term "Soft Robotics" has been proposed. As the materials are soft, this technology been proposed as a good material for dealing with minimally invasive surgery. Unstructured environments or interacting with humans will be easy because these materials can deform around their environment. Soft

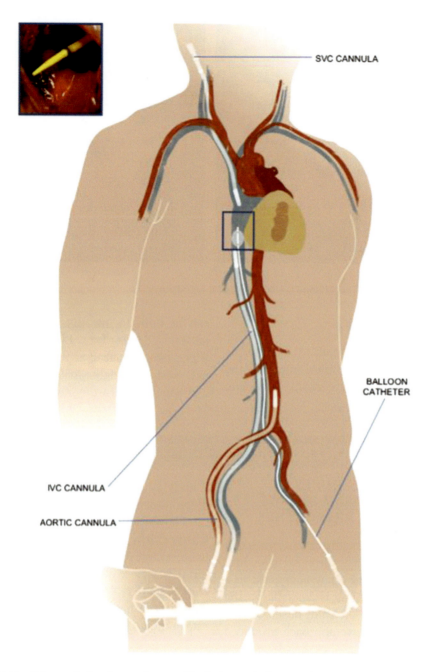

FIGURE 11.13 Schematic for alternative caval isolation technique with the use of Coda balloon catheter. (Reprinted from *Ann Thorac Surg*, 109(4), Sazzad F, Kuzemczak M, Kofidis T et al. A Novel Minimally Invasive Technique of Temporary Caval Occlusion for Right Heart Surgery, e309-e311, courtesy-Weronika Skiba, © 2020 by The Society of Thoracic Surgeons with permission from Elsevier.)

FIGURE 11.14 Combined mitral and aortic valve procedure.

FIGURE 11.16 MITACS by EACTS.

FIGURE 11.15 Soft Robotics in minimally invasive surgery.

FIGURE 11.17 ISMICS courses.

Robotic devices have desirable traits for applications in minimally invasive surgery (MIS), but many interdisciplinary challenges remain unsolved. A report can be found in the link (Figure 11.15).

WHERE AND HOW TO LEARN

MINIMALLY INVASIVE TECHNIQUES IN ADULT CARDIAC SURGERY (MITACS)

Information on the MITACS course can be found in the website linked in Figure 11.16.

INTERNATIONAL SOCIETY FOR MINIMALLY INVASIVE CARDIOTHORACIC SURGERY (ISMICS) COURSES

The ISMICS also offers courses on combined minimally invasive cardiac surgery (Figure 11.17).

REFERENCES

1. Guang Tong, Hao Yu, Xuan Zhou, Ben Zhang, Shenghui Bi, Lin Luo, Tao Yan, Xianyue Wang, Hua Lu, Tao Ma, Xiaowu Wang, Zhongchan Sun, Weida Zhang. Concomitant surgical atrial fibrillation ablation is safe and efficacious in patients undergoing double valve replacement – a cohort study. *International Journal of Surgery* 2018;57:54–59. doi: 10.1016/j.ijsu.2018.04.023.

2. Mahesh Ramchandani, Odeaa Al Jabbari, Walid K. Abu Saleh, Basel Ramlawi. Cannulation strategies and pitfalls in minimally invasive cardiac surgery. *Methodist DeBakey Cardiovascular Journal* 2016;12(1):10–13. doi: 10.14797/mdcj-12-1-10. PMID: 27127556.

3. Joseph Lamelas. Concomitant minithoracotomy aortic and mitral valve surgery: the minimally invasive "Miami

Method". *Annals of Cardiothoracic Surgery* 2015;4(1):85-87. doi: 10.3978/j.issn.2225-319X.2014.09.14.
4. Sazzad F, Kuzemczak M, Kofidis T. A Novel Minimally Invasive Technique of Temporary Caval Occlusion for Right Heart Surgery. *Ann Thorac Surg.* 2020;109(4):e309-e311. doi:10.1016/j.athoracsur.2019.10.033
5. Christidis NK, Fox SA, Swinamer SA, et al. Reason and Timing for Conversion to Sternotomy in Robotic-Assisted Coronary Artery Bypass Grafting and Patient Outcomes. *Innovations (Phila).* 2018;13(6):423–427. doi:10.1097/IMI.0000000000000566
6. Tabata M, Umakanthan R, Khalpey Z, et al. Conversion to full sternotomy during minimal-access cardiac surgery: reasons and results during a 9.5-year experience. *J Thorac Cardiovasc Surg.* 2007;134(1):165–169. doi:10.1016/j.jtcvs.2007.01.077

12.1

THE CORONARIES
Minimally Invasive Coronary Artery Bypass Grafting Surgery

JANET M. C. NGU, MING HAO GUO AND MARC RUEL

HISTORY OR INTRODUCTION

Minimally invasive coronary artery bypass grafting surgery (MICS CABG) was developed by Dr. Joseph T. McGinn Jr and Dr. Marc Ruel in the year 2005. MICS CABG allows for revascularization to all myocardial territories through a small left anterior thoracotomy at the fourth or fifth intercostal space. This operation does not require robotic or thoracoscopic equipment [1], and can be performed with or without the utilization of cardiopulmonary bypass (CPB) [2]. In addition, anastomoses to different coronary territories can be manually constructed under direct vision. Over the years, there have been significant advancements and improvements in this technique. It has been widely adopted by cardiac surgeons worldwide, including North America, Europe and Asia (Figure 12.1.1).

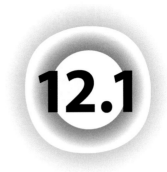

HOW TO DO IT/STEP BY STEP

PATIENT POSITIONING

- ∞ Fifteen- to thirty-degree right lateral decubitus position, using a longitudinal shoulder roll under the left scapula.
- ∞ Left arm may be left on the side or elevated over the head using a Krauss

FIGURE 12.1.1 A presentation on the MICS and robotic CABG.

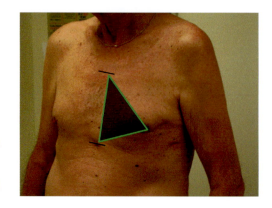

FIGURE 12.1.2 Chest marking for MICS CABG.

- arm support with a protection pad secured to the right side of the operating table.
- ∞ The groins should be accessible for femoral cannulation should CPB be needed.
- ∞ Both legs should be accessible for vein graft harvesting.
- ∞ The use of a radial artery for multiple arterial grafting is desirable. If the right is used, it can be harvested at the same time as the thoracotomy and LITA harvest. If the left radial is used, this should be completed prior to positioning the patient for MICS CABG.

CHEST MARKING AND INCISION

- ∞ The incision is marked using an imaginary triangle that connects the sternal angle and the xyphoid (Figure 12.1.2); this enters the correct space in most cases.
- ∞ A 4–6-cm curvilinear incision is made from the mid-clavicular line of the fourth or fifth intercostal space and extended laterally.
  - ∞ Men: usually just below the nipple.
  - ∞ Women: below the breast along the infra-mammary crease; the dissection is then carried underneath the breast tissue to access the desired intercostal space, usually going one space cephalad.
- ∞ Be cautious when extending the incision medially, as there is a risk of damaging the left internal thoracic artery (LITA).
- ∞ Once the pleural space is entered, use index finger to locate the apex of the heart.
- ∞ It is critically important that the apex be located one intercostal space beneath the incision:
  - ∞ Allows for optimal manipulation of the position of the heart for distal targets.
  - ∞ Simultaneously provides access to the aorta for proximal anastomosis.

HARVESTING THE LEFT INTERNAL THORACIC ARTERY (LITA)

- ∞ A ThoraTrak retractor (Medtronic, Inc, Minneapolis, MN) with #1 and #5 blades is inserted through the incision to spread the intercostal space.
- ∞ The top end of the ThoraTrak retractor track is connected cephalad to a Rultract Skyhook retractor (Rultract, Inc, Independence, OH), which is positioned at the patient's left shoulder.
- ∞ The LITA can be found medial to the intercostal space incision, and it can be harvested from a lateral approach under direct vision using long instruments, in either a skeletonized or non-skeletonized manner.

- ∞ LITA harvesting begins at its mid-portion directly in-line with the incision, and the LITA is dissected proximally to the level of the subclavian vein.
- ∞ After this, the Rultract retractor is connected to the inferior end of the ThoraTrak retractor to elevate the distal end – to facilitate the harvesting of the distal portion of the LITA down to its bifurcation.
- ∞ Other conduits such as the radial artery and saphenous vein grafts can be harvested in the usual fashion.

PROXIMAL ANASTOMOSIS

- ∞ Exposure of the aorta is the key to the proximal anastomoses and can be achieved in a stepwise approach:
  a. Anesthesia:
     i. Maintain a central venous pressure between 8 and 12 mmHg to minimize right ventricular distension.
     ii. Increase the positive end-expiratory pressure (PEEP) on the isolated right lung up to 10–12 cm H_2O to hyperinflate the right lung, which helps push the aorta towards the MICS CABG incision.
  b. The Rultract Skyhook retractor is repositioned to pull the ThoraTrak retractor in a cephalad and rightward direction to expose the aorta.
  c. The pericardial fat on the anterior surface is excised to allow for better exposure.
  d. The pericardium is opened gradually towards and midline anterior to the ascending aorta; multilevel pericardial retraction sutures are placed to bring the superior mediastinum inferiorly and leftward towards the MICS CABG incision; an unfolded 4 × 4 gauze is placed anterior to the superior vena cava to facilitate leftward displacement of the ascending aorta (Ruel technique).
  e. Alternatively, the posterior ascending aorta can be dissected from the pulmonary artery, and an open 4 × 4 gauze or a half-inch Penrose drain can be passed posterior to the aorta for left anterior retraction (McGinn technique).

FIGURE 12.1.3 Proximal anastomosis during MICS CABG.

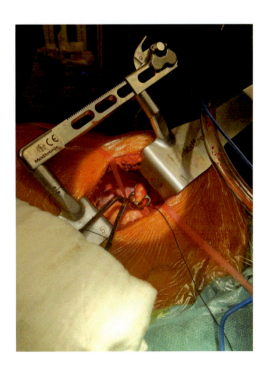

FIGURE 12.1.4 Proximal anastomose in MICS CABG.

f. With either technique, an 8-mm incision is made in the left sixth or seventh intercostal space in the anterior axillary line to allow the introduction of the Octopus Non-Sternotomy Tissue Stabilizer (Medtronic) or equivalent.

g. The right ventricular outflow tract (RVOT) or proximal pulmonary artery is gently flattened and displaced leftward and posteriorly by using an epicardial stabilizer; TEE is critical at this time to ensure that there is not RVOT obstruction
   - After the sequential maneuvers above, the proximal ascending aorta will be well exposed.
   - Target systolic blood pressure to be between 75 and 85 mmHg when applying the side-biting aortic clamp to the aorta.
   - Conduits can be anastomosed to the proximal aorta under direct visualization using long instruments in the usual fashion.
   - After completing the proximal anastomosis, the conduits should be marked to ensure proper orientation (Figure 12.1.3 and Figure 12.1.4.).

DISTAL ANASTOMOSIS

- Anterior wall (i.e. left anterior descending artery LAD)
  - The LAD territory is typically directly visualized underneath the initial MICS CABG incision with minimal movement of the heart.
  - The Octopus Non-Sternotomy Tissue Stabilizer (Medtronic) is re-inserted through the same incision at the left sixth or seventh intercostal space in the anterior axillary line.
  - The Octopus Tissue Stabilizer is applied to the LAD target.
  - Distal anastomosis to LAD is performed under direct vision in the usual fashion.
- Lateral wall (i.e. obtuse marginal OM)
  - The suction cup of a Starfish Non-Sternotomy Heart Positioner

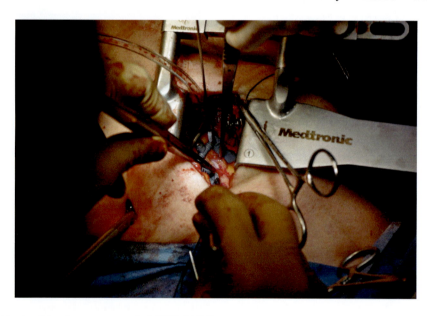

FIGURE 12.1.5 Distal anastomose in MICS CABG.

(Medtronic) is detached from the handle; an umbilical tape is secured to the suction cup to make an "armless Starfish Heart Positioner".
- ∞ The armless Starfish Heart Positioner is applied with suction adjacent to the cardiac apex towards the lateral wall.
- ∞ Using the Starfish Heart Positioner, the apex is retracted inferiorly towards the right hip, and the marginal branches of the circumflex coronary artery can be well visualized.
- ∞ The same Octopus Tissue Stabilizer used previously is applied to the OM target and the distal anastomosis can be performed under direct vision in the usual fashion.
∞ Inferior wall (i.e. posterior descending artery [PDA])
- ∞ Similarly, the retraction of the cardiac apex using the armless Starfish Heart Positioner toward the patient's left shoulder allows visualization of the PDA branch of the right coronary artery.
- ∞ The Octopus Tissue Stabilizer is applied to the PDA target.
- ∞ The distal anastomosis is performed under direct vision in the usual fashion (Figure 12.1.5).

CHEST CLOSURE

∞ One Blake drain is placed into the pericardial space and extended into the left pleural space, through the same incision at the left sixth or seventh intercostal space in which the Octopus Non-Sternotomy Tissue Stabilizer (Medtronic) was inserted.
∞ The left lung is reinflated slowly to ensure proper lies of grafts (especially LITA-LAD) and the Blake drain.
∞ The intercostal space is reapproximated using one or two No. 2 Vicryl sutures in simple interrupted fashion.
∞ The subcutaneous tissue is closed in two layers using 2-0 Monocryl sutures.
∞ The skin is closed using dissolvable sutures in subcuticular fashion (Figure 12.1.6 and Figure 12.1.7).

FIGURE 12.1.6 On MICS CABG, Joseph McGinn.

FIGURE 12.1.7 MICS CABG by Sathyaki Nambala.

POST-OPERATIVE CARE

∞ The drain should stay in the patient for at 3 days post-operatively.
∞ Adequate pain control.
∞ Watch for pleural effusion and rapid atrial fibrillation.

TOOLS/INSTRUMENTS AND DEVICES

- Key instruments:
  - ThoraTrak MICS Retractor System or equivalent
    This device is used for retracting the intercostal space in MICS.
  - Rultract Skyhook retractor or equivalent
    This device can be joined to the ThoraTrak retractor to facilitate the harvesting of the distal portion of the LITA.
  - Octopus Non-Sternotomy Tissue Stabilizer or equivalent
    This device has a three-pod headlink that is small and appropriate for use in MICS CABG. It is also flexible, making it ideal for use through small incisions (Figure 12.1.8).
  - Armless Starfish Heart Positioner or equivalent
    This device comes with flexible suction pods that adapt to the shape of the patient's heart, allowing for better access to any of the coronary arteries in an MICS CABG.
  - Derra aortic clamp or equivalent
    The Derra aortic clamp can be used to control blood flow in vessels.
  - Kay-Lambert aortic clamp or equivalent

This device is used when an anastomosis needs to be performed (Figure 12.1.9).

FIGURE 12.1.8 Medtronic tissue stabilizer.

FIGURE 12.1.9 Atraumatic instrument list, Philing.

FIGURE 12.1.10 MICS CABG using the da Vinci surgical robot.

PERIOPERATIVE CONSIDERATION

A successful MICS CABG requires careful preoperative assessment and planning. Table 12.1.1 summarizes several critical considerations with the related reasons prior to an MICS CABG.

ANESTHESIA

Close collaboration between the anesthesiologist and surgeon is extremely critical to ensure a successful MICS CABG. The following should be established or administered prior to the start of the procedure:

282   Minimally Invasive Cardiac Surgery

FIGURE 12.1.11 Totally endoscopic CABG.

FIGURE 12.1.13 Strategies for MICS CABG, Prem Rabindra.

FIGURE 12.1.12 Procedure video with Joseph T. McGinn.

- ∞ Intubation with a double-lumen endotracheal tube or the utilization of bronchial blockers allows for left-lung ventilation.
- ∞ Transesophageal echocardiography (TEE):
  - ∞ To monitor cardiac function.
  - ∞ To ensure no RVOT obstruction during positioning of the heart for proximal anastomosis (described in the "How to do it" section).
  - ∞ To help position guide, wire-guided femoral arterial and venous cannulas should be used.

- ∞ Routine cardiac surgical monitoring: peripheral arterial line, central venous line and/or pulmonary artery catheter placement.
- ∞ Paravertebral thoracic (T2–T3) blockade can be considered for better post-procedural pain control.

ALTERNATIVE APPROACHES

MICS CABG is certainly an important alternative to conventional sternotomy for coronary revascularization. Other less commonly done approaches include robotic CABG and totally endoscopic CABG (Figure 12.1.10 to Figure 12.1.14).

TABLE 12.1.1 Critical considerations during preparation for an MICS CABG

Consideration	Reasons
Good chest wall anatomy (re: morbid obesity, previous chest trauma)	Allows for good exposure of the heart
Good femoral access	Allows for peripheral cannulation if CPB is needed, either electively or emergently
LV size, performance and hemodynamic stability	Ability to tolerate hemodynamic changes associated with manual manipulation of the heart
Adequate pulmonary function	Ability to tolerate single-lung ventilation and change in positive pressure ventilation
Adequate target vessel size and quality	Small or intramyocardial targets are feasible with higher technical demand
No significant aortic calcification	Allows for side-biting aortic clamp for proximal anastomosis

CAVEATS AND CONTROVERSIES

In our opinion, it appears important that MICS CABG be part of each major cardiac surgery referral center's armamentarium in this day and age so as to better serve the patients who are anatomically suitable for this. Patient selection and an efficient "heart team" are the key to success in the practice of MICS CABG.

FIGURE 12.1.14 How to perform an MIDCAB step-by-step, CTS.net.

RESEARCH, TRENDS AND INNOVATION

McGinn and Ruel, in a seminal paper [3], showed that, with the use of a minimally invasive strategy, it is possible to revascularize multiple myocardial territories, namely the anterior, lateral and inferior myocardial territories. The team successfully showed that multi-vessel minimally invasive CABG can be done safely and effectively with excellent short-term outcomes where perioperative mortality rates and risks of conversion to sternotomy were low.

WHERE AND HOW TO LEARN

In addition to the various online resources it is now possible to learn these techniques from specialized centers worldwide, including the prestigious centers of Marc Ruel (Cardiac Surgery Research at the University of Ottawa Heart Institute), McGinn (Sanger Heart and Vascular Institute, North Carolina) and Theodoros Kofidis (National University Heart Centre, Singapore).

REFERENCES

1. Chan V, Lapierre H, Sohmer B, Mesana TG, Ruel M. Handsewn proximal anastomoses onto the ascending aorta through a small left thoracotomy during minimally invasive multivessel coronary artery bypass grafting: a stepwise approach to safety and reproducibility. *Semin Thorac Cardiovasc Surg.* 2012;24(1):79-83. doi:10.1053/j.semtcvs.2011.12.010.
2. Gothard, J.W.W. (2004). *Minimally Invasive Cardiac Surgery*, 2nd ed. *BJA: British Journal of Anaesthesia* 92(4):607–607. doi: 10.1093/bja/aeh537
3. McGinn, J.T. Jr, Usman, S., Lapierre, H., Pothula, V.R., Mesana, T.G., & Ruel, M. (2009). Minimally invasive coronary artery bypass grafting: dual-center experience in 450 consecutive patients. *Circulation* 120:S78–84.

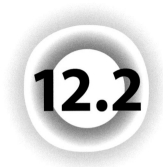

12.2

THE CORONARIES
Robot Facilitated Coronary Artery Bypass Grafting

LÁSZLÓ GÖBÖLÖS AND JOHANNES BONATTI

HISTORY AND INTRODUCTION

The general goal of minimally invasive robotic surgical procedures is to incur the smallest possible trauma during the intervention via a port-only approach, instead of extensive exposures (Figure 12.2.1). After unsuccessful approaches to perform endoscopic coronary bypass surgery by applying long shafted thoracoscopic devices, the ground-breaking total endoscopic coronary bypass grafting (TECAB) was delivered in 1998 utilizing a surgical robot [1,2].

In the past two decades the latter technique has gradually evolved from a single- to a multivessel operation, also practiced on a beating heart or under cardioplegic settings [3–9]. (Figure 12.2.2).

The advancing functionality of the robotic system also facilitated the progression to harvesting bilateral internal thoracic arteries with a view towards total arterial grafting via TECAB [10]. TECAB is often combined with percutaneous coronary intervention techniques – integrated or hybrid procedures. Current surgical robots equipped with procedure-specific robotic adapters ("end effectors") on the medical device market have significantly improved surgical vision, ease of target area exposure and overall operative ergonomics. As with other minimally invasive techniques, a learning curve with robot-facilitated TECAB is unavoidable [11]. However, given

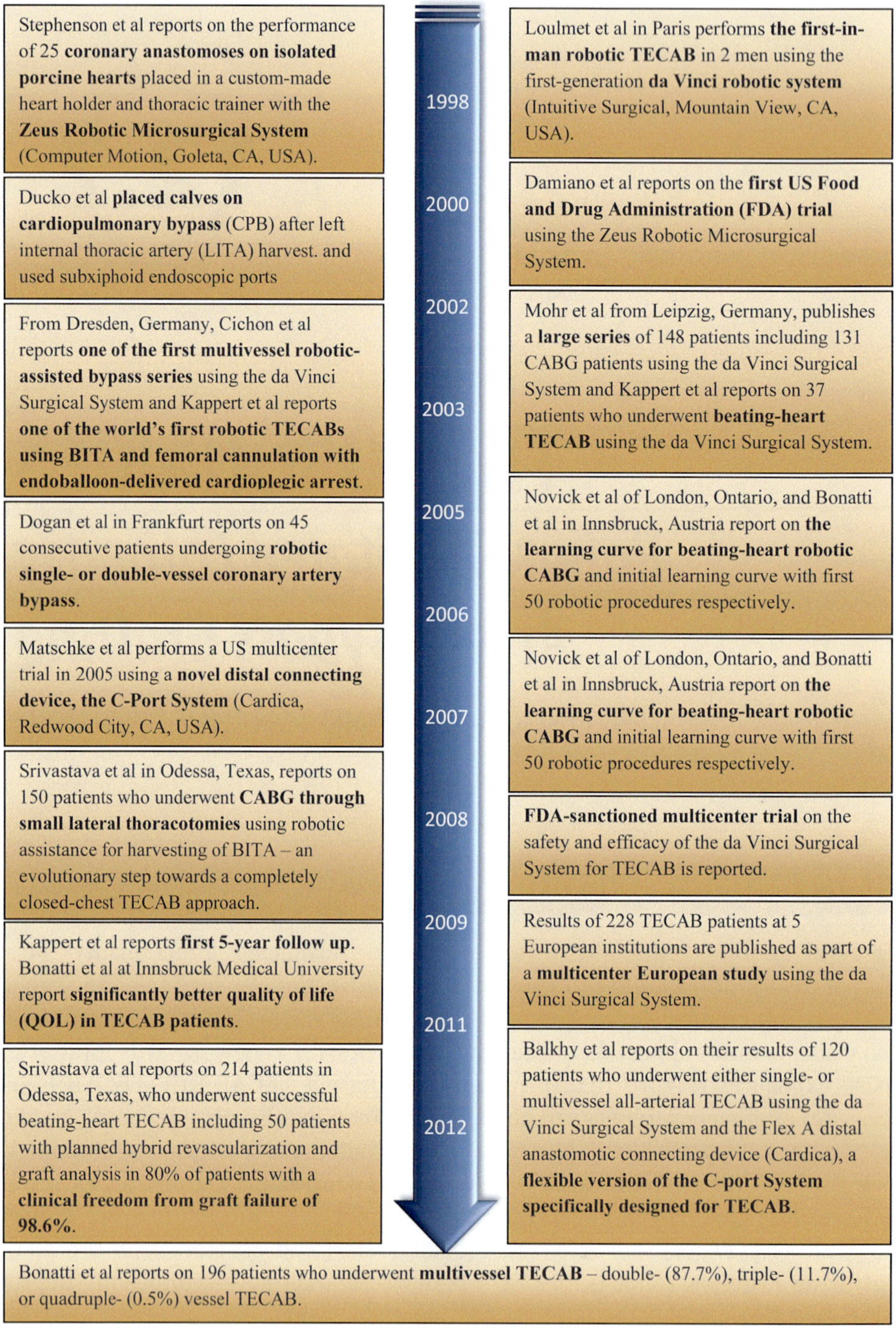

Timeline: Brief history of robotic-assisted CABG

1998
- Stephenson et al reports on the performance of 25 **coronary anastomoses on isolated porcine hearts** placed in a custom-made heart holder and thoracic trainer with the **Zeus Robotic Microsurgical System** (Computer Motion, Goleta, CA, USA).
- Loulmet et al in Paris performs **the first-in-man robotic TECAB** in 2 men using the first-generation **da Vinci robotic system** (Intuitive Surgical, Mountain View, CA, USA).

2000
- Ducko et al **placed calves on cardiopulmonary bypass** (CPB) after left internal thoracic artery (LITA) harvest. and used subxiphoid endoscopic ports
- Damiano et al reports on the **first US Food and Drug Administration (FDA) trial** using the Zeus Robotic Microsurgical System.

2002 / 2003
- From Dresden, Germany, Cichon et al reports **one of the first multivessel robotic-assisted bypass series** using the da Vinci Surgical System and Kappert et al reports **one of the world's first robotic TECABs using BITA and femoral cannulation with endoballoon-delivered cardioplegic arrest**.
- Mohr et al from Leipzig, Germany, publishes a **large series** of 148 patients including 131 CABG patients using the da Vinci Surgical System and Kappert et al reports on 37 patients who underwent **beating-heart TECAB** using the da Vinci Surgical System.

2005 / 2006
- Dogan et al in Frankfurt reports on 45 consecutive patients undergoing **robotic single- or double-vessel coronary artery bypass**.
- Novick et al of London, Ontario, and Bonatti et al in Innsbruck, Austria report on **the learning curve for beating-heart robotic CABG** and initial learning curve with first 50 robotic procedures respectively.

2007
- Matschke et al performs a US multicenter trial in 2005 using a **novel distal connecting device, the C-Port System** (Cardica, Redwood City, CA, USA).
- Novick et al of London, Ontario, and Bonatti et al in Innsbruck, Austria report on **the learning curve for beating-heart robotic CABG** and initial learning curve with first 50 robotic procedures respectively.

2008
- Srivastava et al in Odessa, Texas, reports on 150 patients who underwent **CABG through small lateral thoracotomies** using robotic assistance for harvesting of BITA – an evolutionary step towards a completely closed-chest TECAB approach.
- **FDA-sanctioned multicenter trial** on the safety and efficacy of the da Vinci Surgical System for TECAB is reported.

2009 / 2011
- Kappert et al reports **first 5-year follow up**. Bonatti et al at Innsbruck Medical University report **significantly better quality of life (QOL) in TECAB patients**.
- Results of 228 TECAB patients at 5 European institutions are published as part of a **multicenter European study** using the da Vinci Surgical System.

2012
- Srivastava et al reports on 214 patients in Odessa, Texas, who underwent successful beating-heart TECAB including 50 patients with planned hybrid revascularization and graft analysis in 80% of patients with a **clinical freedom from graft failure of 98.6%**.
- Balkhy et al reports on their results of 120 patients who underwent either single- or multivessel all-arterial TECAB using the da Vinci Surgical System and the Flex A distal anastomotic connecting device (Cardica), a **flexible version of the C-port System specifically designed for TECAB**.

Bonatti et al reports on 196 patients who underwent **multivessel TECAB** – double- (87.7%), triple- (11.7%), or quadruple- (0.5%) vessel TECAB.

FIGURE 12.2.1 Brief history of robotic-assisted CABG [1].

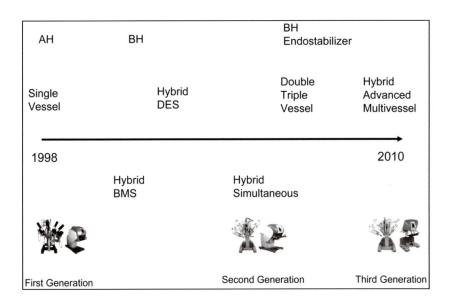

FIGURE 12.2.2 Development of robotic totally endoscopic coronary artery bypass grafting from 1998 to 2010. Note the improvement in performance from single bypass grafting only to complex surgical endoscopic and hybrid interventions. AH indicates arrested heart; BH, beating heart; BMS, bare metal stent; and DES, drug-eluting stent.

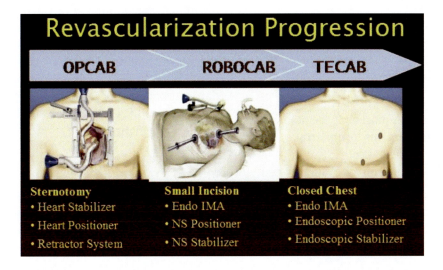

FIGURE 12.2.3 Revascularization progression. IMA = internal mammary artery; NS = non-sternotomy; =OPCAB = off-pump coronary artery bypass; ROBOCAB = robotic-assisted coronary artery bypass; TECAB = totally endoscopic coronary artery bypass. (Reprinted from *Ann Thorac Surg*, 82(3), Turner WF Jr, Sloan JH. Robotic-assisted coronary artery bypass on a beating heart: initial experience and implications for the future, 790–794, © 2006 by The Society of Thoracic Surgeons with permission from Elsevier.)

the intuitive feel of open surgery provided by the modern robot console, a cardiac surgeon in an experienced center may achieve optimal results without a protracted learning curve [12] (Figure 12.2.3).

HOW TO DO IT/STEP BY STEP

PATIENT SELECTION

In our opinion, any patient who presents with clear indication of coronary bypass surgery is a candidate for TECAB. However, it is essential to be aware of major contraindications. Hence TECAB represents an elective surgical approach, and redo procedures would challenge the surgeon by leading to the extensive and tedious procedure of adhesiolysis in the endoscopic setting. Keeping in mind the detailed contraindications, 25–30% of the current coronary artery bypass grafting (CAB) population can in our hands be treated via a robotic endoscopic pathway. As TECAB necessitates significant surgical training, it is strongly recommended to start with simple operations, exclusively in selected low-risk patients.

PREPARATION

Only one surgical robot is available on the medical devices market at the moment that enables the surgeon to undertake TECAB. Robotic surgical units usually possess the third-generation da Vinci system (Si version). Figure 12.2.4 demonstrates the operator's placement at the robotic console maneuvering with so called "masters", translating surgical actions into intrathoracic robotic instrument movements and robotic 3D camera positions. Foot pedals allow instrument and camera control to be swapped, including electrocautery. Surgical vision is maintained by a high-resolution 3D binocular system.

OPERATIVE GUIDE

STEP 1: PATIENT PLACEMENT AND OPERATIVE START-UP

The patient is placed in standard supine position on the operative table with the upper limbs stacked beside the trunk and the left chest side slightly elevated using an antidecubitus jelly-pack. We always have to be aware of the emerging necessity of an urgent sternotomy. Therefore, the patient has to be prepared and draped as for a standard coronary procedure and the equipment for open CAB should always be ready on the spot (Figure 12.2.5).

STEP 2: PORT INSERTION AND ROBOT DOCKING

Ports should be guided into the left pleural cavity by the most experienced team member in an ideal case, as correct port placement is essential for smooth operation (Figure 12.2.6). Port insertion requires complete left lung deflation to avoid organ injury; "lung down" must be clearly reassured by the anesthetic team prior to any insertion attempts.

The camera port is positioned in the fifth intercostal space/anterior axillary line, and CO_2 filling commences at 8–10 mmHg

FIGURE 12.2.4 Operator's placement at the robotic console.

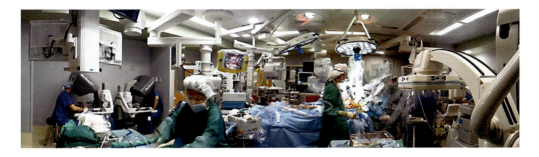

FIGURE 12.2.5 TECAB procedure being performed in the University of Maryland hybrid operating room. TECAB, robotic totally endoscopic coronary artery bypass [1].

pressure. If hemodynamic instability occurs at this step, CO_2 pressure has to be set accordingly to hinder ongoing drop in the central venous return.

The chest cavity is to be visualized under direct scope sight; then the right and left instrument accesses are inserted four fingerbreadths apart cranially and caudally from the camera port, halfway between the anterior axillary and mid-clavicular lines. After all, the surgical robot is docked to the operative table. A special robotic diathermy spatula is mounted onto the right manipulator arm and simultaneously a Debakey forceps on the contralateral side. Figure 12.2.7 demonstrates the correct port arrangement and instrument placement. Figure 12.2.8 shows the docked robotic arms in action.

STEP 3: INTERNAL MAMMARY ARTERY TAKEDOWN

As the next step, the 30° angled robotic camera has to be turned to "camera up" view. The internal mammary artery (IMA) should be clearly identified by its obvious pulsations in the usual anatomic position. Applying the skeletonized IMA harvest method, we recommend setting the diathermy to 15–20 Watts so as not to expose the graft material to excessive heat shock. Side branch cauterization on the adjacent chest wall is usually sufficient throughout IMA takedown (Figure 12.2.9). Rarely, Liga-clipping is necessary to close up significant branches or to control side branch hemorrhage.

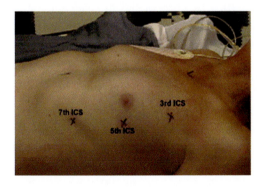

FIGURE 12.2.6 Skin markings showing port positioning for the camera arm in the fifth intercostal space (5th ICS), left instrument arm in the seventh intercostal space (7th ICS) and right instrument arm in the third intercostal space (3rd ICS). (Reprinted from *Ann Thorac Surg*, 81(3), Srivastava S, Gadasalli S, Agusala M, et al. Use of bilateral internal thoracic arteries in CABG through lateral thoracotomy with robotic assistance in 150 patients, 800-806, © 2006 by The Society of Thoracic Surgeons with permission from Elsevier.)

FIGURE 12.2.7 Correct port arrangement and instrument placement.

FIGURE 12.2.8 Docked robotic arms in action.

FIGURE 12.2.11 Utility port placement.

FIGURE 12.2.9 IMA harvesting technique.

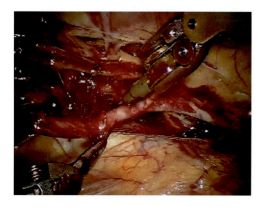

FIGURE 12.2.10 Left IMA harvest.

For bilateral IMA harvesting the right pleural space can be well accessed through extended retrosternal dissection. To simplify the procedure, in case of double IMA takedown, we prepare the right artery before the left one. Otherwise, access and vision might be compromised with a reverse sequence. After heparin administration, the IMA can be clipped distally followed by division with robotic Potts scissors. The completed graft is then sunk into the left pleural cavity, facilitating additional autodilation (Figure 12.2.10).

STEP 4: UTILITY PORT PLACEMENT

After IMA takedown, a 5-mm diameter utility port should be inserted under clear scope vision opposite the camera port in the left parasternal region. This step has significantly reduced procedure durations according to the current medical reports. This port enables seamless surgical material supply and removal, e.g. sutures, bulldogs, silastic tapes, suction tubing (Figure 12.2.11).

STEP 5: PRECORDIAL FAT PAD RESECTION AND PERICARDIAL EXPOSURE

At this step the camera is facing down to visualize the precordial fat pad and pericardium. A diathermy spatula is inserted on the right and long tip forceps on the left side to remove the fat pad in a craniocaudal direction. An oversized pericardial fat pad might require initiating cardiopulmonary bypass first to empty the heart so as to enhance the resection process by exposing further the pleural cavity.

Then, the pericardium is opened just above the right ventricular outflow tract. The incision is extended heading towards the diaphragmatic pericardial fold and then laterally. The aperture is further extended cranially in the direction of the phrenic nerve. The anatomic boundary of the latter must be always identified without any doubt. Mind both the phrenic nerve and left atrial appendage due to their vicinity to the pericardial aperture line (Figure 12.2.12).

FIGURE 12.2.12   Pericardial exposure.

FIGURE 12.2.13   Peripheral vascular cannulation.

STEP 6: PERIPHERAL VASCULAR CANNULATION AND APPLICATION OF ENDOCLAMP (ENDOBALLOON OCCLUSION)

The left groin offers a standard vascular exposure target. A limited perivascular dissection should be performed to avoid postoperative lymphatic leakage. To prevent malperfusion of the corresponding distal vascular territory, an extra recurrent femoral perfusion loop is placed and the peripheral tissue supply is monitored in real-time by near-infrared spectroscopy (NIRS). Venous return is established by a 25 Fr Seldinger-type cannula forwarded to the superior vena cava under TOE guidance. A 21 or 23 Fr arterial line having a sheathed side branch is inserted into the common femoral artery, and the cardiopulmonary bypass circuit is built.

A completely deflated balloon is progressed through the sheathed femoral arterial side branch. Under real-time TEE supervision, the guide wire is propagated towards the aortic root, and the endoballoon is positioned just right above the aortic valve. The cardioplegic line and root

FIGURE 12.2.14   Beating-heart totally endoscopic coronary artery bypass.

vent are connected to the extracorporeal circuit, and aortic root and simultaneous endoballoon pressure measurements are registered by corresponding manometers. If other cannulation approaches are necessitated, the endoballoon catheter can still be inserted in most cases via a separate 19 Fr cannula placed into the common femoral artery (Figure 12.2.13).

STEP 7: CARDIOPULMONARY BYPASS

The extracorporeal circulation in arrested-heart (AH)-TECAB is started gradually under TOE vision of the descending thoracic aorta to allow meticulous inspection for any signs of retrograde aortic dissection as early as possible. At sufficient venous drainage the blood pressure is low and also the lack of ventricular ejections facilitates the endoballoon inflation in the correct position. Correct positioning is monitored by TOE and adequate bilateral radial arterial perfusion pressures is maintained.

After this step, cardioplegia is administered. Rapid cardioplegic induction is facilitated with adenosine administration (6 mg/20 mL of normal saline). If sufficient balloon occlusion is proven, systemic cooling to 34°C is commenced and cardioplegia repeated every 20 minutes.

STEP 8: IDENTIFICATION AND EXPOSURE OF THE TARGET VESSELS

To expose different structures on the heart surface, the robotic endostabilizer provides an effective support in both BH-TECAB

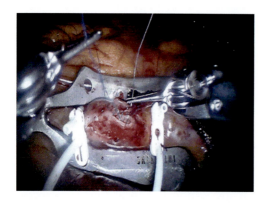

FIGURE 12.2.15 The endostabilizer is placed into the intrathoracic space via a subcostal port docked on the fourth arm of the da Vinci® system right after IMA takedown and heart exposure

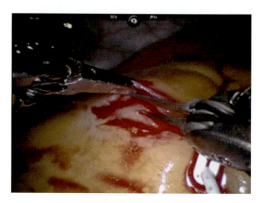

FIGURE 12.2.17 Coronary arteriotomy with endoscopic Potts scissors.

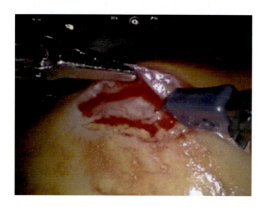

FIGURE 12.2.16 Opening of coronary with endoscopic knife.

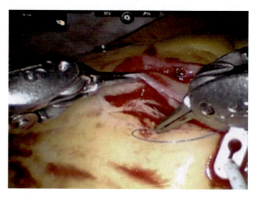

FIGURE 12.2.18 First stitch in the coronary, going from inside to outside, on the toe side.

and AH-TECAB. This device is fed through a 12-mm port situated on the left subcostal space two fingerbreadths lateral to the xiphoid angle. The insertion process is guided by the robotic camera in "up-facing" view and is directed by the patient site surgeon towards the patient's left shoulder. The subcostal port is connected to the fourth arm of the da Vinci system.

To gain an optimal view and access to the targeted coronary arteries, the camera is set "face down" (Figure 12.2.14). With the aid of a subcostal endostabilizer device, the left anterior descending (LAD) and circumflex (Cx) coronary artery branches can be sufficiently reached. The endostabilizer is activated by a dedicated foot pedal and the suction pods are lined up alongside the target area. Local immobilization is achieved in this fashion in beating-heart TECAB, and the target vessel is moved into a comfortable work position in both BH-TECAB and AH-TECAB.

The right coronary artery system can be accessed by inserting the endostabilizer through the 12-mm left-sided instrument port. With this port arrangement the subcostal port can be used as the left robotic instrument arm. The acute margin of the right ventricle is lifted up using the endostabilizer, and excellent access to the posterior descending artery or posterolateral artery can be obtained. To this point, we have applied this

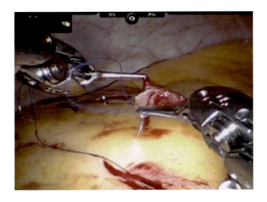

FIGURE 12.2.19 First stitch in the mammary, going from inside to outside.

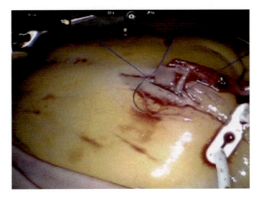

FIGURE 12.2.20 Suture of the back wall of the anastomosis.

method only in arrested-heart TECAB. As appropriate exposure of the target vessel is achieved, the epicardium is opened with robotic Potts scissors (Figure 12.2.15).

STEP 9: ROBOT-FACILITATED ENDOSCOPIC CORONARY ANASTOMOSIS

Prior to start the coronary anastomotic process, final fashioning is undertaken on the bypass graft material. The bulldog occluded graft facet is shaped in an oblique manner and further opened to a total length of 4 mm to create a "cobra head"-type anastomotic profile. Simultaneously the free flow of the vessel has to be ensured. The target coronary artery is dissected for exposure of the target using the robotic instruments. To maintain a bloodless operative field in BH-TECAB, silastic tapes are placed both proximal and distal to the graft landing zone, although on most occasions only the proximal one is going to be obstructed. The target vessel is incised and an appropriately sized intraluminal shunt is guided into the distal segment of the opening; then the contralateral shunt head is passed through the proximal vessel and the silastic tape is released. Similar to conventional bypass grafting, Debakey forceps and a robotic lancet beaver knife open the target area of the vessel (Figure 12.2.16).

The incision is then enlarged to approximately 4 mm in length by robotic Potts scissors to match the previously fashioned graft (Figure 12.2.17).

A 7-cm-long double-armed polypropylene suture is supplied via the parasternal utility port. A pair of robotic black diamond micro forceps facilitates the coronary artery suture process. The initial stitch is placed in a backhand way on the toe of the coronary in an inside-out fashion. The needle is parked safely away in the epicardium (Figure 12.2.18 and Figure 12.2.19).

The suture line is carried on with the contralateral needle, but now from the toe of the graft inside-out, and the coronary artery site will follow as outside-in.

After the first three throws, the graft is parachuted down to the coronary level and the stitching procedure becomes easier. Suturing is continued along the back wall, following which adequate suture line tension is applied then to the heel (Figure 12.2.20). Figure 12.2.21 depicts the suturing sequence completion.

After going around the heel, the needle is parked away and the first needle is taken to carry on from the toe of the anastomosis again to complete the suture line. Lumen patency can be checked with the tips of micro forceps in a gentle manner. The completed suture line has to be meticulously

FIGURE 12.2.21 Video depicts the suturing sequence completion.

FIGURE 12.2.22 Placement of pleural drain through the camera porthole.

inspected for slings. Slings can be corrected with the aid of suture needles.

STEP 10: FINAL ACTIONS

Bypass graft transit time ultrasound flow has to be reassured in all cases by a purpose-made endoscopic flow probe to maintain standard operative results. This specific probe is brought in via the subcostal port. Blood collection in the left pleural cavity is removed by a flexible suction catheter via the utility port or the right instrument port. On completion, the patient is weaned off from cardiopulmonary bypass, but the robot stays docked and the instruments are parked in the LIMA bed. This is a crucial step as the heart is volume loaded after decannulation and the attempted reinsertion of instruments may cause organ injury.

Once the patient's oxygenation is stabilized and the pump function has recovered, protamine is administered. At this stage the last endoscopic inspection of the thoracic cavity commences. Constant thorough attention is paid by both the console surgeon and tableside team. After sufficient hemostasis, the robotic system is undocked, although the ports are still left in position to avoid unnecessary CO_2 loss before the last manual inspections with the robotic camera. Then the ports are removed in a stepwise fashion under constant scope supervision, and the portholes are cauterized and packed with surgical hemostat such as Fibrillar™ or Surgicel™. Finally, a pleural drain is inserted through the camera porthole (Figure 12.2.22). Postoperative additive pain control is provided by local anesthetic infiltration of the portholes (Figure 12.2.23 and Figure 12.2.24).

TOOLS/INSTRUMENTS AND DEVICES

1. Da Vinci Xi Robot (Intuitive, Sunnyvale, CA) (Figure 12.2.25)
2. EndoWrist Stabilizer (Intuitive, Sunnyvale, CA) (Figure 12.2.26)
3. Saddle Loops (Quest Medical, Allen, TX) (Figure 12.2.27)
4. C-Port® Flex-A® distal anastomotic device (Dextera, Redwood City, CA) (Figure 12.2.28)
5. Handless transit time flow probe (MediStim VeriQ, Norway) (Figure 12.2.29)

PERIOPERATIVE CONSIDERATION

PREOPERATIVE ASSESSMENT AND WORK-UP

All patients should undergo a standard preoperative assessment process as for conventional CAB. Standardized preoperative work-up includes past medical and current clinical history, physical examination, standard blood tests (full blood count, renal

TABLE 12.2.1 CT angiography chest/abdomen/pelvis parameter assessment prior to TECAB

Heart	Lungs	Vascular
Heart dimensions (cardiothoracic ratio, LV distance to chest wall)	Lung size (intrathoracic workspace)	Ascending aortic diameter at right pulmonary artery crossing
LIMA and target vessel distance	Lung pathology	Atherosclerotic significance at all levels
Target vessel course (epi- vs. intramyocardial)	Pleural pathology (e.g. adhesions, plaques)	Iliofemoral anatomy and pathologic changes
Pericardial fat pad size		Other vascular pathologies (e.g. aneurysm, dissection)

and hepatic function tests, clotting screen, blood group type and cross-match), carotid Doppler study, ankle-brachial pressure index (ABPI), pulmonary function tests and echocardiography. To be able to determine TECAB suitability, chest-abdomen-pelvis computed tomographic (CT) angiography is required. All necessary CT parameters have to be reviewed not only by the surgeon, but the surgical team and radiologist, as shown in Table 12.2.1.

ANESTHETIC CONSIDERATIONS

Standard cardiac anesthetic principles apply for TECAB cases as well, albeit an experienced cardiac anesthetist with minimally invasive procedures subspecialty should be involved in all cases. Table 12.2.2 reviews specific anesthetic issues in TECAB procedures. Trans-esophageal echocardiography (TOE) is a must to visualize global cardiac function, regional wall motion abnormalities and adequate endo-balloon placement in real-time during arrested-heart TECAB.

TABLE 12.2.2 Specific anesthetic aspects

Double-lumen intubation or bronchial blocker
Percutaneous defibrillator pads
Constant TEE follow-up during procedure
NIRS monitoring for both cerebral and lower extremity

POSTOPERATIVE CARE

TECAB postoperative care is equivalent to the standard post-sternotomy bypass surgery. Atelectatic changes may be extensive resulting from single-lung ventilation, and gradually resolves with standard respiratory physiotherapy. Extra vigilance is suggested to assess the peripheral arterial and venous perfusion on a regular basis during the postoperative course after remote access cannulation. Postoperative pain may be quite intense, especially alongside the camera port sites, but diminishes within the early postoperative days. Sternal precautions are unnecessary as with other minimally invasive sternal-sparing procedures.

TIME DEMAND

TECAB is a complex surgical setting providing only a limited view of the operative field. This and additional factors require more significant time investment than conventional CABG. Table 12.2.3 shows procedure times indicated in the medical literature. Nota bene, most of the published articles contain data including a significant proportion of learning curve procedures. TECAB can be trained at an adequate safety level with a step-by-step approach (port insertion, IMA harvesting, pericardiotomy, anastomosis suturing), with the continuously improving experience and efficacy leading to synthesis of an entire operation.

TABLE 12.2.3 Procedure times for TECAB

Method author	Cases	LIMA-LAD anastomosis (min)	Total OR time (min)
SVST, MVST, RACAB			
Subramanian [6]	30	N/A	444 ± 45 (multivessel)
Turner [7]	70	N/A	356 (first 10 cases)
			232 (second 10 cases)
Srivastava [10]	150	N/A	311 ± 12
Jegaden [13]	78	N/A	204 ± 42
Bayramoglu [14]	100	N/A	166 ± 20
AH-TECAB			
Falk [3]	32	22 (15–34)	330 (220–507)
Dogan [5]	37	18 ± 4	N/A
Bonatti [15]	40	35 (23–66)	366 (including angiography)
Argenziano [16]	85	28 ± 11	260–400 (single vessel)
Bonatti [17]	100	10–100	178–690 (including angiography)
Zaouter [18]	38	60 ± 37	N/A
BH-TECAB			
Kappert [4]	3	37 ± 13	208 ± 42 (single vessel)
Srivastava [8]	108	14 ± 4	273 ± 130 (single and multivessel)
Srivastava [9]	139	13 ± 6	177 ± 53 (single vessel)
Yang [19]	100	N/A	219 ± 58
Dhawan [20]	106	N/A	326 ± 139
Cheng [12]	90	9.6	161

Abbreviations: AH-TECAB – arrested-heart totally endoscopic coronary artery bypass; BH-TECAB – beating heart totally endoscopic coronary artery bypass grafting; CAB – coronary artery bypass grafting; min – minutes; LAD – left anterior descending coronary artery; LIMA – left internal mammary artery; MVST – multivessel small thoracotomy; RACAB – robotic-assisted coronary artery bypass grafting; SVST – single-vessel small thoracotomy.

Learning curve time requirements using the second-generation TECAB robot are lower than in the first, and the same trend can be obviously observed with the third-generation robot [11]. In the near future, realistic time demand for TECAB will probably be between 3 and 5 hours, even with the inclusion of multivessel CAB. Procedural times in this range allow us to complete two procedures daily in one operative theatre. This goal has already been achieved by our team at the Cleveland Clinic, Abu Dhabi.

FIGURE 12.2.23 Robotic CABG by Francis P Sutter.

FIGURE 12.2.24 TECAB by Husam H Balkh.

ALTERNATIVE APPROACHES

CANNULATION

If moderate to severe aortoiliac atherosclerosis is present, we strongly suggest abandoning the femoral approach. Instead, the left subclavian artery is targeted as the arterial perfusion site in the infraclavicular region and an 8-mm prosthetic "chimney anastomosis" is created to connect the arterial line without compromise of the peripheral limb perfusion. Axillary cannulation ensures antegrade perfusion from the descending thoracic aortic level downstream and may also reduce the risk of retrograde aortoiliac dissection.

CARDIOPLEGIA

Percutaneous retrograde cardioplegic cannula can also be inserted on demand after anesthesia induction. In this case both antegrade and retrograde cardioplegia can be administered as per customized protocols.

TECAB APPROACHES

As seen above, TECAB can be performed with or without the aid of cardiopulmonary bypass and also under cardioplegic conditions (AH-TECAB) or on a beating heart (BH). We emphasize the necessity to train both skill sets as it adds enormous flexibility for the robotic surgical team to customize the procedural efficacy to the particular patient demand.

BH-TECAB has the advantage of avoiding the side effects of cardiopulmonary bypass, albeit the target vessel visualization and anastomotic technique require finer operative skills compared to AH-TECAB. Surgeons should have full command of the anastomotic techniques under cardioplegic conditions prior to switching to a beating-heart setting.

It is also beneficial to standardize the peripheral stand-by cannulation for potential cardiopulmonary bypass even in beating-heart TECAB, which might emerge as a safety net in case of hemodynamic instability, severe ventricular arrhythmia or sudden myocardial ischemia.

AH-TECAB allows the creation of coronary anastomoses with an increased comfort level, although this approach demands extra training in remote access perfusion and the safe application of an endoballoon or transthoracic cross-clamp. These skills should be gained stepwise in operations other than TECAB such as mini-thoracotomy mitral valve or ASD II repair, before embarking on total endoscopic CABG. In our experience, circumflex or right coronary territory bypass grafting in a reliable fashion should commence first on the arrested heart as the target area has to be completely off-loaded for sufficient rotation and placement.

FIGURE 12.2.25   Da Vinci Xi surgical system.

FIGURE 12.2.26   EndoWrist Stabilizer by Intuitive Surgical

FIGURE 12.2.27 Saddle Loops by Quest Medical, Allen, TX

FIGURE 12.2.28 C-Port® Flex-A® distal anastomotic device.

CORONARY GRAFTING OPTIONS

All coronary territories can be robotically revascularized without any compromise. The most common TECAB procedures include left internal mammary to the left anterior descending artery (LIMA to LAD), right internal mammary artery (RIMA) to LAD in combination with LIMA to the diagonal and/or circumflex territory grafts and LIMA to LAD combined with RIMA to the RCA branches. The latter procedure requires a Y-graft anastomosis construction.

TECAB AS HYBRID CORONARY PROCEDURE

LIMA to LAD or bilateral IMA endoscopic bypass grafts represent a well-founded long-term therapeutic solution with increased survival rates, and thus remain valuable components of hybrid coronary revascularizations. Hybrid coronary interventions merge minimally invasive surgical and percutaneous intervention techniques into reliable alternatives to multivessel open CAB or PCI. TECAB in combination with PCI is one of the early birds of hybrid procedures. An international multicentric trial revealed no stroke or mortality with robotic TECAB [21]. Early graft patency rates of LIMA grafts measured 96.3%. Bonatti et al. performed the initial single-session robotic hybrid coronary interventions [22]. An emerging number of advanced and complex hybrid coronary interventions, including multivessel TECAB and/or multivessel PCI, followed and have also been reported by other workgroups in further publications [23, 24]. The revascularization sequence does not have a major effect on clinical results, although patients having PCI first showed shorter ICU and hospital length of stay than patients undergoing surgery first [25].

CAVEATS AND CONTROVERSIES

CONTRAINDICATIONS TO TECAB

Multivessel TECAB and advanced hybrid PCI have evolved to become standardized, well-established procedures. Any clinical indication for CAB can be evaluated for a robotic-assisted minimally invasive approach. The major contraindications are listed in Table 12.2.4. A multidisciplinary team consisting of cardiac surgeons and cardiologists should assess suitability on a case-by-case basis (Figure 12.2.30).

Major pulmonary pathology is a challenge for extended single-lung ventilation. Hemodynamic instability is a clear contraindication to robotic surgery. Endothoracic scar tissue formation resulting from irradiation, trauma, previous thoracic surgery or

TABLE 12.2.4 Contraindications to TECAB

Absolute	Relative
Cardiogenic shock	Unstable patient on IABP
Hemodynamic instability	Severe left ventricular function (EF <30%)
Severe lung function impairment (FEV1 <70%, VC <2.5 L)	Bovine heart (<25 mm between LV and chest wall)
Pulmonary hypertension	Previous heart surgery
Chest deformities (e.g. pectus excavatum)	Previous severe chest trauma
Multimorbid patient	Previous chest irradiation
Significant generalized vasculopathy	
Diffusely diseased or small coronaries	
Intramyocardial coronaries for BH-TECAB	
Ascending aortic diameter >3.8 cm and severe aortoiliac calcification for AH-TECAB	

inflammatory disease is manageable with advanced robotic experience, albeit technically very demanding. Any factor that reduces or distorts the pleural space, such as cor bovinum and chest cavity deformities, has to be considered as an additional risk factor, as well as poor target vessel quality and systemic atherosclerotic disease.

Preoperative chest-abdomen-pelvis CT angiogram is an essential assessment component of aortic and iliofemoral atherosclerotic burden. If non-significant aortoiliac atherosclerosis is present, femoro-femoral cannulation for cardiopulmonary bypass can be established at low risk. Advanced aortoiliac vascular pathology precludes remote access perfusion. If moderate to severe aortoiliac atherosclerosis is present, we strongly suggest abandoning the femoral approach. Heavily calcified, minute or widely diseased targets are not suited for TECAB.

Thorough preoperative assessment of pros and cons has to be conducted to assess whether it is beneficial to expose the patient to a potentially longer cardiopulmonary bypass time, myocardial ischemia and overall procedural duration in contrast to the benefits of a minimally invasive method. The above dilemma exponentially matches patients carrying additional comorbidities on board.

ENDOBALLOON

Freedom of atherosclerotic debris in aortic arch and descending thoracic aorta is necessary for safe endoballoon application in AH-TECAB. A 38-mm maximal ascending

FIGURE 12.2.29 MediStim, VeriQ, Norway.

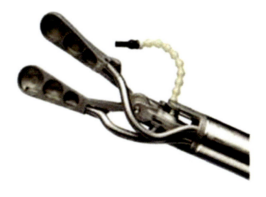

FIGURE 12.2.30 Da Vinci Xi endowrist. © 2020, Intuitive Surgical, Inc.

FIGURE 12.2.31 Anastomotic techniques for robotic beating-heart TECAB.

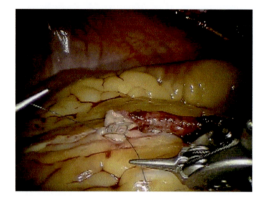

FIGURE 12.2.32 Putting tension on suture of back wall.

aortic diameter is a cornerstone, but the aortic valve must also show structural integrity and functional competency. It has to be ensured that a completely deflated balloon is progressed through the sheathed femoral arterial side branch. If severe aortoiliac calcification is present or a descending or arch protruding/mobile aortic atheroma is detected on TOE, the endoballoon application is contraindicated. In these cases, we choose a beating-heart TECAB procedure (Figure 12.2.31).

EXTRACORPOREAL CIRCULATION

The extracorporeal circulation in AH-TECAB is started gradually under TOE vision of the descending thoracic aorta to allow meticulous inspection for any signs of retrograde aortic dissection as early as possible. Exceptional attention has to be paid to avoid accidental air injection through the cardioplegic line.

We prophylactically cannulate BH-TECAB patients for safety reasons. The cannulas are placed at an ACT level of 300 s and flushed with heparin saline solution. Should cardiopulmonary bypass become necessary, the ACT is raised to 480 s. Cardiopulmonary bypass backup is extremely helpful in the following scenarios:

- ∞ In BH multivessel TECAB for adequate exposure of the lateral and back wall of the heart.
- ∞ When ischemia occurs during target vessel occlusion.
- ∞ If intrathoracic space is limited.
- ∞ If uncontrolled bleeding emerges.

The rapid establishment of perfusion in acute and potentially life-threatening complications poses an extremely challenging task with a robot docked to the patient. Also, the importance of the time factor should never be underestimated, and hasty actions may lead to collateral, but otherwise preventable, vascular injury. Instant cardiopulmonary bypass backup grants valuable peace of mind in our experience.

During supportive pump runs, significant diffuse bleeding might be encountered through portholes, the IMA bed and other structures, which may require intermittent transthoracic suction to evacuate the pool of blood in the left pleural space.

CORONARY ANASTOMOSIS

Further technical challenges have to be considered when finalizing the anastomoses in both AH and BH cases. In AH-TECAB, the target coronary should already be incised at the end stage of cardioplegia administration to reduce the possibility of vascular back wall injury. It is essential to apply adequate suture line tension in order to avoid leaks on the back wall, which are quite

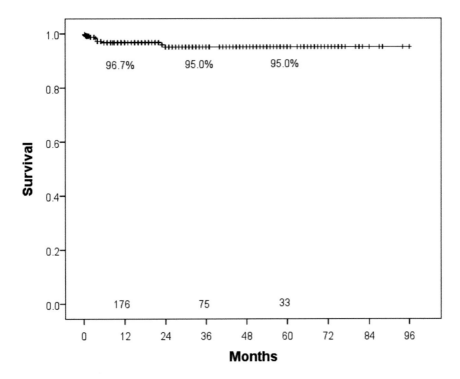

FIGURE 12.2.33　Cumulative survival.

challenging to correct compared to those on the facing front side.

Retrograde bleeding of the target vessel could indicate either retrograde aortic root flow as a consequence of low endoaortic balloon pressure or inadequate venous drainage. Venous cannula adjustment facilitates the overall drainage. Further controlled endoballoon inflation or silastic tape insertion around the target vessel will ameliorate operative field flooding. A clear operative field is a must for further safe anastomosis.

In the beating-heart setting the endostabilizer has to be applied carefully on the right ventricular surface, as accidental perforation poses a potential challenge. Suturing maneuvers must be well controlled and carried out with caution in order to avoid accidental injuries on the coronary wall (Figure 12.2.32). Esmolol administration provides effective heart rate reduction to facilitate the anastomotic process. As manipulations on a magnified bouncing operative field pose a technical challenge, intensive simulator training and dry and wet lab settings are key elements of preparation to move into a clinical setting. Bonatti et al. in 2006 depicted the technical challenges faced during AH-TECAB [15]. It will be prudent to undertake more advanced techniques of TECAB including multivessel TECAB on low-risk patients [20].

OTHER CAVEATS

Following weaning from cardiopulmonary bypass, it is crucial to keep the robot docked and the instruments parked in the LIMA bed, as the heart is volume loaded after decannulation and the attempted reinsertion of instruments may cause organ injury. Single-lung ventilation and cardiopulmonary bypass may result in transient respiratory compromise, which should resolve rapidly in response to respiratory physiotherapy. The pleural drain should be inserted during left lung inflation in order to avoid accidental graft injuries in the final stage of the surgery.

The importance of continuous excellent bilateral communication with the anesthetic team throughout the operation cannot be overstated, especially regarding the following:

- ∞ Initiation of single-lung ventilation.
- ∞ Regulating CO_2 insufflation pressure.
- ∞ Detecting signs of peripheral ischemia in the case of a femoral cardiopulmonary bypass approach.
- ∞ Correcting incidental endoballoon migration at cardioplegic TECAB.
- ∞ Establishing adequate heart rate control.
- ∞ Reviewing eventual regional wall motion abnormalities in beating-heart procedures.
- ∞ Respiratory management after a longer cardiopulmonary bypass run on single-lung ventilation.

RESEARCH, TRENDS AND INNOVATION

REDUCED SURGICAL TRAUMA ADVANTAGES

All current versions of TECAB result in a shortened length of hospital stay and a reduced postoperative recovery period. DeRose et al. found, in a mini-thoracotomy robotic-assisted coronary artery bypass (RACAB) series, that 82% of patients resumed normal daily routine within 10 days [26].

Kon et al. showed it took 1.8 months on average to return to full activities following robotic-assisted CAB via mini-thoracotomy compared to 4.4 months with full sternotomy OPCAB [27]. Bonaros et al. analyzed Short Form 36 scores at AH-TECAB vs. conversion to full sternotomy and primary sternotomy. Thirty-day postoperative scores indicating general health ranked higher with TECAB. Three-month scores assessing physical power and bodily pain were also superior in this group [28]. The study also demonstrated that post-TECAB patients restarted outdoor biking or hiking within 30 days, whereas following sternotomy the above physical activities returned 1 month later. Establishing a safe enhanced recovery after surgery (ERAS) path can also reduce postoperative mechanical ventilation time, transfusion rate and both intensive care unit and hospital stays [18].

INTERMEDIATE- AND LONG-TERM OUTCOMES

An increasing number of publications analyze TECAB intermediate- and long-term outcomes. DeCanniere reported 94.9% freedom from major adverse cardiac or cerebral events (MACCE) at 6 months in BH-TECAB and 91.2% in AH-TECAB in a multicenter study on early TECAB experience [29]. The Dresden experience showed 75.7% freedom from major adverse events in their first 41 patients after 5 years. Overall survival was 92.7%, and freedom from reintervention of the left anterior descending artery was 82.9% [30].

Bonatti et al. revealed a similar incidence of major adverse events among the first 25 single-vessel AH-TECAB patients, although the Innsbruck Medical University series discovered dramatic improvement regarding freedom from MACCE in the second to fourth cohorts consisting of 25 patients each [17]. Jegaden et al. described their 3-year experience with 96.0% survival [13]. Currie et al. showed that 8-year graft patency was 92.7% [31].

Yang et al. showed that patency rates of the LIMA graft at short-term (up to 1 year), mid-term (between 1 and 3 years) and long-term (over 3 years) after surgery in the TECAB group were 98.8%, 97.8% and 97.1%, and those for MINICAB were 98.5%, 97.1% and 96.4%, respectively [19]. Combined Innsbruck Medical University and University of Maryland 5-year hybrid TECAB outcomes reviewed in 226 patients had a survival rate of 92.9% and 83.1/75.2% (single-/multivessel) freedom from MACCE; 2.7% of bypass grafts and 14.2% of PCI necessitated reintervention in the mid-term results. The average length of hospital stay was 6 days. General household duties could be resumed within a fortnight and full daily activity in 42 days [32].

Cumulative survival, freedom from angina and freedom from MACCE in 410 patients undergoing totally endoscopic coronary artery bypass grafting from 2001 to 2010 at the University of Maryland and at Innsbruck Medical University are shown in in Figure 12.2.33, Figure 12.2.34 and Figure 12.2.35 [33].

PREDICTORS OF SUCCESS AND SAFETY, FURTHER PATIENT ASPECTS

Progression in robotic technology has enabled TECAB to emerge as an established procedure worldwide in specialized centers. Bonaros et al. have analyzed the 10-year multicentric outcomes of 500 TECAB cases regarding predictors of success and safety. Success was defined as freedom from any adverse events or conversions, and safety as freedom from MACCE, major vascular injuries or long-term ventilation. Success and safety rates measured 80% (400 patients) and 95% (474 patients), respectively. Independent predictors of success were AH-TECAB, single-vessel TECAB, thoracic assistance and non-learning curve cases. The only independent predictor

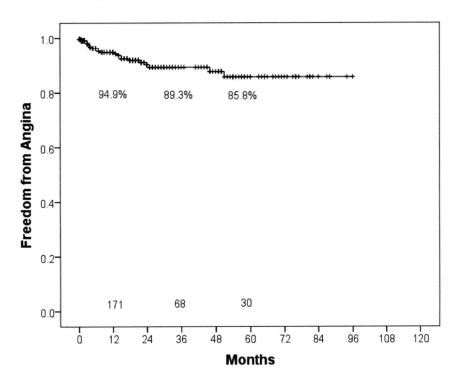

FIGURE 12.2.34 Cumulative freedom from angina.

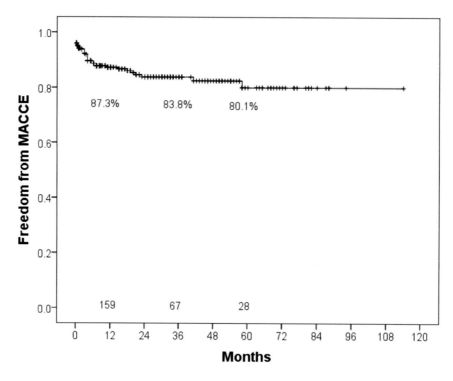

FIGURE 12.2.35 Cumulative freedom from MACCE.

for safety was the EuroSCORE. The above results well highlight that success is characterized by simplicity and established surgical technique, while safety is determined by correct patient selection [34].

Hemli et al. evaluated whether body mass index has an effect on short-term outcomes in robotic-assisted coronary surgery. Although LIMA takedown time and total operative time were extended in the obese, there was no difference in non-obese and obese patients in terms of mortality or MACCE [35]. Wiedemann et al. investigated if sex differences affect TECAB outcomes in 500 consecutive patients and concluded that gender had no influence on robotic postoperative outcomes [36].

SUMMARY AND FUTURE ASPECTS

Robotic TECAB has been proven to be a safe and reliable surgical procedure in several centers worldwide in the past decade in both beating- and arrested-heart settings. Total endoscopic port access operations lower surgical trauma, preserve thoracic structural integrity and simultaneously result in cosmetic advantages. Several publications undoubtedly show encouraging early postoperative recovery and rapid return to full functional activity without needing 3 months' sternal precautions. The price to pay for this is the extended operative time. With the exclusion of learning-curve cases, the initial annual freedom from MACCE in TECAB patients is definitely above 90% [37, 38].

With the constant development of surgical techniques and improving software and hardware support, a further broad application spectrum of robotic-facilitated CAB is likely. Special demand for surgeon and team training in the field will probably focus these procedures in specific centers. Simulation sessions are undoubtedly key components of surgical team education. Complex procedures are already performed on a regular

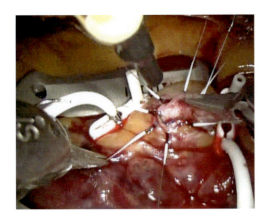

FIGURE 12.2.36 Left internal mammary artery to left anterior descending artery distal anastomosis using interrupted S18-U clips (Medtronic, Minneapolis, MN) in TECAB. (Reprinted from *Ann Thorac Surg*, 100(4), Yang M, Wu Y, Wang G, Xiao C, Zhang H, Gao C. Robotic Total Arterial Off-Pump Coronary Artery Bypass Grafting: Seven-Year Single-Center Experience and Long-Term Follow-Up of Graft Patency, 1367-1373, © 2015 by The Society of Thoracic Surgeons with permission from Elsevier.)

FIGURE 12.2.37 STS workshop.

FIGURE 12.2.38 STS/TSF Advanced Robotic Cardiac Surgery Fellowship.

FIGURE 12.2.39 AATS cardiac surgery robotic program.

FIGURE 12.2.40 EACTS courses.

FIGURE 12.2.41 ISMICS cardiac surgery courses.

basis, and a significant proportion of standard operations via sternotomy is expected to be replaced step by step by minimally invasive robotic procedures in the near future. Hybrid methods are increasingly incorporated into the robotic armamentarium, and recent developments of procedure-specific robotic instruments will optimize exposure of the cardiac back wall (Figure 12.2.36). Single-port access is under further expansion in endoscopic surgical fields, and will soon offer new prospect in TECAB techniques. Automatic anastomotic devices offer another novel future pathway, although further clinical tests have to commence to warrant safe daily application [39].

Long-distance telesurgical procedures may emerge as sustainable, but the effective action range is limited by the speed and quality of the signal transfer. The latest technical projects address problems with virtual target vessel immobilization in beating-heart settings to facilitate seamless anastomosis construction. Theoretically, completely automated robotic TECAB operations are possible, and it reveals the future generations of heart surgeons and medical engineers. We can conclude that robotics definitely offers exciting prospects for the surgical treatment of ischemic heart disease [40].

WHERE AND HOW TO LEARN

1. **The Society of Thoracic Surgeons Workshop on Robotic Cardiac Surgery**

The society offers a broad range of educational programs and activities, including the STS Workshop on Robotic Cardiac Surgery (Figure 12.2.37).

2. **The Thoracic Surgery Foundation Advanced Robotic Cardiac Surgery Fellowship**

This $25,000 advanced fellowship opportunity will be awarded to a surgeon and their institution to support and facilitate the successful initiation of a high-quality robotic cardiac surgery program at his/her home institution. Applicants must attend the STS Workshop on Robotic Cardiac Surgery (Figure 12.2.38).

3. **The American Association for Thoracic Surgery Cardiac Surgical Robotics Program**

AATS Foundation Fellowship and Research Scholarships aimed to bring the community of cardiothoracic surgeons together (Figure 12.2.39).

4. **European Association for Cardio-Thoracic Surgery Courses on minimally invasive techniques**

EACTS provides high-quality training courses that are attended by delegates from all over the world. As an educational institution, their goal is to promote a non-dogmatic learning environment (Figure 12.2.40).

5. **International Society of Minimally Invasive Cardiac Surgery courses**

The International Society for Minimally Invasive Cardiothoracic Surgery (ISMICS) offers co-sponsorship for qualified educational programs in the cardiothoracic and cardiovascular specialties (Figure 12.2.41).

REFERENCES

1. Lee JD, Srivastava M, Bonatti J. History and current status of robotic totally endoscopic coronary artery bypass. *Circ J* 2012;76(9):2058–65.
2. Stephenson ER Jr, Sankholkar S, Ducko CT, Damiano RJ Jr. Robotically assisted microsurgery for endoscopic coronary artery bypass grafting. *Ann Thorac Surg*. 1998;66(3):1064-1067. doi:10.1016/s0003-4975(98)00656-0.
3. Falk V, Diegeler A, Walther T, Banusch J, Brucerius J, Raumans J, et al. Total endoscopic computer enhanced coronary artery bypass grafting. *Eur J Cardio-thorac Surg* 2000;17:38–45.

4. Kappert U, Cichon R, Tugtekin SM, Schueler S. Closed chest coronary artery bypass on the beating heart. *Heart Surg Forum* 2001;4:89–90.
5. Dogan S, Aybek T, Andressen E, Byhahn C, Mierdl S, Westphal K, et al. Totally endoscopic coronary artery bypass grafting on cardiopulmonary bypass with robotically enhanced telemanipulation: report of forty-five cases. *J Thorac Cardiovasc Surg* 2002;123:1125–1131.
6. Subramanian V, Patel N, Patel N, Loulmet D. Robotic assisted multivessel minimally invasive direct coronary artery bypass with port-access stabilization and cardiac positioning: paving the way for outpatient coronary surgery? *Ann Thorac Surg* 2005;79:1590–1596.
7. Turner WF, Sloan JH. Robotic-assisted coronary artery bypass on a beating heart: initial experience and implications for the future. *Ann Thorac Surg* 2006;82:790–794.
8. Srivastava S, Gadasalli S, Agusala M, Kolluru R, Barrera R, Quismundo S, et al. Robotically assisted beating heart totally endoscopic coronary artery bypass (TECAB). Is there a future? *Innovations* 2008;3:52–58.
9. Srivastava S, Gadasalli S, Agusala M, Kolluru R, Barrera R, Quismundo S, et al. Beating heart totally endoscopic coronary artery bypass. *Ann Thorac Surg* 2010;89:1873–1880.
10. Srivastava S, Gadasalli S, Agusala M, Kolluru R, Naidu J, Shroff M, et al. Use of bilateral internal thoracic arteries in CABG through lateral thoracotomy with robotic assistance in 150 patients. *Ann Thorac Surg* 2006;81:800–806.
11. Schachner T, Bonaros N, Wiedemann D, Weidinger F, Feuchtner G, Friedrich G, et al. Training surgeons to perform robotically assisted totally endoscopic coronary surgery. *Ann Thorac Surg* 2009;88(2):523–7.
12. Cheng N, Gao C, Yang M, Wu Y, Wang G, Xiao C. Analysis of the learning curve for beating heart, totally endoscopic, coronary artery bypass grafting. *J Thorac Cardiovasc Surg* 2014;148:1832–1836.
13. Jegaden O, Wautot F, Sassard T, Szymanik I, Shafy A, Lapeze J, et al. Is there an optimal minimally invasive technique for left anterior descending coronary artery bypass? *J Cardiothorac Surg* 2011;6:37.
14. Bayramoglu Z, Caynak B, Ezelsoy M, Oral K, Sagbas E, Akpınar B. Angiographic evaluation of graft patency in robotic-assisted coronary artery bypass surgery: 8-year follow-up. *Int J Med Robot* 2014;10:121–127.
15. Bonatti J, Schachner T, Bonaros N, Ohlinger A, Danzmayr M, Jonetzko P, et al. Technical challenges in totally endoscopic robotic coronary artery bypass grafting. *J Thorac Cardiovasc Surg* 2006;131:146–153.
16. Argenziano M, Katz M, Bonatti J, Srivastava S, Murphy D, Poirier R, et al. Results of the prospective multicenter trial of robotically assisted totally endoscopic coronary artery bypass grafting. *Ann Thorac Surg* 2006;81:1666–1674.
17. Bonatti J, Schachner T, Bonaros N, Oehlinger A, Wiedemann D, Ruetzler E, et al. Effectiveness and safety of total endoscopic left internal mammary artery bypass graft to the left anterior descending artery. *Am. J. Cardiol.* 2009;104(12):1684–1688.
18. Zaouter C, Imbault J, Labrousse L, Abdelmoumen Y, Coiffic A, Colonna G, et al. Association of robotic totally endoscopic coronary artery bypass graft surgery associated with a preliminary cardiac enhanced recovery after surgery program: a retrospective analysis. *J Cardiothorac Vasc Anesth* 2015;29:1489–1497.
19. Yang M, Wu Y, Wang G, Xiao C, Zhang H, Gao C. Robotic total arterial off-pump coronary artery bypass grafting: seven-year single-center experience and long-term follow-up of graft patency. *Ann Thorac Surg* 2015;100:1367–1373.
20. Dhawan R, Roberts JD, Wroblewski K, Katz JA, Raman J, Chaney MA. Multivessel beating heart robotic myocardial revascularization increases morbidity and mortality. *J Thorac Cardiovasc Surg* 2012;143:1056–1061.
21. Katz M, Van Praet F, de Canniere D, Murphy D, Siwek L, Seshadri-Kreaden U, et al. Integrated coronary revascularization: percutaneous coronary intervention plus robotic totally endoscopic coronary artery bypass. *Circulation* 2006;114(1 Suppl):I473–I476.
22. Bonatti J, Schachner T, Bonaros N, Jonetzko P, Ohlinger A, Löckinger A, et al. Treatment of double vessel coronary artery disease by totally endoscopic bypass

surgery and drug-eluting stent placement in one simultaneous hybrid session. *Heart Surg Forum.* 2005;8(4):E284–286.
23. Jansens J, De Croly P, De Cannière D. Robotic hybrid procedure and triple-vessel disease. *J Cardiac Surg* 2009;24(4):449–450.
24. Bonatti J, Lehr E, Vesely MR, Friedrich G, Bonaros N, Zimrin D. Hybrid coronary revascularization: which patients? when? how? *Curr Opin Cardiol* 2010;25(6):568–574.
25. Srivastava MC, Vesely MR, Lee JD, Lehr EJ, Wehman B, Bonaros N, et al. Robotically assisted hybrid coronary revascularisation: does sequence of intervention matter? *Innovations.* 2013;8(3):177–183.
26. Derose JJ, Balaram SK, Ro C, Swistel DG, Singh V, Wilentz JR, et al. Mid-term results and patient perceptions of robotically-assisted coronary artery bypass grafting. *Interact Cardiovasc Thorac Surg* 2005;4(5):406–411.
27. Kon ZN, Brown EN, Tran R, Joshi A, Reicher B, Grant MC, et al. Simultaneous hybrid coronary revascularization reduces postoperative morbidity compared with results from conventional off-pump coronary artery bypass. *J Thorac Cardiovasc Surg* 2008;135(2):367–375.
28. Bonaros N, Schachner T, Wiedemann D, Oehlinger A, Ruetzler E, Feuchtner G, et al. Quality of life improvement after robotically assisted coronary artery bypass grafting. *Cardiology.* 2009;114(1):59–66.
29. de Canniere D, Wimmer-Greinecker G, Cichon R, Gulielmos V, Van Praet F, Seshadri-Kreaden U, et al. Feasibility, safety, and efficacy of totally endoscopic coronary artery bypass grafting: multicenter European experience. *J Thorac Cardiovasc Surg* 2007;134(3):710–716.
30. Kappert U, Tugtekin S, Cichon R, Braun M, Matschke K. Robotic totally endoscopic coronary artery bypass: a word of caution implicated by a five-year follow-up. *J Thorac Cardiovasc Surg* 2008;135(4):857–862.
31. Currie ME, Romsa J, Fox SA, Vezina WC, Akincioglu C, Warrington JC, et al. Long-term angiographic follow-up of robotic-assisted coronary artery revascularization. *Ann Thorac Surg* 2012;93(5):1426–1431.
32. Bonatti OJ, Zimrin D, Lehr EJ, Vesely M, Kon ZN, Wehman B, et al. Hybrid coronary revascularisation using robotic totally endoscopic surgery; perioperative outcomes and 5-year results. *Ann Thorac Surg* 2012;94(6):1920–1926.
33. Bonatti J, Schachner T, Bonaros N, Lehr EJ, Zimrin D, Griffith B. Robotically assisted totally endoscopic coronary bypass surgery. *Circulation* 2011;124(2):236–44.
34. Bonaros N, Schachner T, Lehr E, Kofler M, Wiedemann D, Hong P, et al. Five hundred cases of robotic totally endoscopic coronary artery bypass grafting: predictors of success and safety. *Ann Thorac Surg* 2013;95(3):803–812.
35. Hemli JM, Darla LS, Panetta CR, Jennings J, Subramanian VA, Patel NC. Does body mass index affect outcomes in robotic-assisted coronary artery bypass procedures? *Innovations* 2012;7(5):350–353.
36. Wiedemann D, Schachner T, Bonaros N, Lehr EJ, Wehman B, Hong P, et al. Robotic totally endoscopic coronary artery bypass grafting in men and women: are there sex differences in outcome? *Ann Thorac Surg* 2013;96(5):1643–1647.
37. Cao C, Indraratna P, Doyle M, Tian DH, Liou K, Munkholm-Larsen S, et al. A systematic review on robotic coronary artery bypass graft surgery. *Ann Cardiothorac Surg* 2016;5(6):530–543.
38. Seco M, Edelman JJ, Yan TD, Wilson MK, Bannon PG, Vallely MP. Systematic review of robotic-assisted, totally endoscopic coronary artery bypass grafting. *Ann Cardiothorac Surg* 2013;2(4):408–418.
39. Canale LS, Mick S, Mihaljevic T, Nair R, Bonatti J. Robotically assisted totally endoscopic coronary artery bypass surgery. *J Thorac Dis* 2013;5(Suppl 6):S641–649.
40. Göbölös L, Ramahi J, Obeso A, Bartel Th, Traina M, Edris A, et al. Robot assisted totally endoscopic coronary bypass surgery. *Ind J Thorac Cardiovasc Surg* 2018;34(Supplement 2):94–104.

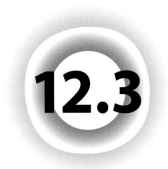

ANAORTIC, OFF-PUMP, TOTAL-ARTERIAL CORONARY ARTERY BYPASS GRAFTING SURGERY
The Coronaries

MICHAEL SECO, J JAMES B EDELMAN, FABIO RAMPONI, MICHAEL K WILSON, AND MICHAEL P VALLELY

HISTORY AND INTRODUCTION

INTRODUCTION

The debate of on-pump versus off-pump coronary artery bypass grafting (CABG) has been continuing as long as surgical revascularization has been performed. This has been fueled by a number of randomized controlled trials that have seen no improvement and even harm associated with an off-pump technique, but a multitude of observational studies demonstrating significant benefit. Whilst the most common CABG technique used today remains cardiopulmonary bypass with an arrested heart, many centers pursue off-pump CABG (OPCAB) and continue to refine the surgical technique.

HISTORY OF OPCAB AND TECHNICAL INNOVATION

The first direct coronary revascularization procedures in the early 1960s were performed on the beating heart without cardiopulmonary bypass [1], however rapid developments in extracorporeal circulation and myocardial protection were soon adopted as they made the operations safer, more standardized and reproducible. In the 1980s Buffolo and Benetti published their extensive series on OPCAB, in which most patients received grafts to the LAD and right coronary artery, but with more limited and difficult grafting of the posterior and lateral wall vessels [2,3]. In the 1990s, hybrid coronary revascularization was also proposed, involving a LIMA-LAD graft performed through a mini-thoracotomy off-pump, and percutaneous coronary intervention for the non-LAD targets [4].

Innovative technology has played a key role in the development of OPCAB. Initially, stabilization of the target coronary vessel was obtained by stay sutures, but the advent of mechanical stabilizers transformed the way OPCAB was performed, and was accompanied by an evident improvement in surgical results [5]. The critical challenge was the exposure of the lateral and inferior walls, which was further improved with the use of pressure and vacuum-assisted positioners that caused less hemodynamic instability.

RESEARCH, TRENDS AND INNOVATION

STROKE AND OTHER PERI-OPERATIVE COMPLICATIONS

Neurologic injury is a major peri-operative complication of coronary surgery, which can manifest in the short term as coma and impaired motor function or confusional state, and in the long term as a decline in cognitive function, behavioral changes or physical dysfunction [6]. More recently, the high incidence of psychiatric issues following coronary surgery has also been recognized; these issues potentially share a common etiology with more overt neurologic injury [7].

A variety of mechanisms has been proposed to contribute to neurologic injury in this setting. The primary mechanism is embolic injury, which can arise from both micro- and macro-embolization of atheromatous plaque, air, debris or clot. Atheromatous plaque can be dislodged through clamping of the aorta, aortic cannulation and through the high-velocity jet of blood from the aortic cannula against the vessel wall. Other mechanisms include many of the possible effects of cardiopulmonary bypass, such as systemic inflammatory responses, hypoperfusion and hyperperfusion. The theorized reduction in neurologic injury with off-pump surgery is therefore two-fold: [1] a reduction in embolic events by avoidance of aortic manipulation and cardiopulmonary bypass; and [2] avoidance of the deleterious effects of cardiopulmonary bypass.

An alternative to the dichotomous on- and off-pump groups is to consider the range of coronary bypass techniques in relation to their degree of aortic manipulation. In this way they can be categorized into on-pump CABG with multiple clamps (cross-clamp plus partial-clamp) (i.e. the most aortic manipulation); on-pump CABG with a single cross-clamp; OPCAB with a partial-clamp for proximal anastomosis (OPCAB-PC); OPCAB using a "clampless" proximal anastomotic device, for example the Heartstring device (OPCAB-HS, Maquet

Cardiovascular, San Jose, California); and finally "anaortic" or "no-touch" OPCAB (anOPCAB) (i.e. no aortic manipulation).

A network meta-analysis including 13 observational studies and >37,000 patients has been performed by our group to compare these various techniques simultaneously [8]. AnOPCAB was the most effective method for decreasing the risk of post-operative stroke (−78% vs. CABG, −66% vs. OPCAB-PC, −52% vs. OPCAB-HS). AnOPCAB was also the most effective at reducing mortality (−50% vs. CABG, −40% vs. OPCAB-HS), renal failure (−53% vs. CABG), bleeding complications (−48% vs. OPCAB-HS, −36% vs. CABG), atrial fibrillation (−34% vs. OPCAB-HS, −29% vs. CABG, −20% vs. OPCAB-PC) and shortening the length of intensive care unit stay (−13.3 h). Figure 12.3.1 contains Forrest plots comparing the major peri-operative complication for each technique. As a result, the latest 2018 ESC/EACTS myocardial revascularization guidelines include a Class I recommendation for minimizing aortic manipulation where possible [9]. Whilst the anOPCAB technique carried the least risk in most endpoints, "Rankograms" demonstrated that OPCAB-PC and OPCAB-HS also carried less risk than on-pump CABG [8]. This further demonstrates the importance of avoiding cardiopulmonary bypass as well as aortic manipulation.

Unlike the meta-analysis, the large randomized trials comparing on- and off-pump CABG in low-risk (Randomized On/Off Bypass [ROOBY] trial) [10], moderate-risk (CABG Off- or On-Pump Revascularization Study [CORONARY] trial) [11] and high-risk (Off-Pump versus On-Pump Coronary-Artery Bypass Grafting in Elderly Patients [GOPCABE] trial) [12] patients have not found a similar reduction in the rate of post-operative stroke. However, these trials have not reported the degree of aortic manipulation, and the proportion of anOPCAB patients is unknown (though likely low).

Other groups have looked at the effect of introducing an anOPCAB technique on peri-operative outcomes over time. Albert and colleagues established anOPCAB routinely from 2005 onwards, and saw a significant decrease in the risk of stroke (0.64% post-adoption vs. 1.40% pre-adoption, $p < 0.0001$) [13]. This difference was mostly driven by a decrease in early strokes (i.e. a deficit apparent after emerging from anesthesia), whilst the incidence of delayed stroke was similar (i.e. after first awaking without any deficit). This is, again, consistent with the hypothesized mechanisms of reduction in intra-operative embolic events.

In addition, one of the major driving factors for the recommendation for PCI over CABG in many patients is the high risk of stroke associated with surgical revascularization. A recent meta-analysis of patient-level data found that the 30-day stroke rate was 0.4% in PCI vs. 1.1% in CABG (with all subgroups of aortic manipulation combined) (HR 0.33, $p < 0.001$), although the rate of stroke between 30 days and 5 years was comparable (2.2% vs. 2.1%, $p = 0.72$) [14]. Patients who experience a stroke within 30 days also have a significantly higher risk of 5-year mortality. However, the network meta-analysis has demonstrated that there is no difference in 30-day stroke risk between anOPCAB and PCI (OR 0.92) [15].

Compared to on-pump CABG, anOPCAB and PCI both reduce the risk of stroke by a similar amount (72% and 69% reductions, respectively). If confirmed in a direct comparative study, these results would suggest that many more patients could benefit from the superior long-term revascularization of coronary surgery.

HIGH-RISK PATIENTS

Multiple studies have suggested that high-risk patients, such as those with chronic

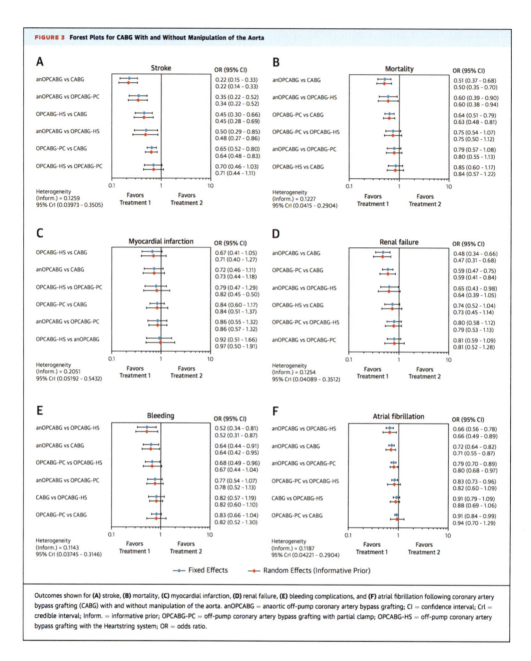

FIGURE 12.3.1 Forrest plots comparing major complications following CABG with various degrees of aortic manipulation. (Reprinted from *J Am Coll Cardiol*, 69(8), Zhao DF, Edelman JJ, Seco M, et al. Coronary Artery Bypass Grafting with and without Manipulation of the Ascending Aorta: A Network Meta-Analysis, 924-936, © 2017, with permission from Elsevier.)

kidney disease, diabetes or advanced age, disproportionately benefit from OPCAB techniques. A recent meta-analysis of randomized controlled trials demonstrated a significant linear relationship with the patients' risk profile and the benefit derived from OPCAB in terms of mortality, myocardial infarction and stroke [16]. Similarly, data from the Society of Thoracic Surgeons (STS) National Database demonstrated that

OPCAB patients in the third and fourth highest risk quartiles had significantly lower mortality than predicted (38% and 55% reduction, respectively), but patients in the first and second lowest risk quartiles did not [17]. The benefit was most significant for patients with an STS-PROM score above 2.5 to 3% [17].

Patients with peripheral vascular disease involving the ascending aorta or carotid arteries are also at much higher risk for neurologic injury given the mechanisms described in the section titled, "Research, trend and innovation". This risk factor is unfortunately relatively common in patients undergoing CABG, occurring in an estimated 10–30% [18]. OPCAB that avoids aortic manipulation is therefore of particular benefit to these patients. Computed tomography is often used in patients aged over 70 years to identify the presence of significant aortic atherosclerosis pre-operatively, and epi-aortic ultrasound can be used intra-operatively to further assess the aorta [9]. Multiple observational studies have confirmed lower mortality and lower peri-operative stroke in this patient group [18,19], and the latest myocardial revascularization guidelines also reflect this [9].

CAVEATS AND CONTROVERSIES

COMPLETE REVASCULARIZATION AND LONG-TERM OUTCOMES

One of the main criticisms of OPCAB surgery has been that the increased technical difficulty may result in reduced graft patency and fewer graft numbers, leading to incomplete surgical revascularization and worse long-term outcomes (Figure 12.3.2).

The results of the ROOBY trial demonstrated reduced 5-year survival [10] and reduced angiographic patency at 1 year in the OPCAB group [20]. However, this trial has been criticized for including relatively inexperienced OPCAB surgeons. The trials where surgery was performed only by experienced surgeons reported small increases in the need for repeat revascularization at 30 days (CORONARY: OPCAB 0.7% vs. CABG 0.2%; and GOPCABE: OPCAB 1.3% vs. 0.4%), that reflect the difficulty of the technique. However, this difference was not reflected in the rate of myocardial infarction, which did not differ between techniques at 30 days and 1 year in these trials.

A recent retrospective cohort study, limited to surgeons with a minimum of 100 completed off-pump cases, also found reduced 10-year survival (33.4% vs. 29.6%, HR 1.11), higher risk of incomplete revascularization (15.7% vs. 8.8%) and higher rates of repeat revascularization (15.4% vs. 14.0%) with OPCAB [21], further supporting this argument. The higher rate of incomplete revascularization is significant, as this is a known factor that negatively affects the long-term outcome [22].

In contrast, a number of studies have found no difference in the graft patency rate following OPCAB surgery [23–25]. A meta-analysis (including both the ROOBY and CORONARY trials) also found no difference in mid- to long-term outcomes between OPCAB and CABG (HR 1.06) [26] Differences in surgeons' experience, varying completeness of follow-up and angiographic definitions are possible explanations for differences in results. Thus, more evidence is required before drawing conclusions about patency rate and long-term outcome. Nonetheless, a surgical technique for OPCAB that enables the reliable performance of distal anastomoses and achieves complete revascularization is crucial and described in detail next.

HOW TO DO IT/STEP BY STEP

ANAORTIC OPCAB SURGICAL TECHNIQUE

There are numerous methods of configuring grafts in order to achieve complete revascularization whilst minimizing or indeed eliminating aortic manipulation. In practice this is achieved through utilizing in situ grafts and extension or y-grafts. One standard approach is to revascularize the LAD with an in situ skeletonized LIMA (Figure 12.3.3), and the lateral and inferior walls with an in situ skeletonized RIMA/radial tandem graft and sequential anastomoses (Figure 12.3.4A) (27). This utilizes dual inflows and separates the anterior wall blood supply from the rest of the heart, thus protecting the integrity of the LIMA to LAD graft. An alternative is an in situ LIMA to LAD, with a radial artery or RIMA y-graft to the lateral and inferior walls (Figure 12.3.4B) (28).

The positioning of the heart is a key component of performing off-pump surgery, as a balance of optimal exposure for anastomosis and hemodynamic stability is needed. This is achieved through a combination of pericardial release, "pericardial heart strings" and the off-pump stabilizer. The pericardium is opened longitudinally and the incision extended near the diaphragm laterally in both directions, towards the RA/SVC junction, and obliquely at the pulmonary valve. This allows for exposure of the lateral wall vessels by rolling the heart on the caval axis into the right pleural space, providing maximum exposure with minimal effect on venous return. Care must be taken not to injure the phrenic nerve. Pericardial heart strings are then placed in the left lateral inferior pericardial recess (Heartstring 1), and the diaphragmatic surface just medial to the IVC (Heartstring 2) (Figure 12.3.5). Tension on these strings can help to position the heart.

An off-pump stabilizer is used to perform the anastomoses. There are four major cardiac positions used (Figure 12.3.6):

1. High-lateral wall vessels (first diagonal, intermediate, first obtuse marginal). The table is rolled towards the surgeon with the patient's head down. Heartstring 1 is placed on tension with wet sponges behind the heart as required. The heart is rolled across and vertically towards the right chest (Figure 12.3.7).
2. Low-lateral wall vessels (second/third marginal, posterolateral circumflex). The table remains in the same position as above. Heartstring 1 is tightened across the arm of the sternal retractor, with Heartstring 2 pulled inferiorly. The stabilizer is moved down to the target vessel with the heart remaining in the right chest.

FIGURE 12.3.2　Off-pump CABG: 30 years of debate.

FIGURE 12.3.3　Skeletonized bilateral IMA harvest video.

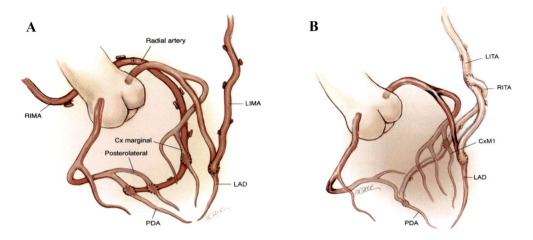

FIGURE 12.3.4 Configuration of grafts to achieve anaortic off-pump CABG with complete revascularization using (A) LIMA-LAD and RIMA-radial artery tandem graft to lateral and inferior walls, or (B) LIMA-LAD and LIMA-RIMA (or radial artery) y-graft. Reprinted with permission, © Beth Croce, Bioperspective.com

3. Inferior wall vessels (posterolateral right and right posterior descending). The heart is positioned "apex-up". The table is centered, remaining head-down. Heartstring 2 is used, with a wet pack placed medial to the IVC. If the heart moves across to the left, then lateral tension on Heartstring 1 and placing an additional wet sponge against the lateral wall can help to prevent this (Figure 12.3.8).
4. Anterior wall vessels (second/third diagonal, left anterior descending). Often a wet pack behind the heart is all that is required. Some tension on Heartstring 1 laterally can be helpful (Figure 12.3.9).

The anastomoses are completed in the order of the four positions listed above (high-lateral wall first, anterior wall last). Silastic intracoronary shunts are used when performing all distal anastomoses (Figure 12.3.10 and Figure 12.3.11).

These provide a number of advantages, including maintaining some distal coronary artery flow during grafting, providing a bloodless field to operate in and to help prevent technical errors such as catching the back wall of the coronary artery with a suture. Once the anastomosis is near complete, the soft shunt is removed before pulling the suture tight and securing it. Silastic

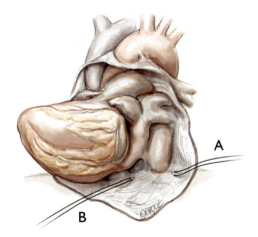

FIGURE 12.3.5 Pericardial heart strings placed to assist positioning of the heart: (A) left lateral inferior pericardial recess; (B) diaphragmatic surface medial to the inferior vena cava. Reprinted with permission, © Beth Croce, Bioperspective.com

FIGURE 12.3.6 Preparing the pericardium.

FIGURE 12.3.8 Access to inferior wall vessel.

FIGURE 12.3.7 How to approach high-lateral wall vessels.

FIGURE 12.3.9 Addressing anterior wall vessel.

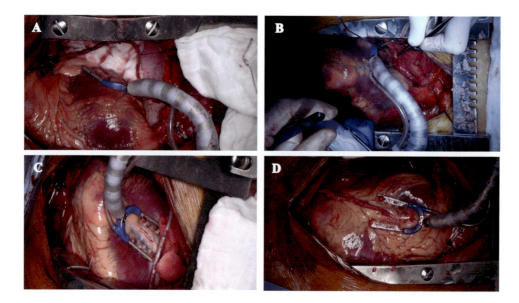

FIGURE 12.3.10 Four major cardiac positions stabilized and exposed during off-pump anastomoses: (A) high-lateral wall vessels, (B) low-lateral wall vessels, (C) inferior wall vessels, (D) anterior wall vessels.

slings or bulldog clamps can also be applied to the coronary artery proximal to the anastomosis to help create a bloodless field, but should be used sparingly in an effort to reduce inadvertent injury to the coronary artery or ventricular wall. Assessing grafts intraoperatively using transit flow time measurement is useful and can assist in detecting conduit or anastomotic issues [9]. This is particularly important in off-pump surgery, with the concern regarding graft patency. Detailed discussion of the utility and application of transit flow time measurement can be found in the literature [29] (Figure 12.3.12).

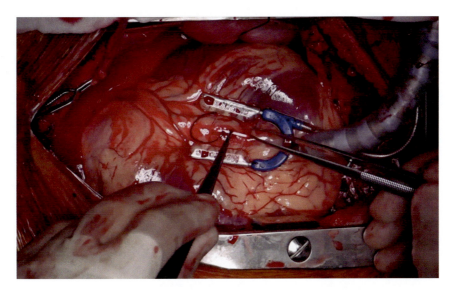

FIGURE 12.3.11 Off-pump anastomosis setup utilizing myocardial stabilizer and insertion of intracoronary shunt.

FIGURE 12.3.12 Anaortic OPCAB technique summary video.

TOOLS/INSTRUMENTS AND DEVICES

1. Off-pump revascularization tissue stabilizers (Figure 12.3.13):
   - ∞ Octopus and Octopus Nuvo stabilizers (Medtronic, Minnesota, USA)
   - ∞ Acrobat-i stabilizer (Getinge, Gothenburg, Sweden)
   - ∞ Platypus stabilizer (Beating Heart, Sydney, Australia)

2. Intracoronary shunts:
   - ∞ ClearView Intracoronary Shunt (Medtronic, Minnesota, USA)
   - ∞ "Homemade" silastic shunts
3. MiraQ Cardiac transit time flow measurement (Medistim, Oslo, Norway)

For more details please see Figure 12.3.14 to Figure 12.3.19.

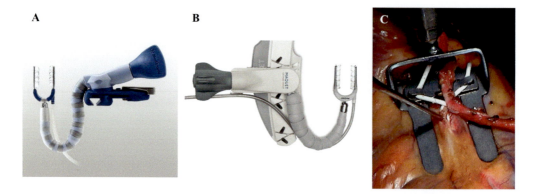

FIGURE 12.3.13 Off-pump stabilizers help in both stabilizing the coronary artery for grafting and positioning the heart: (A) Octopus® Evolution Tissue Stabilizer [Reproduced with permission of Medtronic, Inc.] and (B) Acrobat-i® both utilize suction along the stabilizer feet and are single-patient use [© 2020 Getinge AB, with permission]; (C) the Platypus® stabilizer does not utilize suction and instead relies on mechanical traction, though can be re-sterilized for multiple use [© 2020 Beating Heart Pty Ltd, with permission].

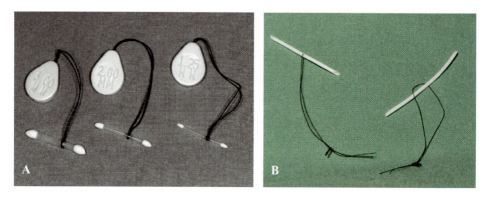

FIGURE 12.3.14 Intracoronary shunts have multiple benefits during off-pump surgery, including providing a clear view of the anastomotic site, providing blood flow to the distal myocardium during grafting and helping to prevent technical errors. (A) Commercially available ClearView shunt [Reproduced with permission of Medtronic, Inc.], (B) "Homemade" shunt. These are constructed at the beginning of each case by trimming a section of silastic tubing and passing a silk stitch through it. They have the advantage of being relatively inexpensive; the length can be adjusted as desired; and the silastic tubing is soft and flexible, aiding insertion.

FIGURE 12.3.15 Octopus and Octopus Nuvo stabilizers, Medtronic.

FIGURE 12.3.16 Acrobat-i stabilizer, Getinge AB.

318   Minimally Invasive Cardiac Surgery

FIGURE 12.3.17 Platypus stabilizer, Beating Heart, Sydney, Australia.

FIGURE 12.3.19 MiraQ Cardiac, Medistim.

FIGURE 12.3.18 ClearView Intracoronary Shunt, Medtronic.

ALTERNATIVE APPROACHES

Other methods of coronary artery bypass grafting include conventional CABG, MIDCAB, minimally invasive CABG, robotic CABG and hybrid CABG. The details of these bypass technique can be found in the other chapters of the book.

WHERE AND HOW TO LEARN

EACTS OPCAB FELLOWSHIP

The fellowship's goal is to provide newly graduated cardiothoracic surgeons from around the world with an educational opportunity to enhance their clinical understanding and to acquire theoretical and practical knowledge in the surgical management of patients with coronary artery disease, with special interest in off-pump and minimally invasive techniques. This will be under the guidance of leading surgeon-educators in this field (Figure 12.3.20).

EBM BEAT + YOUCAN SIMULATOR

It is a step before WETLAB and refers to practice of using artificial objects such as a simulator. Because WETLAB uses actual biological tissue, realistic skill practice that is possible; however, due to individual differences, repeated practice using the exact same tissue is not possible (Figure 12.3.21).

FIGURE 12.3.20 EACTS OPCAB fellowship.

FIGURE 12.3.21   EBM Beat + Youcan simulator.

SUMMARY

OPCAB, and in particular the anaortic approach that avoids all aortic manipulation, is a reproducible technique that is capable of achieving complete revascularization using multi-arterial and in situ grafts. It reduces the risk of peri-operative complications, including neurological injury, by avoiding the deleterious effect of cardiopulmonary bypass and manipulation and clamping of the ascending aorta. The technique may provide the most benefit to high-risk patients. There are some concerns regarding long-term outcomes, and therefore surgeons must assess graft patency intra-operatively and strive for complete revascularization.

REFERENCES

1. Goetz RH, Rohman M, Haller JD, Dee R, Rosenak SS. Internal mammary-coronary artery anastomosis. A nonsuture method employing tantalum rings. *J Thorac Cardiovasc Surg* 1961;41:378–86.
2. Buffolo E, Andrade JC, Succi JE, Leão LE, Cueva C, Branco JN, et al. Direct myocardial revascularization without extracorporeal circulation: technique and initial results. *Tex Heart Inst J* Texas Heart Institute; 1985;12(1):33–41.
3. Benetti FJ, Naselli G, Wood M, Geffner L. Direct myocardial revascularization without extracorporeal circulation. Experience in 700 patients. *Chest* 1991;100(2):312–6.
4. Angelini GD, Wilde P, Salerno TA, Bosco G, Calafiore AM. Integrated left small thoracotomy and angioplasty for multivessel coronary artery revascularisation. *Lancet* 1996;347(9003):757–8.
5. Calafiore AM, Vitolla G, Mazzei V, Teodori G, Di Giammarco G, Iovino T, et al. The LAST operation: techniques and results before and after the stabilization era. *Ann Thorac Surg* 1998;66(3):998–1001.
6. Seco M, Edelman JJB, Van Boxtel B, Forrest P, Byrom MJ, Wilson MK, et al. Neurologic injury and protection in adult cardiac and aortic surgery. *J Cardiothorac Vasc Anesth* 2015;29(1):185–95.
7. Indja B, Seco M, Seamark R, Kaplan J, Bannon PG, Grieve SM, et al. Neurocognitive and psychiatric issues post cardiac surgery. *Heart Lung Circ* 2017;26(8):779–85.
8. Zhao DF, Edelman JJ, Seco M, Bannon PG, Wilson MK, Byrom MJ, et al. Coronary artery bypass grafting with and without manipulation of the ascending aorta: a network meta-analysis. *J Am Coll Cardiol* 2017;69(8):924–36.
9. Sousa Uva M, Neumann F-J, Ahlsson A, Alfonso F, Banning AP, Benedetto U, et al. 2018 ESC/EACTS guidelines on myocardial revascularization. *Eur J Cardio-Thorac Surg* 2018;34(15):2949.
10. Shroyer AL, Grover FL, Hattler B, Collins JF, McDonald GO, Kozora E, et al. On-pump versus off-pump coronary-artery bypass surgery. *N Engl J Med* 2009;361(19):1827–37.

11. Lamy A, Devereaux PJ, Prabhakaran D, Taggart DP, Hu S, Paolasso E, et al. Effects of off-pump and on-pump coronary-artery bypass grafting at 1 year. *N Engl J Med* 2013;368(13):1179–88.
12. Diegeler A, Börgermann J, Kappert U, Breuer M, Böning A, Ursulescu A, et al. Off-pump versus on-pump coronary-artery bypass grafting in elderly patients. *N Engl J Med* 2013;368(13):1189–98.
13. Albert A, Ennker J, Hegazy Y, Ullrich S, Petrov G, Akhyari P, et al. Implementation of the aortic no-touch technique to reduce stroke after off-pump coronary surgery. *J Thorac Cardiovasc Surg* 2018;156(2):544–4.
14. Head SJ, Milojevic M, Daemen J, Ahn J-M, Boersma E, Christiansen EH, et al. Stroke rates following surgical versus percutaneous coronary revascularization. *J Am Coll Cardiol* 2018;72(4):386–98.
15. Zhao DF, Edelman JJB, Seco M, Bannon PG, Vallely MP. Stroke risk following anaortic off-pump coronary artery bypass grafting versus percutaneous coronary intervention: a network meta-analysis. *J Am Coll Cardiol* 2018;72 (21): 2679–2680.
16. Kowalewski M, Pawliszak W, Malvindi PG, Bokszanski MP, Perlinski D, Raffa GM, et al. Off-pump coronary artery bypass grafting improves short-term outcomes in high-risk patients compared with on-pump coronary artery bypass grafting: meta-analysis. *J Thorac Cardiovasc Surg* 2016;151(1):60–77.e1–58.
17. Puskas JD, Thourani VH, Kilgo P, Cooper W, Vassiliades T, Vega JD, et al. Off-pump coronary artery bypass disproportionately benefits high-risk patients. *Ann Thorac Surg* 2009;88(4):1142–7.
18. Karthik S, Musleh G, Grayson AD, Keenan DJM, Pullan DM, Dihmis WC, et al. Coronary surgery in patients with peripheral vascular disease: effect of avoiding cardiopulmonary bypass. *Annals Thorac Surg* 2004;77(4):1245–9.
19. Mishra M, Malhotra R, Karlekar A, Mishra Y, Trehan N. Propensity case-matched analysis of off-pump versus on-pump coronary artery bypass grafting in patients with atheromatous aorta. *Ann Thorac Surg* 2006;82(2):608–14.
20. Hattler B, Messenger JC, Shroyer AL, Collins JF, Haugen SJ, Garcia JA, et al. Off-pump coronary artery bypass surgery is associated with worse arterial and saphenous vein graft patency and less effective revascularization: results from the veterans affairs randomized on/off bypass (ROOBY) trial. *Circulation* 2012;125(23):2827–35.
21. Chikwe J, Lee T, Itagaki S, Adams DH, Egorova NN. Long-term outcomes after off-pump versus on-pump coronary artery bypass grafting by experienced surgeons. *J Am Coll Cardiol* Elsevier; 2018;72(13):1478–86.
22. Garcia S, Sandoval Y, Roukoz H, Adabag S, Canoniero M, Yannopoulos D, et al. Outcomes after complete versus incomplete revascularization of patients with multivessel coronary artery disease: a meta-analysis of 89,883 patients enrolled in randomized clinical trials and observational studies. *J Am Coll Cardiol* 2013;62(16):1421–31.
23. Puskas JD, Williams WH, O'Donnell R, Patterson RE, Sigman SR, Smith AS, et al. Off-pump and on-pump coronary artery bypass grafting are associated with similar graft patency, myocardial ischemia, and freedom from reintervention: long-term follow-up of a randomized trial. *Ann Thorac Surg* 2011;91(6):1836–42; discussion 1842–3.
24. Kobayashi J, Tashiro T, Ochi M, Yaku H, Watanabe G, Satoh T, et al. Early outcome of a randomized comparison of off-pump and on-pump multiple arterial coronary revascularization. *Circulation* 2005;112(9 Suppl):I338–43.
25. Magee MJ, Alexander JH, Hafley G, Ferguson TB, Gibson CM, Harrington RA, et al. Coronary artery bypass graft failure after on-pump and off-pump coronary artery bypass: findings from PREVENT IV. *Ann Thorac Surg* 2008;85(2):494–9; discussion 499–500.
26. Zhao DF, Edelman JJ, Seco M, Bannon PG, Vallely MP. Long-term outcomes following off-pump coronary artery bypass grafting: fixed-effects versus random-effects models. *J Am Coll Cardiol* 2018;72(3):345–7.
27. Ramponi F, Seco M, Edelman JB, Sherrah AG, Bannon PG, Brereton RJL, et al. Dual inflow, total-arterial, anaortic, off-pump coronary artery bypass grafting: how to do it. *Ann Cardiothorac Surg* 2018;7(4):552–60.

28. Royse AG, Brennan AP, Ou-Young J, Pawanis Z, Canty DJ, Royse CF. 21-year survival of left internal mammary artery-radial artery-Y graft. *J Am Coll Cardiol* 2018;72(12):1332–40.

29. Amin S, Werner RS, Madsen PL, Krasopoulos G, Taggart DP. Intraoperative bypass graft flow measurement with transit time flowmetry: a clinical assessment. *Ann Thorac Surg* 2018.

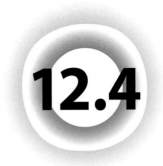

THE CORONARIES
Hybrid Coronary Artery Bypass Grafting Surgery

CLAUDIO MUNERETTO, CHANG GUOHAO AND THEO KOFIDIS

HISTORY AND INTRODUCTION

Cardiac surgery has made many giant leaps of advancements since the first CPB machine was designed and used in 1953 by John Gibbons. The birth of coronary artery bypass graft surgery (CABG) took root when Alexis Carrel first described operating on the coronary circulation in 1910. Being the first surgeon to appreciate the relationship between angina and stenotic coronary artery disease, he performed "complementary circulation" for diseased native coronary arteries in canine experiments. Since then, CABG underwent three distinct eras in its evolution – the "experimental" pioneering era and the era of "vein grafting" followed by the era of "mixed grafting – arterial and venous". These all fall within the era of conventional median sternotomy. Today, we have moved into the fourth era, perhaps even more advanced, where the field of minimally invasive coronary revascularization presents a viable and attractive option, or even the default modality in today's age of hybrid coronary revascularization, further enhancing the partnership between cardiac surgeons and interventional cardiologists to bring about optimal patient outcomes.

Hybrid coronary revascularization (HCR) is a one-stop service provided by cardiac surgeons and cardiologists. This modern concept was first described by Angelini et al. in the mid-1990s, and several patient series using HCR have been

FIGURE 12.4.1 On the experimental surgery of the thoracic aorta and heart.

FIGURE 12.4.2 HCR, clinical benefits and technologies.

published since then [1]. HCR enables the surgeon to perform, within the patient's closed anterior chest, a revascularization configuration equivalent to that of a regular coronary artery bypass graft surgery without the need for a sternotomy, and in most patients, without the use of CPB, in a minimally invasive fashion. In this chapter, we present various considerations, techniques and equipment available for hybrid coronary revascularization (Figure 12.4.1, Figure 12.4.2 and Figure 12.4.3).

HOW TO DO IT/STEP BY STEP

According to the definition from the American Heart Association and the European Society for Cardiology, HCR for multi-vessel disease is defined as a planned, intentional combination of the LIMA to LAD grafting and a catheter-based intervention to one or more non-LAD coronary arteries during the same hospital stay. This

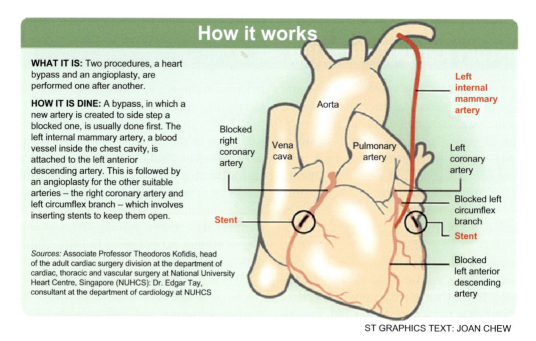

FIGURE 12.4.3 Summary of hybrid coronary revascularization. The Straits Times © Singapore Press Holdings Limited. Reprinted with permission.

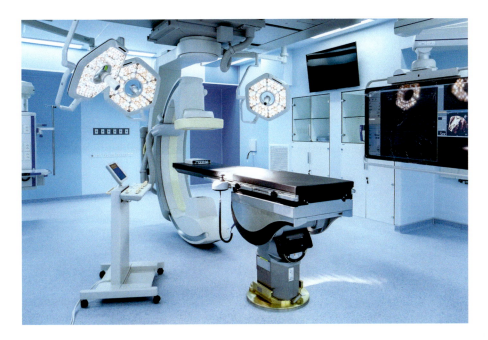

FIGURE 12.4.4 Setup of a hybrid operating theatre.

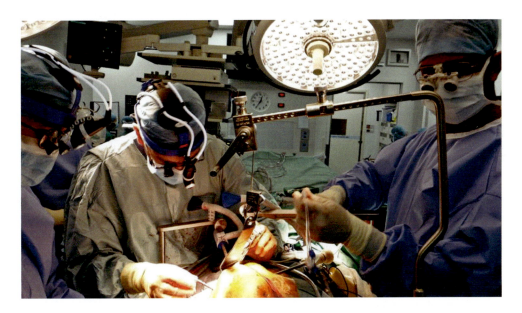

FIGURE 12.4.5 Hybrid revascularization with minimally invasive staged CABG; LIMA anastomosis to LAD followed by PCI.

can be performed concurrently in a hybrid operating room in a single operative setting (same-stop hybrid revascularization) or can be performed in two different stages, separated by a period of hours to a few weeks, often during the same hospital stay [2] (Figure 12.4.4). This hybrid approach is especially useful in patients with multi-vessel coronary artery disease.

FIGURE 12.4.6 Introduction and key procedural steps to HCR.

FIGURE 12.4.7 Robot-assisted heart bypass with cardiac catheterization.

McGinn et al. [3] demonstrated the use of a minimally invasive strategy to revascularize multiple myocardial territories, namely the anterior, lateral and inferior myocardial territories. This allows for the feasibility of surgical revascularization of the vessels, which may not be amenable to PCI, thereby offering an expansion of the types of patients suitable for the hybrid revascularization program. The ability to surgically revascularize the artery (other than the LAD) allows PCI to be carried out on one vessel, with the remaining two receiving internal mammary artery/saphenous vein grafts (Figure 12.4.5, Figure 12.4.6 and Figure 12.4.7). These territories were accessed via the fifth left intercostal space through a 4–6-cm thoracotomy. The coronary targets were stabilized using a positioner and epicardial stabilizer. The team successfully showed that multi-vessel minimally invasive CABG can be done safely and effectively with excellent short-term outcomes. In the first 450 consecutive patients treated via this technique, complete revascularization was achieved in 95% of patients. Perioperative mortality was 1.3% (compared to 2.5% in conventional CABG) and the risks of conversion to sternotomy and cardiopulmonary bypass were 3.8% and 7.6%, respectively.

TOOLS/INSTRUMENTS AND DEVICES

The concept of HCR combines the advantages of PCI and CABG. Percutaneous intervention in non-LAD lesions enables full revascularization despite minimal invasive surgical access to address the left-sided stenoses. The performance of coronary anastomoses via the left anterior thoracotomy requires a variety of instruments, from patient positioning, to the harvesting of the left internal thoracic artery and fashioning of the distal and proximal anastomoses.

PERIOPERATIVE CONSIDERATION

Patient selection is important for hybrid revascularization. To date, CABG is the preferred option for patients with chronic total occlusions, highly calcified lesions and diffusely diseased and bifurcation coronary lesions. In patients for whom CABG is not an option, HCR offers the LIMA survival benefit beyond PCI. This is a reasonable option in patients with at least double vessel disease (LAD and a non-LAD lesion), who are not suitable surgical candidates. In these patients, the non-LAD lesion can be dealt with by PCI. Such patients include those with a lack of suitable bypass conduits, ascending aortic disease or a nongraftable coronary vessel which may still be amenable to PCI. In addition, patients with multiple comorbidities that will increase the risk of CABG will benefit from the minimally invasive techniques employed in HCR. This includes patients with a recent history of AMI, poor LVEF, previous cardiac surgery or severe extra-cardiac arteriopathy [4].

ALTERNATIVE APPROACHES

Hybrid coronary revascularization is the planned use of minimally invasive LIMA-LAD revascularization and PCI. There are various approaches a surgeon can adopt by using this concept; ranging from the simplest MIDCAB and PCI to non-LAD lesions to the complex robotic-assisted revascularization of the left-sided coronary stenoses via the left anterior thoracotomy followed by PCI to the right-sided coronary stenoses. The sequence at which this is carried out has its pros and cons, which will be further elaborated on in the section below on "caveats and controversies".

CAVEATS AND CONTROVERSIES

In the field of hybrid revascularization, there remains the question of a single-stage versus a double-stage procedure. Theoretically, concurrent hybrid revascularization with PCI should first result in a shorter length of stay and is safer as it allows for conversion to CABG should complications of PCI occur. However, there are associated risks of bleeding due to the use of dual antiplatelet therapy and incomplete heparin reversal, as well as acute stent thrombosis due to the proinflammatory status directly after surgery. In addition, by doing PCI after CABG in a single-stage procedure in the hybrid operating theatre, the angiography offers confirmation of LIMA-LAD patency. Other challenges that limit the practice of single-stage HCR are increased costs, need for a hybrid operating suite with trained personnel and the logistical difficulties of coordinating two different teams in the same operating theatre at different times.

In performing the simultaneous HCR, revascularization of the LAD coronary artery can be performed by the conventional minimally invasive direct coronary artery bypass (MIDCAB) technique (Figure 12.4.8 and Figure 12.4.9), or ideally by a robotically assisted endoscopic approach after the LIMA has been harvested as a

FIGURE 12.4.8 How to perform an MIDCAB.

FIGURE 12.4.9 Presentation on the MIDCAB and hybrid revascularization.

FIGURE 12.4.10 Optimal strategy for high-risk coronary patients for HCR.

FIGURE 12.4.12 Hybrid revascularization: why, when and how.

FIGURE 12.4.11 HCR with robotic LIMA to LAD and PCI.

FIGURE 12.4.13 ISMICS 2014 annual meeting presentation.

pedicle under direct vision (Figure 12.4.10 and Figure 12.4.11). The PCI is performed after closure of the thoracotomy, and angiography is then done to confirm patency of the LIMA-LAD graft, followed by PCI to the non-LAD lesions.

A double-stage procedure with PCI followed by CABG is currently reserved for patients with acute coronary syndrome with a non-LAD culprit. This approach may complicate the surgery due to bleeding risks associated with the need for continued use of dual antiplatelet therapy and the sequence of intervention does not allow angiographical assessment of the patency of the LIMA to LAD graft. By far, the double-stage LIMA to LAD graft and PCI (drug-eluting stents) for non-LAD lesions is currently the most adopted approach. Similar to single-stage HCR, the patency of the LIMA to LAD graft can be confirmed with coronary angiography during the time of PCI. This strategy also has the advantage of operating on the patient before the commencement of antiplatelet treatment. However, in the event of a complication or failure of PCI, emergent CABG with a higher risk of mortality will be required (Figure 12.4.12).

RESEARCH, TRENDS AND INNOVATION

ISMICS 2014 ANNUAL MEETING PRESENTATION

A Paradigm shift in Coronary Revascularization – 1021 Consecutive Robot Assisted Coronary Artery Bypass Procedures (Figure 12.4.13).

REFERENCES

1. Angelini GD, Wilde P, Salerno TA, Bosco G, Calafiore AM. Integrated left small thoracotomy and angioplasty for multivessel coronary artery revascularisation. *Lancet* 1996;347(9003):757–8.
2. Harskamp RE, Bonatti JO, Zhao DX, et al. Standardizing definitions for hybrid coronary revascularization. *J Thorac Cardiovasc Surg* 2014;147(2):556–60.
3. McGinn JT Jr., Usman S, Lapierre H, et al. Minimally invasive coronary artery bypass grafting: dual-center experience in 450 consecutive patients. *Circulation* 2009;120(11 Suppl):S78–84.
4. Us MH, Basaran M, Yilmaz M, et al. Hybrid coronary revascularization in high-risk patients. *Tex Heart Inst J* 2006;33(4):458–62.

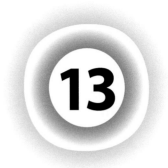

MINIMALLY INVASIVE ATRIAL ABLATION SURGERY

ANIL K GEHI, AND ANDY C KISER

HISTORY AND INTRODUCTION

Atrial fibrillation (AF) is the most common clinical arrhythmia and is associated with significant morbidity and mortality. The incidence of AF continues to rise, likely attributable to the aging of the patient population and the rising prevalence of chronic cardiac disease. As the overall prevalence of AF rises, it continues to be a great burden on the healthcare system.

Surgical techniques for the rhythm control of AF emerged in the 1980s. The "Corridor" procedure, described by Guiraudon et al. in 1985, isolated the sinus node along with a small corridor of atrium from the rest of the atrium, giving the patient normal sinus rhythm (NSR), while the rest of the atrium was still fibrillating [1, 2].

The pioneering work of James Cox led to the Cox maze procedure in the late 1980s [3]. Dividing the atria into smaller segments with a cut-and-sew technique meant fewer re-entrant circuits were maintained. The principles of the "Cox maze III" procedure remain the gold standard for all ablative interventions for AF with long-term success rates of >90% as assessed by symptom guidance alone [4].

Damiano et al. described the "cut-and-sew maze IV" to replace some incisions with RF and cryothermal energy sources to reduce operative time while preserving procedural success [5] (Figure 13.1). However, open surgery for standalone AF never gained popularity given its complexity and significant morbidity.

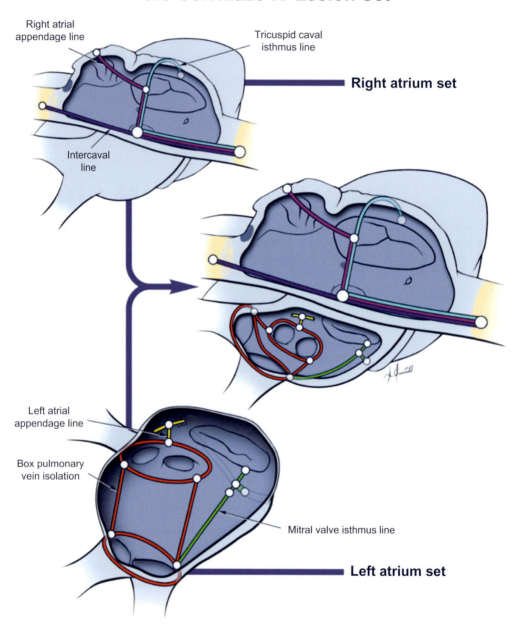

FIGURE 13.1 Six circuit interruption lines of Cox maze. (Reprinted from Surgical Treatment of Atrial Fibrillation, 1st edition, Jonathan P, Christian Z. Ralph D, Foundation and Fundamentals, Page 15, © 2017 with permission from Elsevier.)

FIGURE 13.2 STS University Course 10: Atrial Fibrillation.

FIGURE 13.3 Conventional concomitant Cox maze IV procedure.

Since its advent in the late 1990s, radiofrequency (RF) endocardial catheter ablation has emerged as a less invasive tool for the management of symptomatic AF. The improved efficacy of endocardial catheter ablation over antiarrhythmic drug therapy has been established in several randomized controlled trials. However, longer-term data have proved to be less encouraging [6, 7].

Multiple factors likely contribute to AF recurrence after catheter ablation including progression of the underlying disease processes, inadequate ablation of important targets for therapy and reversibly injured sites of ablation. When followed over several years, it is clear that recurrence of AF after endocardial catheter ablation is relentless, often warranting repeat ablation procedures. With the goal of improving efficacy, particularly in those patients with risk factors for poor outcomes using a standard catheter ablation technique, less invasive surgical ablation techniques have emerged as an alternative to the "cut-and-sew" procedures. Although the Cox maze surgery is highly effective, its complexity and associated morbidity have limited its adoption as a widespread standalone treatment for AF. Alternative minimally invasive surgical procedures have been developed for those not requiring concomitant cardiac surgery.

HOW TO DO IT/STEP BY STEP

The advancement of minimally invasive approaches, with and without the use of cardiopulmonary bypass, has reduced the trauma of the surgical procedure, thereby expanding the number of patients experiencing this therapy. Some minimally invasive approaches replicate the maze procedure better than others, with some compromising procedural completeness for less invasive techniques. However, the guiding principles of a surgical therapy for AF remain the same: complete isolation of the four pulmonary veins, electrical isolation of the posterior left atrium, management of the left atrial appendage and appropriate ablation of the right atrium (Figure 13.2).

MINIMALLY INVASIVE COX MAZE PROCEDURE

Lee et al. and Ad et al. have described a minimally invasive Cox maze III/IV procedure that is perhaps most similar to the conventional Cox maze procedure. The procedure is performed with cardiopulmonary bypass (CPB) via a right minithoracotomy, and creates a lesion pattern that closely mimics the original maze III pattern using cryotherapy [8, 9] (Figure 13.3 to Figure 13.5.6).

PULMONARY VEIN ISOLATION

Epicardial off-pump pulmonary vein isolation became important after pulmonary

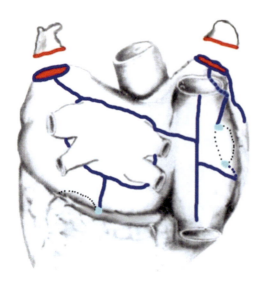

FIGURE 13.4 Typical lesion set of the Cox maze III procedure. Incisions encircle the pulmonary veins with connecting lesions to the mitral annulus and the left atrial appendage. An incision across the atrial septum crosses from the left to the right atrium. The right atrial incisions are from the superior to the inferior vena cava; to the right atrial appendage, which is excised, and further to the tricuspid annulus; and along the lateral right atrial free wall to the posterior annulus of the tricuspid valve. (Incisions = dark blue; excision = red; cryo = light blue). (Reprinted from *Prog Cardiovasc Dis,* 58(2), Kumar P, Kiser AC, Gehi AK. Hybrid treatment of atrial fibrillation, 213–220, © 2015, with permission from Elsevier.)

FIGURE 13.5 Maze procedure, Cleveland Clinic.

FIGURE 13.6 ACS how I do it: minimally invasive Cox maze IV procedure.

veins were identified as an important source triggering AF [10]. With ablation of the pulmonary veins, 62% patients failed to return to AF at 8 months. Saltman initially described a bilateral thoracoscopic approach using microwave energy to create a box lesion around the pulmonary veins [11].

PRUITT BOX LESION

Pruitt et al. subsequently described using microwave energy via bilateral thoracoscopy to create a box lesion around the pulmonary veins, a right atrial lesion to the atrial appendage and another from the superior to the inferior vena cava and staple occlusion of the left atrial appendage (LAA) [12] (Figure 13.7).

WOLF MINI MAZE

The bipolar radiofrequency clamp was introduced in the mid-2000, and in 2005 Wolf described an epicardial off-pump pulmonary vein isolation procedure performed via thoracoscopy or minithoracotomy [13]. It is now known as the Wolf mini maze procedure [14] (Figure 13.8).

PVI VIA RIGHT MINITHORACOTOMY

Speziale et al. described the use of an alternative surgical technique for pulmonary vein isolation through only a right minithoracotomy. A linear vacuum-assisted unipolar RF ablation catheter was looped around the pulmonary veins by way of the transverse and oblique pericardial sinuses using a magnet-tipped introducer [15]. While there is an advantage of using only a right thoracic incision for Speziale's approach, the left atrial appendage is not addressed (Figure 13.9 and Figure 13.10).

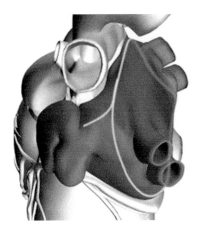
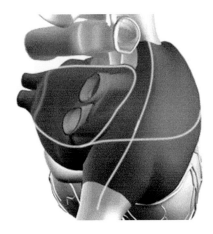

FIGURE 13.7 Completed left atrial lesion set for intermittent atrial fibrillation and biatrial lesion set for continuous atrial fibrillation respectively. (Reprinted from *Ann Thorac Surg*, 81(4), Pruitt JC, Lazzara RR, Dworkin GH, Badhwar V, Kuma C, Ebra G. Totally endoscopic ablation of lone atrial fibrillation: initial clinical experience, 1325-1331, © 2006, with permission from Elsevier.)

PULMONARY VEIN ISOLATION AND AUTONOMIC DENERVATION

As the role of ganglionated plexi (GP) in the initiation and maintenance of AF became apparent, GP ablation emerged as a potential ancillary strategy for surgical AF ablation. Patients underwent bilateral mini-thoracotomies with GPs identified by vagal response to high-frequency stimulation. Bipolar radiofrequency clamps were used to isolate the pulmonary vein antra and GP ablation was performed [16] (Figure 13.11). A left atrial appendage exclusion procedure may be performed via excision or stapling.

DALLAS LESION SET

Edgerton et al. developed a beating-heart procedure using minimally invasive techniques known as the "Dallas" lesion set [17]. This approach was designed to make a connection to the left fibrous trigone at the aortic valve root and involved totally thoracoscopic isolation of bilateral pulmonary vein antra using a bipolar RF clamp. Additionally, the GP were interrogated and ablated, the LAA was excised and a connecting lesion was added between the pulmonary veins at the LA roof, which was also extended to the fibrous aortic valve annulus and to the excised LAA base. The conduction block across the roof and anterior trigone lines was verified by pacing techniques (Figure 13.12 and Figure 13.13).

The minimally invasive, beating heart approach to AF treatment enables real-time interrogation of the surgical ablations because the heart remains electrically active. It is therefore important to interrogate the integrity of the ablation lines to confirm transmurality AND to eliminate gaps.

FIVE BOX ABLATION

There is ongoing dialogue concerning the validity of lesion interrogation acutely versus delayed lesion interrogation to allow

FIGURE 13.8 Wolf mini maze procedure.

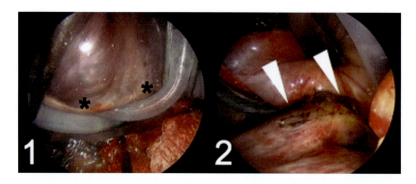

FIGURE 13.9 Intraoperative videoscopic views: (1) The branches of the ablation probe (asterisks) are tightened in place around the orifices of the four pulmonary veins. (2) The ablation line can be inspected at the end of the energy delivery, and appears uniform (arrowheads). (Reprinted from *Ann Thorac Surg,* 90(1), Speziale G, Bonifazi R, Nasso G, et al. Minimally invasive radiofrequency ablation of lone atrial fibrillation by monolateral right minithoracotomy: operative and early follow-up results, 161-167, © 2010, with permission from Elsevier.)

any acute and temporally non-conductive injuries to recover. The five-box thoracoscopic maze procedure described by Sirak critically interrogates the ablation lines to confirm the epicardial electrical isolation of five segments of the left and right atrium [18, 19] (Figure 13.14 to Figure 13.18).

TOOLS/INSTRUMENTS AND DEVICES

- AtriCure, West Chester, OH (Figure 13.19)
- RF ablation clamps (Synergy, AtriCure, West Chester, OH)
- Surgical ablation pens
    - Bipolar pen and physiologic recorder (AtriCure, West Chester, OH) (Figure 13.20)
    - Bipolar unidirectional ablation device (CoolRail, AtriCure) (Figure 13.21)
- The Cobra Fusion Ablation System
- AtriClip (AtriCure Inc, West Chester Township, OH)
- Other devices:
    - Temporary external pacemaker (Oscor, Oscor INC., Palm Harbor, FL)
    - Monopolar radiofrequency device with suction adherence and internal cooling (Cobra Adhere XL; Estech, San Ramon, Calif) (Figure 13.22 and Figure 13.23)

FIGURE 13.10 Atrial fibrillation PVI with GP ablation.

FIGURE 13.11 Cardiac electrophysiology epicardial GP ablation.

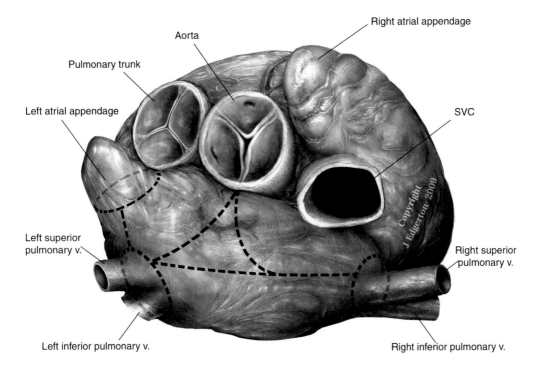

FIGURE 13.12 The Dallas lesion set. SVC = superior vena cava; v. = vein. (Reprinted from *Operative Techniques in Thoracic and Cardiovascular Surgery*, 14(3), James R. Edgerton, Total Thorascopic Ablation of Atrial Fibrillation Using the Dallas Lesion Set, Partial Autonomic Denervation, and Left Atrial Appendectomy, 224-242, © 2009, with permission from Elsevier.)

- Tetrapolar EP catheter (Avail, Josephson Curve, type A; Biosense Webster)
- F decapolar electrode endocardial catheter (P-Supra CS; Biosense Webster, Diamond Bar, Calif)
- Cannula designed for pericardioscopic access (nContact Surgical, Morrisville, NC, USA)
- Irrigated, unipolar RF ablation device (Visitrax, nContact Surgical, Morrisville, NC)
- Endoscopic 10-mm/5-mm laparoscopic ports (Karl Storz Endoscopy, Tuttlingen, Germany)
- Numeris Guided Coagulation System (nContact, Inc)
- Teflon monopolar electrocautery hook probe (ATC Technologies, Wilmington, Mass)

PERIOPERATIVE CONSIDERATIONS

PAROXYSMAL VERSUS PERSISTENT AF

The majority of patients in the initial studies had paroxysmal AF. Because endocardial catheter ablation can be highly effective for paroxysmal AF and is a much less invasive procedure, standalone epicardial ablation for paroxysmal AF has not gained widespread acceptance. Follow-up studies have demonstrated that pulmonary vein isolation alone is insufficient for the treatment

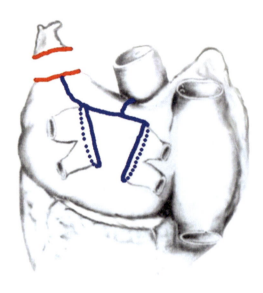

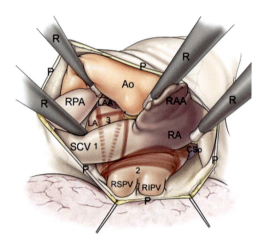

FIGURE 13.13 The "Dallas" epicardial lesion set. Blue lines indicate epicardial ablation lesions (AtriCure). Red lines indicate surgical lines. (Reprinted from *Prog Cardiovasc Dis*, 58(2), Kumar P, Kiser AC, Gehi AK. Hybrid treatment of atrial fibrillation, 213-220, © 2015, with permission from Elsevier.)

FIGURE 13.14 Five-box thoracoscopic maze.

FIGURE 13.15 A large enclosed triangle is created on the dome of the left atrium (LA) posterior to the interatrial septum, consisting of a transmitral line originating from the noncoronary aortic root, a transverse roof line between the superior pulmonary antra and a line from the apex of the transmitral line to the right pulmonary antrum. Note the ablations isolating the superior vena cava and distal coronary sinus. (Reprinted from *Ann Thorac Surg*, 90(3), Sirak J, Jones D, Schwartzman D. The five-box thoracoscopic maze procedure, 986-989, © 2010, with permission from Elsevier.) (Ao = aorta; CSo = coronary sinus; LAA = left atrial appendage; P = pericardium; R = retractor; RA = right atrium; RAA = right atrial appendage; RIPV = right inferior pulmonary vein; RPA = right pulmonary artery; RSPV = right superior pulmonary vein.)

of persistent AF [20]. Additionally, the particular role of ganglionated plexi ablation is unclear, and no randomized studies have specifically evaluated its benefit. In those with persistent AF, adding linear ablation to pulmonary vein isolation, specifically isolating the posterior left atrium, has proven to be beneficial [21]. However, the creation of ablations that connect to the cytoskeleton of the heart, thus closing electrical gaps that may persist near the mitral and tricuspid valve, remains difficult, if not impossible, with existing energy sources on the beating heart.

MINIMALLY INVASIVE SURGICAL VERSUS CATHETER ABLATION

The advances in technology since the original maze procedure have facilitated the expansion of a minimally invasive surgical option to many patients with non-paroxysmal AF. Yet despite these advances, none approach the low level of invasiveness of catheter ablation. To evaluate the differences in catheter and surgical ablation for AF, Boersma et al. compared the efficacy and safety of catheter ablation and minimally invasive surgical ablation in 124 patients with drug-refractory

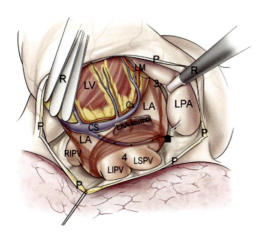

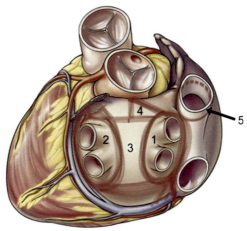

FIGURE 13.16 With the apex elevated, the enclosure of the posterior left atrium is completed with linear ablations connecting the inferior pulmonary veins. The ablations on the dome of the left atrium, including the junction of the transmitral line with the superior interantral line, and traversing the distal coronary sinus, are easily visualized. (Reprinted from *Ann Thorac Surg*, 90(3), Sirak J, Jones D, Schwartzman D. The five-box thoracoscopic maze procedure, 986-989, © 2010, with permission from Elsevier.) (CS = coronary sinus; Cx = circumflex; LA = left atrium; LAA = left atrial appendage; LIPV = left inferior pulmonary vein; LM = left main; LPA = left pulmonary artery; LSPV = left superior pulmonary vein; LV = left ventricle; P = pericardium; R = retractor; RIPV = right inferior pulmonary vein.)

FIGURE 13.17 The complete five-box lesion pattern encompasses four contiguous compartments: the two pulmonary antra (1,2), the posterior left atrium (3) and an enclosed triangle on the dome of the left atrium incorporating the connection the anterior trigone of the mitral annulus (4), as well as the superior vena cava (5). Additional linear lesions connect both the left pulmonary antrum and the transmitral line to the base of the left atrial appendage, and the right pulmonary antrum to the coronary sinus. (Reprinted from *Ann Thorac Surg*, 90(3), Sirak J, Jones D, Schwartzman D. The five-box thoracoscopic maze procedure, 986-989, © 2010, with permission from Elsevier.)

AF, left atrial dilatation (>4 cm) and hypertension [22]. AF was paroxysmal (67%), persistent (33%) or long-standing persistent (8%). The surgical ablation consisted of the Dallas lesion set as described by Edgerton. Catheter ablation consisted of wide-area linear antrum ablation with PV isolation guided by circular mapping catheter. Additional lines were made at the discretion of the operator. Patients were followed with ECG and 7-day Holter monitoring at 6 and 12 months. The median length of stay was 5.5 days vs 2 days for surgical or catheter ablation, respectively.

In the surgical group, complications included one patient requiring conversion to median sternotomy, one patient requiring pacemaker implantation, six patients with pneumothorax, one with hemothorax, one with stroke, one tamponade and one rib fracture. In the catheter group, complications included one transient ischemic attack and four groin hematomas. However, at 12 months, freedom from AF >30 seconds in the absence of antiarrhythmic drugs was 66% in the surgical group vs 37% in the catheter group (p = 0.0022).

COMORBIDITIES

Patients considered for surgery should also be screened for other cardiac disease prior to intervention based on thorough history

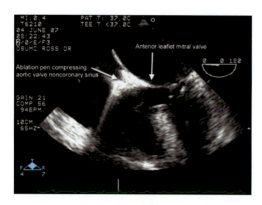

FIGURE 13.18 Ablation of the anterior mitral trigone is verified by demonstration on transesophageal echocardiography of compression of the noncoronary sinus of aorta. (Reprinted from *Ann Thorac Surg*, 90(3), Sirak J, Jones D, Schwartzman D. The five-box thoracoscopic maze procedure, 986-989, © 2010, with permission from Elsevier.)

FIGURE 13.19 AtriCure, West Chester, OH.

and physical examination. An echocardiogram should be performed to assess for valvular heart disease and regional wall motion abnormalities. Older patients and those with cardiovascular risk factors may warrant a diagnostic coronary angiogram.

FIGURE 13.20 Cardioblate surgical ablation pens.

FIGURE 13.21 Bipolar unidirectional ablation device (CoolRail, AtriCure).

FIGURE 13.22 Atrial clipping for atrial fibrillation – case report.

Patients with severe lung disease or chronic smoking history should have pulmonary function assessment to determine suitability for single-lung ventilation.

ALTERNATIVE APPROACHES

HYBRID ABLATION

Hybrid ablation is a useful alternative for patients with persistent AF. The endocardial catheter ablation may supplement the gaps in ablation lines performed epicardially. The epicardial and endocardial ablation may be done as a convergent (simultaneous epicardial-endocardial ablation) or staged procedure. The epicardial ablation may be performed via thoracoscopic (bilateral or monolateral) or transdiaphragmatic (either isolated subxiphoid pericardioscopic or with laparoscopic aid) approaches.

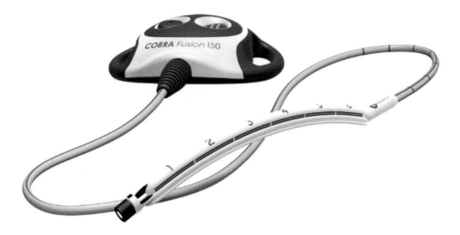

FIGURE 13.23   Cobra Fusion 150 Ablation System. Reproduced with permission of AtriCure, Inc.

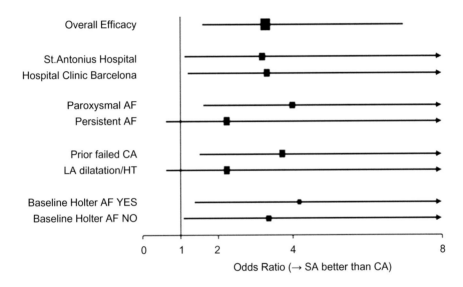

FIGURE 13.24   Forest plot of subgroup analysis for surgical ablation (SA) vs catheter ablation (CA) efficacy. AF indicates atrial fibrillation; LA, left atrium; and HT, hypertension. (Reprinted with permission from Boersma LV, Castella M, van Boven W, et al. Atrial fibrillation catheter ablation versus surgical ablation treatment (FAST): a 2-center randomized clinical trial. *Circulation* 125(1), 23-30, © 2012 American Heart Association, Inc.)

THORACOSCOPIC APPROACH

Mahapatra et al. reported their experience with a hybrid epicardial and endocardial ablation in 15 patients with persistent or long-standing persistent AF who had failed at least 1 attempt at endocardial ablation and antiarrhythmic drug therapy [23]. Patients were excluded if they had another indication for cardiac surgery or a prior history of cardiac surgery. Bilateral thoracoscopic off-pump epicardial ablation was performed using the Dallas lesion set (pulmonary vein isolation, SVC isolation, roof and mitral line, elimination of ganglia response, ligament of Marshall ablation and left atrial appendage exclusion). Patients

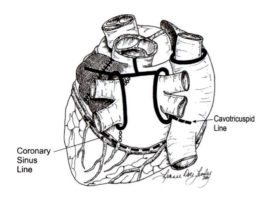

FIGURE 13.25 Schematic representation of epicardial (bold) and endocardial (dashed) ablation lines for sequential procedure. (Reprinted from *Ann Thorac Surg*, 19(6), Mahapatra S, LaPar DJ, Kamath S, et al. Initial experience of sequential surgical epicardial-catheter endocardial ablation for persistent and long-standing persistent atrial fibrillation with long-term follow-up, 1890-1898, © 2011, with permission from Elsevier.)

FIGURE 13.26 Thoracoscopic maze (TT maze/hybrid maze)

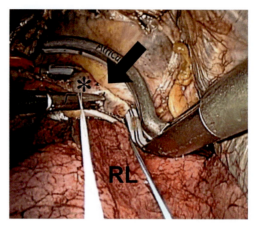

FIGURE 13.27 Right pulmonary vein isolation. A large antral lesion (arrow) is created using a bipolar radiofrequency clamp, resulting in complete isolation of the right pulmonary veins (PVs). The antrum of the right PVs (*) is clearly visible. RL = right lung. (Reprinted from *J Am Coll Cardiol*, 60(1), Pison L, La Meir M, van Opstal J, Blaauw Y, Maessen J, Crijns HJ. Hybrid thoracoscopic surgical and transvenous catheter ablation of atrial fibrillation, 54-61, © 2012 American College of Cardiology Foundation, with permission from Elsevier.)

were cardioverted, and PV and SVC isolation was confirmed by an electrophysiologist in the operating room. Endocardial ablation was performed an average of 4 days later as a staged procedure (Figure 13.24, Figure 13.25 and Figure 13.26).

During endocardial ablation, SVC isolation was confirmed, a cavotricuspid isthmus line was created, and PV isolation and block across the roof and mitral line were confirmed (Figure 13.27). Finally, high-dose isoproterenol was used for induction. Any atrial flutter induced was mapped and ablated. If AF was induced, additional complex fractionated atrial electrogram ablation was performed. All patients were treated with amiodarone or dofetilide for 3 months post-procedure. Routine 7-day or 24-hour continuous monitoring was performed.

La Meir described a hybrid bilateral thoracoscopic approach that included patients with paroxysmal AF. The epicardial ablation included pulmonary vein isolation, roof and inferior LA ablation targeting a posterior "box" and GP ablation. Entrance and exit blocks across the PV and posterior box lines were checked. In the hybrid group of patients, PV isolation and block across the lines were checked endocardially. The induction of AF was performed during endocardial ablation with rapid pacing and/or isoproterenol infusion. In the case of persistent AF, a mitral line was created. Additional SVC isolation was added in those with persistent or long-standing persistent AF, and cavotricuspid isthmus ablation was performed in those with a history of typical right atrial flutter or

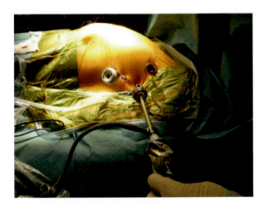

FIGURE 13.28 Placement of ports on the left side of the patient. (Reprinted from *J Am Coll Cardiol*, 60(1), Pison L, La Meir M, van Opstal J, Blaauw Y, Maessen J, Crijns HJ. Hybrid thoracoscopic surgical and transvenous catheter ablation of atrial fibrillation, 54-61, © 2012 American College of Cardiology Foundation, with permission from Elsevier.)

FIGURE 13.29 Stand-alone ablation with Cobra Adhere XL – Claudio Muneretto.

FIGURE 13.30 Hybrid thoracoscopic epicardial and catheter-based endocardial ablation.

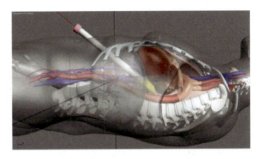

FIGURE 13.31 Transabdominal, transdiaphragmatic access to the pericardium. (Reprinted from *Heart Rhythm* 10(1), Gehi AK, Mounsey JP, Pursell I, et al. Hybrid epicardial-endocardial ablation using a pericardioscopic technique for the treatment of atrial fibrillation, 22-28, © 2013, with permission from Elsevier.)

if it became apparent during the procedure (Figure 13.28). Finally, LAA exclusion was performed in those with an LAA tachycardia or a CHADS2 score ≥1 [24].

Pison et al. reported their experience in 26 patients undergoing hybrid thoracoscopic and transvenous ablation for AF in patients who had either failed prior catheter ablation, had an enlarged left atrial volume (≥29 ml/m^2) or had persistent or long-standing persistent AF [25]. Similar to Mahapatra and La Meir, the pulmonary veins were isolated at the antra using a bipolar RF clamp and confirmed endocardially. In those with persistent AF, a roof line and posterior LA line (box lesion), SVC isolation and intercaval lines were created. Epicardial and endocardial mitral lines were created. A cavotricuspid isthmus line was made in those with a prior history of atrial flutter or flutter during the procedure. Finally, the LAA was excluded in a subset.

Muneretto et al. described a durable hybrid monolateral right-sided thoracoscopic ablation technique with staged transcatheter electrophysiologic evaluation in patients with lone persistent or longstanding persistent AF. The catheter procedure was done 30–45 days after the surgical ablation [26]. This was initially performed using the Cobra Adhere XL and later using the Cobra Fusion device in the multicenter HISTORIC-AF trial [27]. The protocol involved evaluation following surgical ablation with a 6F decapolar electrode endocardial catheter inserted prior at the EP laboratory into the coronary

FIGURE 13.32 The hybrid convergent procedure transabdominal access.

sinus (sensing probe) and a tetrapolar EP catheter introduced through a port, then advanced epicardially within the box lesion (pacing probe) connected to an EP workstation (Figure 13.29).

SUBXIPHOID PERICARDIOSCOPIC APPROACH

Zembala et al. reported their outcomes in Poland using a staged hybrid ablation technique in 27 patients with persistent AF (5 patients) or long-standing persistent AF (22 patients) and a left atrium less than 6 cm in diameter. The epicardial portion of the procedure was performed by way of subxiphoid pericardioscopic access through the diaphragm. An irrigated, unipolar, vacuum-assisted RF linear ablation catheter was utilized through a pericardioscopic access cannula. The epicardial lesion set included a posterior box (roof and low posterior LA lines), antral PV ablation and connecting lesions to the coronary sinus. Endocardial ablation was performed 15 to 20 days later. The endocardial lesion set included the completion of antral PV isolation, mitral isthmus ablation and cavotricuspid isthmus ablation (Figure 13.30, Figure 13.31 and Figure 13.32). Patients were maintained on antiarrhythmic drug therapy for 3 months post-ablation [28].

Gehi et al. described simultaneous hybrid epicardial-endocardial ablation also using a pericardioscopic technique. The majority of patients had persistent (47%) or long-standing persistent (37%) AF (Figure 13.33). Patients with paroxysmal AF had failed at

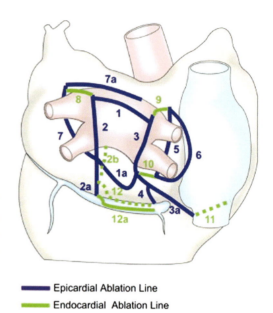

FIGURE 13.33 Epicardial and endocardial ablation lines performed by the surgeon (blue) and by the electrophysiologist (green). 1. Cephalad posterior left atrium. 1a. Caudal posterior left atrium. 2. Left posterior left atrium. 2a. Left inferior pulmonary vein to coronary sinus. 2b. Left inferior pulmonary vein to mitral annulus. 3. Right posterior left atrium. 3a. Right inferior pulmonary vein to inferior vena cava. 4. Right inferior pulmonary vein to right atrium. 5. Right anterior pulmonary veins. 6. Waterston's groove and right atrium. 7. Left anterior pulmonary veins. 7a. Left atrial roof. 8. Connection ablation at left superior pulmonary vein. 9. Connection ablation at right superior pulmonary vein. 10. Connection ablation at right inferior pulmonary vein. 11. Cavotricuspid isthmus. 12. Left atrial coronary sinus. 12a. Internal coronary sinus. (Reprinted from *Heart Rhythm* 10(1), Gehi AK, Mounsey JP, Pursell I, et al. Hybrid epicardial-endocardial ablation using a pericardioscopic technique for the treatment of atrial fibrillation, 22-28, © 2013, with permission from Elsevier.)

least one attempt at endocardial ablation alone. Epicardial ablation was performed through a subxiphoid pericardioscopic technique using an irrigated, unipolar RF linear ablation device [29]. The epicardial lesion set included antral PV ablation, posterior LA box ablation and connecting lesions to the coronary sinus. The posterior LA was mapped during the epicardial portion of ablation to ensure electrical silence. Immediately following epicardial ablation, endocardial ablation was performed to complete antral PV isolation and mitral isthmus ablation. Additional complex fractional atrial electrogram ablation, superior vena cava ablation and cavotricuspid isthmus ablation was left to the discretion of the electrophysiologist. Any atrial flutter or atrial tachycardia was mapped and ablated (Figure 13.34).

Gersak et al. compiled the experience of 4 European centers performing the combined epicardial and endocardial ablation via the pericardioscopic approach in 73 consecutive patients as a convergent procedure. All patients had persistent or long-standing persistent AF with an average AF duration of >4 years. Using a similar lesion set to that of Gehi et al., epicardial ablation included antral PV ablation and posterior LA box ablation. Immediately following epicardial ablation, endocardial ablation included confirming isolation of the PVs and the posterior atria [30].

TRANSDIAPHRAGMATIC COMBINED SUBXIPHOID AND LAPAROSCOPIC APPROACH

Civello described patients (27% paroxysmal, 30% persistent, 43% long-standing persistent) undergoing convergent hybrid ablation using a separate transdiaphragmatic approach. Access to the posterior surface of the heart was achieved via a transdiaphragmatic pericardial window created endoscopically under CO_2 insufflation using a 5-mm Optiview trocar inserted in the left upper quadrant of the abdomen for laparoscopic exploration, an additional trocar (10/12 mm) in the subxyphoid region and a 5-mm trocar in the right upper quadrant [31] (Figure 13.35 and Figure 13.36).

CONCOMITANT MINIMALLY INVASIVE AF ABLATION AND MITRAL VALVE SURGERY

Mitral valve surgery is more commonly associated with AF. In practice, any of the standalone epicardial ablation techniques and hybrid techniques either via minithoracotomy or thoracoscopic approaches may be applied during minimally invasive mitral valve surgery (Figure 13.37 to Figure 13.40).

LEFT ATRIAL APPENDAGE EXCLUSION

Initial studies reported excluding the LAA with endoscopic surgical staplers that could be inserted through a thoracoscope. Currently, the Atriclip is a specialized FDA-approved device designed for LAA exclusion that can be used via minimally invasive approaches (Figure 13.41 and Figure 13.42).

CAVEATS AND CONTROVERSIES

EPICARDIAL ABLATION FOR AF

There are several potential advantages and disadvantages to epicardial ablation techniques for AF. Epicardial ablation offers the opportunity for direct visualization of the atrium and ablation lesions. Even though endocardial ablation technological advances may improve the likelihood of

FIGURE 13.34 Hybrid maze ablation for atrial fibrillation.

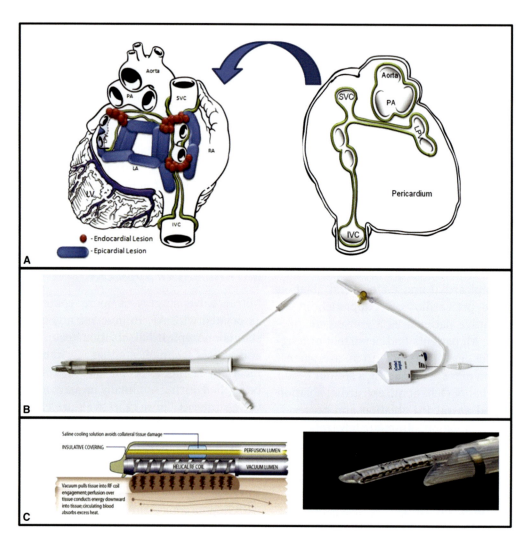

FIGURE 13.35 A. Base lesion pattern. B. Epicardial coagulation device with cannula. C. Cross-section and close-up of the epicardial coagulation device electrode. SVC, superior vena cava; RA, right atrium; IVC, inferior vena cava; LA, left atrium; LPV, left pulmonary vein; PA, pulmonary artery; RF, radio frequency. (Reprinted from *J Thorac Cardiovasc Surg,* 147(4), Geršak B, Zembala MO, Müller D, et al. European experience of the convergent atrial fibrillation procedure: multi-center outcomes in consecutive patients, 1411-1416, © 2014 The American Association for Thoracic Surgery, with permission from Elsevier.)

robust antral isolation (e.g. balloon ablation), linear epicardial ablation, particularly in the atrial body, may be more consistent and result in long-standing, transmural, high-quality lesions.

Ablation from the direction of epicardium to the endocardium allows one to avoid injury to the esophagus when performing ablation on the posterior LA, a potentially critical region for the maintenance of AF. It allows simultaneous LAA exclusion to mitigate stroke risk if necessary. However, approaches using a standalone minimally invasive epicardial approach have their limitations as well as significant anatomic considerations.

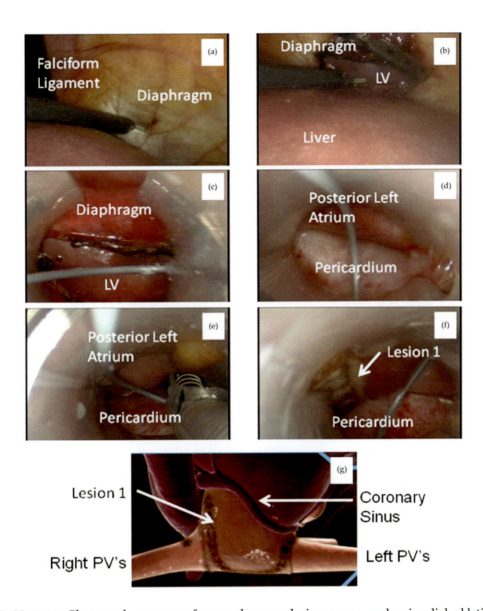

FIGURE 13.36 Photograph sequence from endoscope during access and epicardial ablation. (a) Using an electrocautery tool to create an incision in the central tendon of the diaphragm. (b) Endograsper sizing the width of the incision created in the central tendon of the diaphragm. (c) View from inside the cannula as it is being introduced through the incision created in the diaphragm. (d) Visualization of the posterior left atrium with the left pulmonary veins visible in the bottom right corner. (e) Positioning the epicardial coagulation device with the exposed radiofrequency coil adjacent to the target posterior left atrial tissue. (f) Visualization of the lesion created and tissue discoloration resulting from the application of radiofrequency energy using the epicardial coagulation device. (g) Anatomical drawing illustrating the location of lesions created by the epicardial coagulation device. (Reprinted from Ciello KC, Smith CA, Boedefeld W. Combined endocardial and epicardial ablation for symptomatic atrial fibrillation: single center experience in 100+ consecutive patients. *J Innov Cardiac Rhythm Manage*. 2013;4(9):1367–1373, © 2020, with permission from MediaSphere Medical, LLC.)

FIGURE 13.37 Concomitant ablation – Claudio Muneretto.

FIGURE 13.39 Minimally invasive maze and MVR.

FIGURE 13.38 Concomitant AF ablation during MiMVR – SCTS.

FIGURE 13.40 Combined cryo-maze procedure and mitral valve repair through a ministernotomy.

Beating heart epicardial ablation does not consistently create lesions that extend to the mitral or tricuspid annulus, leaving an opportunity for iatrogenic circuits causing recurrent AF or flutter. The detailed mapping of ablation lines including antral PVI lines and other left or right atrial lines can be challenging in the operating room but is critical to improving success rates. Surgical risk with epicardial ablation is sufficiently higher than with endocardial ablation approaches, with the potential for catastrophic complications.

HYBRID ABLATION FOR AF

Hybrid (epicardial and endocardial) ablation, either simultaneous or staged, offers significant improvements to a standalone epicardial approach. Fundamentally, catheter-based ablation has the advantage of mapping techniques to ensure bidirectional electrical isolation of pulmonary veins or other linear ablation. In addition, certain areas of the atria (e.g. mitral isthmus, cavotricuspid isthmus) are more accessible from an endocardial approach. Catheter ablation techniques also offer the opportunity for detailed mapping of atypical flutters or atrial tachycardia. However, point-by-point ablation can be cumbersome and may not be durable. Surgical ablation offers an anatomic approach with direct visual guidance but no electrophysiologic guidance. Overall, patients undergoing hybrid ablation had better outcomes. However, no cost-effectiveness study has yet been performed to justify the significant additive cost of the hybrid procedure.

Several factors must be considered when building a hybrid ablation program. The approach for epicardial ablation needs to be decided and mastered. Several tools have been developed, each with their advantages and disadvantages. The surgical approach should be tailored to the patient based on prior surgeries or other anatomic considerations. Ultimately, the comfort level and skill of the cardiac surgeon are the most important factors in choosing an epicardial ablation tool.

Hybrid AF ablation changes the working relationship between the electrophysiologist, the cardiac surgeon and the patient. A multidisciplinary approach benefits all

FIGURE 13.41   Atriclip by Dr. A. Marc Gillinov.

FIGURE 13.42   Thoracoscopic left atrial appendage closure.

those involved but can be a significant change to the current working environment. Considerations include the location for the ablation procedure (hybrid surgical suite or staged operating room, then EP laboratory), personnel involved during the epicardial and endocardial portions of the procedure (single dedicated team or multiple teams), anesthesia care (dedicated cardiac anesthesia or not) and postoperative care team (cardiac surgery team, electrophysiology team or a combination) (Figure 13.43).

The potential for complications, particularly during the epicardial portion of the procedure, must be considered and a clear plan must be in place to intervene quickly.

In addition, communication and planning are critical to preoperative, perioperative and postoperative care. This includes issues regarding antiarrhythmic drug use, anticoagulant use and management of any postoperative arrhythmia.

There are significant challenges to a hybrid ablation procedure including multidisciplinary team availability, requirement of a hybrid laboratory, sequence of the procedure and anticoagulation strategy. However, the potential benefits of a hybrid approach can outweigh these challenges, particularly in patients whose outcomes may be more limited with a traditional catheter-based procedure.

RESEARCH, TRENDS AND INNOVATION

MINIMALLY INVASIVE COX MAZE

Ad et al. reported the outcomes of a minimally invasive standalone Cox maze procedure for 104 patients with non-paroxysmal AF. At 3 years, 92% of the patients were in sinus rhythm and 80% in sinus rhythm without anti-arrhythmic medications. There was no operative mortality and only one stroke [32]. Hospital stay was reduced to 4 days, but the procedure requires cardiopulmonary bypass with or without cardiac arrest.

MINIMALLY INVASIVE PULMONARY VEIN ISOLATION

PRUITT BOX LESION

The 50 patients treated by Pruitt had a rapid return to normal activity and an average hospital stay of 3.7 days [12]. However, late follow-up revealed failure of the procedure to electrically isolate the pulmonary veins, with more than 50% returning to AF [33]. Devices using microwave energy have since been removed from the market.

WOLF MINI MAZE

The results for the initial 27 patients were promising, with 91% free from AF at 3-month follow-up. LAA removal reduced stroke risk. This minimally invasive beating heart procedure opened the door for a less invasive surgical approach but avoided many of the lesions initially described by Cox, specifically lesions connecting to the annulus of the mitral and tricuspid valves [13].

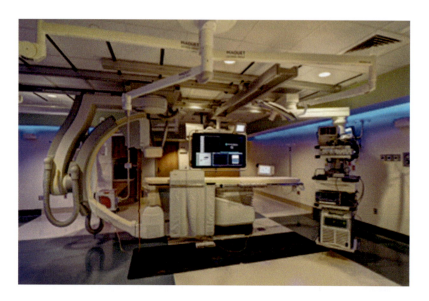

FIGURE 13.43 Hybrid Electrophysiology Laboratory at University of North Carolina.

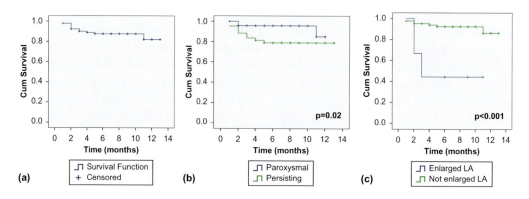

FIGURE 13.44 A. Recurrent atrial fibrillation–free survival in the overall study population. B. Recurrent atrial fibrillation–free survival in patients with preoperative diagnosis of paroxysmal atrial fibrillation (upper line) versus persisting atrial fibrillation (lower line log-rank p = 0.02). C. Recurrent atrial fibrillation–free survival in patients with preoperative demonstration of enlarged left atrium (LA, lower line) versus patients without significantly increased left atrial dimension (upper line, log-rank p < 0.001). Cum, Cumulative. (Reprinted from *J Thorac Cardiovasc Surg*, 142(2), Nasso G, Bonifazi R, Del Prete A, et al. Long-term results of ablation for isolated atrial fibrillation through a right minithoracotomy: toward a rational revision of treatment protocols, e41-e46, © 2011 The American Association for Thoracic Surgery, with permission from Elsevier.)

PULMONARY VEIN ISOLATION VIA RIGHT MINITHORACOTOMY

One hundred and four patients treated with Speziale's technique were followed up with 24-hour Holter monitoring [34]. Periprocedural complications included one case of intraoperative LA rupture requiring sternotomy for repair, one case of hemorrhagic stroke 4 days postoperatively and one transient ischemic attack in the early postoperative period. At an average 17-month follow-up, 89% were free of AF (96% with paroxysmal AF and 80% with persistent AF).

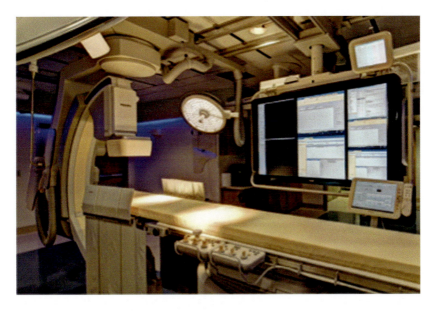

FIGURE 13.45 University of North Carolina Hybrid EP laboratory with fully integrated OR1 Digital Technologies (KARL STORZ Endoscopy-America, Inc.).

PULMONARY VEIN ISOLATION AND AUTONOMIC DENERVATION

Several studies evaluated the benefit of standalone epicardial pulmonary vein isolation with GP ablation on the maintenance of sinus rhythm. Edgerton et al. reported outcomes in 52 patients with symptomatic paroxysmal AF [16]. The LAA was excised or stapled in 88%. Patients were followed with 24-hour Holter or 2-week monitoring at 6 and 12 months. The average hospital length of stay was 5 days. Three patients required postoperative pacemaker implantation. At 12-month follow-up, 80% of patients were in sinus rhythm (Figure 13.44).

DALLAS LESION SET

Edgerton et al. reported 30 patients (10 persistent, 20 long-standing persistent) who were followed for 6 months with ECG and 14- to 21-day auto-triggered monitors. Three (10%) patients required pacemakers. At 6 months, the overall success rate was 58% off antiarrhythmic drugs and 80% with or without antiarrhythmic drugs, as assessed by long-term (14- to 21-day) event monitoring [17].

Weimar et al. reported a larger study of 89 patients with paroxysmal (35%), persistent (24%) or long-standing persistent (42%) AF undergoing the Dallas epicardial lesion set. The mean hospital length of stay was 8 days. One patient required conversion to extracorporeal circulation. Freedom from AF and antiarrhythmic drug therapy was 71%, 82% and 90% at 6, 12 and 24 months, respectively, with no difference in those with paroxysmal or persistent AF. However, 5% of patients required subsequent catheter ablation for recurrent AF or atrial flutter [35].

FIGURE 13.46 Hybrid maze procedure by Richard Lee.

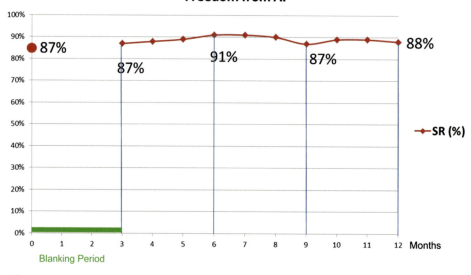

FIGURE 13.47 Freedom from AF at 12 months in patients who underwent hybrid ablation. AF: atrial fibrillation. (Reprinted from Muneretto C, Bisleri G, Rosati F, et al. European prospective multicentre study of hybrid thoracoscopic and transcatheter ablation of persistent atrial fibrillation: the HISTORIC-AF trial. *Eur J Cardiothorac Surg.* 2017;52(4):740-745, with permission from Oxford University Press.)

FIVE-BOX ABLATION

In Sirak's interim follow up, patients fared well with the meticulous thoracoscopic dissection and lesion placement, with an average hospital stay of 3.9 days and 92% freedom from tachyarrhythmias and AAD at 24 months by 7-day event monitoring [36]. Of the 179 patients, 2 required conversion to sternotomy and 2 had catheter ablation of the cavotricuspid isthmus at 13 months and remain in normal rhythm.

HYBRID SURGERY FOR AF

Combined endocardial and epicardial ablation is an intriguing option, which can take advantage of the strengths of surgical and catheter-based ablation (Figure 13.45).

Following epicardial with endocardial ablation offers the opportunity to verify epicardial lesions and approach territories that are inaccessible epicardially. As in endocardial ablation, epicardial ablation often has gaps in lines no matter what tool is used to create these. Endocardial mapping following epicardial ablation allows gaps in epicardial ablation lines to be identified and completed. Endocardial "touch up" of epicardial ablation lines is typically easier and likely more durable after epicardial ablation than after endocardial ablation. Thus, hybrid ablation offers the potential for more robust linear ablation and a lower likelihood of iatrogenic flutter. In addition, the electrophysiologist is ready to map and ablate arrhythmias encountered during ablation including atrial flutter or atrial tachycardia. Additional complex fractionated electrogram ablation is also possible with endocardial ablation (Figure 13.46).

The hybrid approach has demonstrated improved efficacy compared with isolated endocardial or epicardial approaches.

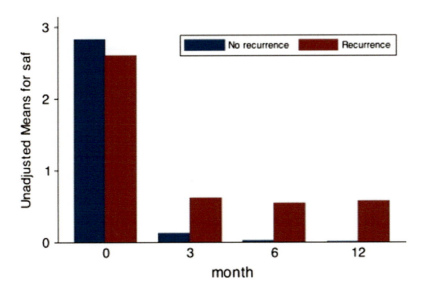

FIGURE 13.48 Symptom relief over time in patients with or without atrial fibrillation (AF) recurrence (Canadian Cardiovascular Society Severity of Atrial Fibrillation [CCS-SAF] score 0–4; higher score indicates more severe symptoms). CCS-SAF significantly improved after ablation regardless of recurrence (p < 0.001). Those without recurrence significantly improved compared with those with recurrence at 3-month follow-up (p = 0.048), 6-month follow-up (P = 0.003) and 12-month follow-up (p < 0.001). (Reprinted from *Heart Rhythm* 10(1), Gehi AK, Mounsey JP, Pursell I, et al. Hybrid epicardial-endocardial ablation using a pericardioscopic technique for the treatment of atrial fibrillation, 22-28, © 2013, with permission from Elsevier.)

However, no study to date has compared a hybrid approach with multiple endocardial ablations in a randomized controlled design (Figure 13.47). It is likely that multiple, staged endocardial ablations will also improve outcomes. This is highlighted by the fact that staged endocardial ablation reveals a high likelihood of pulmonary vein reconnection [37].

The only study approaching this comparison is the study of Mahapatra et al. comparing redo endocardial ablation with simultaneous hybrid ablation in those who had failed prior endocardial ablation [23].

THORACOSCOPIC APPROACH

Mahapatra's study compared outcomes to a matched control group with catheter ablation alone. Overall, the hospital length of stay in the hybrid group was longer but otherwise there were no acute complications in either group aside from a tamponade in the catheter-alone group. At 20 months of follow-up, more patients in the hybrid group were free of atrial arrhythmias off antiarrhythmic drugs (87% vs 53%, p = 0.04) [23].

La Meir et al. reported their experience comparing a hybrid epicardial and endocardial ablation in 35 patients with epicardial-only ablation in 28 patients (45%–50% paroxysmal, 18%–23% persistent, 31%–32% long-standing persistent). Patients were followed with 7-day continuous monitoring at 3, 6 and 12 months post-procedure. There were no complications including mortality, stroke or reoperation for bleeding in the two groups. The median length of hospital stay was 3 to 4 days. At 1-year follow-up, success rates free of atrial arrhythmia >30 seconds off antiarrhythmic drug therapy were higher in those undergoing hybrid ablation compared to epicardial alone (91% vs 82%,

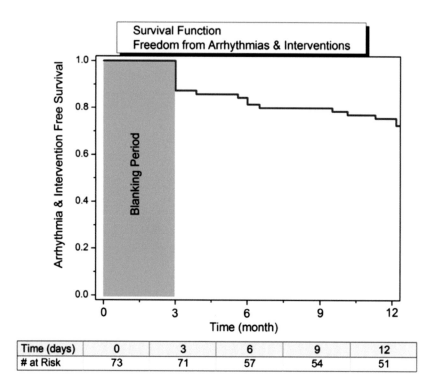

FIGURE 13.49 Arrhythmia and intervention-free survival analysis. (Reprinted from *J Thorac Cardiovasc Surg,* 147(4), Geršak B, Zembala MO, Müller D, et al. European experience of the convergent atrial fibrillation procedure: multicenter outcomes in consecutive patients, 1411-1416, © 2014 The American Association for Thoracic Surgery, with permission from Elsevier.)

p = 0.07), particularly in those with persistent or long-standing persistent AF [24].

In Pison's study, patients underwent 7-day continuous monitoring at 3, 6, 9 and 12 months post-procedure and antiarrhythmics were discontinued at 6 months. Ten of 26 patients had persistent AF, 1 had long-standing persistent AF, and the remainder had paroxysmal AF. The mean hospital length of stay was 7 days. There were no major complications. At 1-year follow-up, the success rate (no atrial arrhythmia >30 seconds without antiarrhythmic drugs) was 93% in those with paroxysmal AF and 90% in those with persistent AF with two patients requiring redo catheter ablation after the hybrid procedure [25].

In the European prospective multicenter HISTORIC-AF trial, following surgical ablation, a stable restoration of sinus rhythm was achieved in 77% and 75% of patients at 6- and 12-month follow-up respectively whereas, following hybrid ablation, sinus rhythm was restored in 91% and 88% of patients at 6- and 12-month follow-up respectively. Despite the box lesion set reproducing only part of the original lesion set of the maze III and IV, the rate of sinus rhythm restoration in combination with a sequential staged transcatheter approach led to an encouraging 80% freedom from

FIGURE 13.50 ISMICS workshop.

anti-arrhythmic drugs. The combination of uni-bipolar RF including the Cobra Fusion device was able to provide a continuous transmural ablation line [27].

SUBXIPHOID PERICARDIOSCOPIC APPROACH

In Zembala's patients, 24-hour Holter monitoring was performed at 6 and 12 months postoperatively. Complications included one patient with tamponade, a second patient requiring sternotomy due to bleeding from an inferior vena cava laceration and a third patient who died 27 days after discharge of unclear cause. At 6 months post-procedure, 72% of patients were in sinus rhythm, 67% without antiarrhythmic drug therapy. At 1-year post-procedure, 80% of patients were in sinus rhythm and off antiarrhythmic drug therapy [28].

Gehi's cohort of 101 patients was followed by 24-hour Holter monitoring or implantable looping monitor at 3, 6 and 12 months. Complications included two patients with tamponade, two patients with bleeding (one requiring surgical intervention) and two deaths (one atrialesophageal fistula and one sudden and unexplained, with unrevealing autopsy) (Figure 13.48). Repeat endocardial ablation was performed in 6% of patients. Including repeat ablation, 12-month arrhythmia-free survival was 73% without concomitant antiarrhythmic drug therapy [29].

Gersak's patients were followed with regular 24-hour Holter monitoring or an implantable loop recorder. Adverse events included one stroke, one tamponade, two with bleeding requiring transfusion and two with bleeding requiring conversion to sternotomy. Over 1-year follow-up, 4% required repeat endocardial ablation and arrhythmia-free survival was 73% [30].

TRANSDIAPHRAGMATIC COMBINED SUBXIPHOID AND LAPAROSCOPIC APPROACH

Civello et al. reported their single-center experience in 104 patients who were followed with 72-hour Holter at 6- and 12-months post-procedure. Complications included one cerebrovascular accident, one pericardial effusion, two pleural effusions and one pulmonary vein stenosis requiring stenting. Repeat procedures were performed in 5% of patients (Figure 13.49). Twelve months post-procedure, 73% were in sinus rhythm without antiarrhythmic drug therapy and 89% with or without antiarrhythmic drug therapy [31].

CONCOMITANT ATRIAL ABLATION WITH MINIMALLY INVASIVE MITRAL SURGERY

Mitral valve surgery is the most common concomitant surgery during which ablation procedures for atrial fibrillation are performed. Minimally invasive mitral valve surgery extends this opportunity to the myriad of ablation procedures that can be performed through a less invasive surgical approach [38]. Jeanmart et al. showed that the use of unipolar RF ablation to perform a mini maze during minimally invasive mitral valve surgery is a safe procedure and is associated with good early results [39].

FIGURE 13.51   AtriCure education and training.

FIGURE 13.52   JICRM.

CONCLUSION

Epicardial AF ablation has come a long way since the initial techniques developed by James Cox. Although the development of epicardial and endocardial ablation techniques had largely occurred in parallel, we are seeing a merging of approaches that offers the potential for significant synergistic benefits. Given the potential risk of epicardial ablation, currently its role is best suited to those in whom endocardial ablation alone may have more limited benefit. This includes patients with persistent or long-standing persistent AF, those with significant structural cardiac disease or those with prior failed attempts at endocardial ablation. But in these populations, hybrid ablation in particular offers distinct advantages, which make it an exciting and promising approach.

WHERE AND HOW TO LEARN

INTERNATIONAL SOCIETY OF MINIMALLY INVASIVE CARDIAC SURGERY (ISMICS) WORKSHOP

ISMICS arranges and patronizes regular meeting, training sessions and workshops around the year in different part of the world (Figure 13.50).

ATRICURE EDUCATION AND TRAINING

AtriCure provides healthcare professionals with training to adapt to evolving techniques. The training programs are designed with the guidance of an education steering committee comprised of key opinion leaders to help individuals at all experience levels learn more about the surgical treatment of atrial fibrillation (Figure 13.51).

THE JOURNAL OF INNOVATIONS IN CARDIAC RHYTHM MANAGEMENT

JICRM is an international open-access peer-reviewed journal. It is a good source of online resources (Figure 13.52).

REFERENCES

1. James W Leitch, George Klein, Raymond Yee, and Gerard Guiraudon. "Sinus Node-Atrioventricular Node Isolation: Long-Term Results with the "Corridor" Operation for Atrial Fibrillation." *Journal of the American College of Cardiology* 17 (1991): 970–975.
2. NM van Hemel, JJ Defauw, JH Kingma, et al. "Long-Term Results of the Corridor Operation for Atrial Fibrillation." *British Heart Journal* 71(2) (1994): 170–6.
3. James L Cox. "The Surgical Treatment of Atrial Fibrillation. IV. Surgical Technique." *Journal of Thoracic and Cardiovascular Surgery* 101 (1991): 584–592.
4. RJ Damiano Jr, L Sydney, Gaynor SL, Bailey M, Prasad S, Cox JL, Boineau JP, Schuessler RP "The Long-Term Outcome of Patients with Coronary Disease and Atrial Fibrillation Undergoing the Cox Maze Procedure." *Journal of Thoracic and Cardiovascular Surgery* 126 (2003): 2016–2021.
5. Sydney L Gaynor, Michael D DiodatoPrasad, S. M., Ishii, Y., Schuessler, R. B., Bailey, M. S., Damiano, N. R., Bloch, J. B., Moon, M. R., & Damiano, R. J., Jr. "A Prospective, Single-Center Clinical Trial of a Modified Cox Maze Procedure with Bipolar Radiofrequency Ablation." *Journal of Thoracic and Cardiovascular Surgery* 128 (2004): 535–542.

6. Wendy S Tzou, Francis E Marchlinski, Erica S Zado, et al. "Long-Term Outcome after Successful Catheter Ablation of Atrial Fibrillation." *Circulation: Arrhythmia and Electrophysiology* 3 (2010): 237–242.
7. Rukshen Weerasooriya, Paul Khairy, Litalien, J., Macle, L., Hocini, M., Sacher, F., Lellouche, N., Knecht, S., Wright, M., Nault, I., Miyazaki, S., Scavee, C., Clementy, J., Haissaguerre, M., & Jais, P. "Catheter Ablation for Atrial Fibrillation: Are Results Maintained at 5 Years of Follow-Up?" *Journal of the American College of Cardiology* 57 (2011): 160–166.
8. Anson M Lee, Kal Clark, Marci S Bailey, et al. "A Minimally Invasive Cox-Maze Procedure: Operative Technique and Results." *Innovations (Philadelphia)* 5 (2010): 281–286.
9. Niv Ad and James L Cox. "The Maze Procedure for the Treatment of Atrial Fibrillation: A Minimally Invasive Approach." *Journal of Cardiac Surgery* 19 (2004): 196–200.
10. Michel Haissaguerre, Pierre Jais, Dipen C Shah, et al. "Spontaneous Initiation of Atrial Fibrillation by Ectopic Beats Originating in the Pulmonary Veins." *New England Journal of Medicine* 339 (1998): 659–666.
11. Adam E Saltman, Lawrence S Rosenthal, Francalancia, N. A., & Lahey, S. J. "A Completely Endoscopic Approach to Microwave Ablation for Atrial Fibrillation." *Heart Surgery Forum* 6 (2003): E38–41.
12. J Crayton Pruitt, Robert R Lazzara, Dworkin, G. H., Badhwar, V., Kuma, C., & Ebra, G. "Totally Endoscopic Ablation of Lone Atrial Fibrillation: Initial Clinical Experience." *Annals of Thoracic Surgery* 81 (2006): 1325–1331.
13. Randall K Wolf, E William Schneeberger, Robert Osterday, et al. "Video-Assisted Bilateral Pulmonary Vein Isolation and Left Atrial Appendage Exclusion for Atrial Fibrillation." *Journal of Thoracic and Cardiovascular Surgery* 130 (2005): 797–802.
14. Randall K Wolf, and Sandra Burgess. "Minimally Invasive Surgery for Atrial Fibrillation-Wolf Mini Maze Procedure." *Annals of Cardiothoracic Surgery* 3 (2014): 122–123.
15. G Speziale, R Bonifazi, G Nasso, et al. "Minimally Invasive Radiofrequency Ablation of Lone Atrial Fibrillation by Monolateral Right Minithoracotomy: Operative and Early Follow-Up Results." *The Annals of Thoracic Surgery* 90(1) (2010): 161–7.
16. James R Edgerton, William T Brinkman, Weaver, T., Prince, S. L., Culica, D., Herbert, M. A., & Mack, M. J. "Pulmonary Vein Isolation and Autonomic Denervation for the Management of Paroxysmal Atrial Fibrillation by a Minimally Invasive Surgical Approach." *Journal of Thoracic and Cardiovascular Surgery* 140 (2010): 823–828.
17. James R Edgerton. "Total Thorascopic Ablation of Atrial Fibrillation Using the Dallas Lesion Set, Partial Autonomic Denervation, and Left Atrial Appendectomy." *Operative Techniques in Thoracic and Cardiovascular Surgery* 14(3) (2009): 224–242.
18. John Sirak, Danielle Jones, Benjamin Sun, et al. "Toward a Definitive, Totally Thoracoscopic Procedure for Atrial Fibrillation." *Annals of Thoracic Surgery* 86 (2008): 1960–1964.
19. John Sirak, Danielle Jones, and David Schwartzman. "The Five-Box Thoracoscopic Maze Procedure." *Annals of Thoracic Surgery* 90 (2010): 986–989.
20. Daniel Scherr, Paul Khairy, Shinsuke Miyazaki, et al. "Five-Year Outcome of Catheter Ablation of Persistent Atrial Fibrillation Using Termination of Atrial Fibrillation as a Procedural Endpoint." *Circulation: Arrhythmia and Electrophysiology* 8 (2015): 18–24.
21. Rochus K Voeller, Marci S Bailey, Andreas Zierer, et al. "Isolating the Entire Posterior Left Atrium Improves Surgical Outcomes after the Cox Maze Procedure." *Journal of Thoracic and Cardiovascular Surgery* 135 (2008): 870–877.
22. Lucas VA Boersma, Manuel Castella, Wimjan van Boven, et al. "Atrial Fibrillation Catheter Ablation Versus Surgical Ablation Treatment (FAST): A 2-Center Randomized Clinical Trial." *Circulation* 125 (2012): 23–30.
23. Srijoy Mahapatra, Damien J LaPar, Sandeep Kamath, et al. "Initial Experience of Sequential Surgical Epicardial-Catheter Endocardial Ablation for Persistent and Long-Standing Persistent Atrial Fibrillation with Long-Term Follow-Up." *Annals of Thoracic Surgery* 91 (2011): 1890–1898.

24. Mark La Meir, Sandro Gelsomino, Fabiana Luca, et al. "Minimally Invasive Surgical Treatment of Lone Atrial Fibrillation: Early Results of Hybrid Versus Standard Minimally Invasive Approach Employing Radiofrequency Sources." *International Journal of Cardiology* 167 (2013): 1469–1475.
25. Laurent Pison, Mark La Meir, Jurren van Opstal, et al. "Hybrid Thoracoscopic Surgical and Transvenous Catheter Ablation of Atrial Fibrillation." *Journal of the American College of Cardiology* 60 (2012): 54–61.
26. C Muneretto, G Bisleri, L Bontempi, and A Curnis. "Durable Staged Hybrid Ablation with Thoracoscopic and Percutaneous Approach for Treatment of Long-Standing Atrial Fibrillation: A 30-Month Assessment with Continuous Monitoring." *The Journal of Thoracic and Cardiovascular Surgery* 144(6) (2012): 1460–5; discussion 1465.
27. C Muneretto, G Bisleri, F Rosati, et al. "European Prospective Multicentre Study of Hybrid Thoracoscopic and Transcatheter Ablation of Persistent Atrial Fibrillation: The HISTORIC-AF Trial." *European Journal of Cardio-Thoracic Surgery* 52(4) (2017): 740–745.
28. Mechal Zembala, Krzystof Filipiak, Oskar Kowalski, et al. "Minimally Invasive Hybrid Ablation Procedure for the Treatment of Persistent Atrial Fibrillation: One Year Results." *Kardiologia Polska* 70 (2012): 819–828.
29. Anil K Gehi, J Paul Mounsey, Irion Pursell, et al. "Hybrid Epicardial-Endocardial Ablation Using a Pericardioscopic Technique for the Treatment of Atrial Fibrillation." *Heart Rhythm* 10 (2013): 22–28.
30. Borut Gersak, Michael O Zembala, Dirk Muller, et al. "European Experience of the Convergent Atrial Fibrillation Procedure: Multicenter Outcomes in Consecutive Patients." *Journal of Thoracic and Cardiovascular Surgery* 147 (2014): 1411–1416.
31. Kenneth C Civello, Charles Andrew Smith, and William Boedefeld. "Combined Endocardial and Epicardial Ablation for Symptomatic Atrial Fibrillation: Single Center Experience in 100+ Consecutive Patients." *Journal of Innovations in Cardiac Rhythm Management* (2013): 1–7. DOI: 10.19102/icrm.2013.040 09 6.
32. Niv Ad, Linda Henry, Ted Friehling, Marc Wish, and Sari D Holmes. "Minimally Invasive Stand-Alone Cox-Maze Procedure for Patients with Nonparoxysmal Atrial Fibrillation." *Annals of Thoracic Surgery* 96 (2013): 792–799.
33. J Crayton Pruitt, Robert R Lazzara, and George Ebra. "Minimally Invasive Surgical Ablation of Atrial Fibrillation: The Thoracoscopic Box Lesion Approach." *Journal of Interventional Cardiac Electrophysiology* 20 (2007): 83–87.
34. Giuseppe Nasso, Raffaele Bonifazi, Armando Del Prete, et al. "Long-Term Results of Ablation for Isolated Atrial Fibrillation through a Right Minithoracotomy: Toward a Rational Revision of Treatment Protocols." *Journal of Thoracic and Cardiovascular Surgery* 142 (2011): e41–46.
35. Timo Weimar, Martina Vosseler, Markus Czesla, et al. "Approaching a Paradigm Shift: Endoscopic Ablation of Lone Atrial Fibrillation on the Beating Heart." *Annals of Thoracic Surgery* 94 (2012): 1886–1892.
36. John H Sirak and David Schwartzman. "Interim Results of the 5-Box Thoracoscopic Maze Procedure." *Annals of Thoracic Surgery* 94 (2012): 1880–1884.
37. Petr Neuzil, Vivek Y Reddy, Josef Kautzner, et al. "Electrical Reconnection after Pulmonary Vein Isolation Is Contingent on Contact Force During Initial Treatment: Results from the EFFICAS I Study." *Circulation: Arrhythmia and Electrophysiology* 6 (2013): 327–333.
38. Anson M Lee. "Maze Permutations during Minimally Invasive Mitral Valve Surgery." *Annals of Cardiothoracic Surgery* 4(5) (2015): 463–468.
39. Hugues Jeanmart, Filip Casselman, Roel Beelen, et al. "Modified Maze during Endoscopic Mitral Valve Surgery: The OLV Clinic Experience." *Annals of Thoracic Surgery* 82 (2006): 1765–9.

14.1

AORTIC SURGERY
Minimally Invasive Ascending Aortic Surgery

OURANIA PREVENTZA

HISTORY OR INTRODUCTION

MINIMALLY INVASIVE AORTIC SURGERY FOR CARDIOVASCULAR SURGEONS

Traditional open aortic surgery procedures for pathologies involving the ascending aorta, aortic arch and descending thoracic aorta can be performed with excellent and durable results. Patient selection is nonetheless very important because some patients who require arch operations or procedures involving the descending thoracic aorta cannot tolerate full median sternotomy or left thoracotomy/thoracoabdominal incisions with cardiopulmonary bypass (CPB) and circulatory arrest. In cardiac surgery, minimally invasive technologies have emerged over the past few years to treat heart valve disease percutaneously and endovascular technologies to treat infrarenal aortic pathologies. As a result, minimally invasive procedures by means of surgical access are now considered alternative options for treating proximal aortic, arch and descending thoracic pathologies.

HISTORY

1983: Prof Nikolay L Volodos and colleagues invented a radial cylindrical stent with a Z-shaped design for the self-fixing expandable vascular endograft (Figure 14.1.1).

1985: Iliac artery stent grafting was performed for the first time in modern

FIGURE 14.1.1 First step in endovascular aortic repair – how it all began.

FIGURE 14.1.2 First clinical application of endovascular stent graft.

history by Volodos and team (clinical observation was published in *Vestnik Khirurgii im I.I. Grekova* in 1986). Volodos NL, Shekhanin VE, Karpovich IP, et al. A self-fixing synthetic blood vessel endoprosthetics (in Russian) *Vestn Khir.* 1986;137:123–125 PMID: 3824776 [1].

1987: Volodos and team inserted a stent graft into the descending thoracic aorta via the femoral artery (Figure 14.1.2). The patient lived for 18 years with no graft malfunction or endoleaks. Volodos NL, Karpovich IP, Shekhanin VE, Troian VI, and Iakovenko LF. A case of distant transfemoral endoprosthesis of the thoracic aorta using a self-fixing synthetic prosthesis in traumatic aneurysm. ([in Russian]) *Grudn Khir.* 1988;6:84–86 [2].

1991: The first hybrid approach was developed for treating complex pathology of the aortic arch. It was used to treat an arch aneurysm that had developed after coarctation repair and that involved the origins of the left subclavian and left carotid arteries. [3].

1991: Endograft placement for abdominal aortic aneurysm performed by Parodi, Palmaz and Barone [4] (Figure 14.1.3).

1994: Thirteen patients undergo thoracic endovascular aortic repair (TEVAR) with physician-made devices in the United States (Figure 14.1.4); reported by Dake and colleagues [5].

2005: First US Food and Drug Administration (FDA) approval of a thoracic endovascular device to treat descending thoracic aortic aneurysm (Figure 14.1.5).

2013: First FDA approval of an endovascular device to repair acute and chronic Type B aortic dissection (Figure 14.1.6).

HOW TO DO IT/STEP BY STEP

SURGICAL APPROACH

AORTIC ROOT, ASCENDING AORTA WITH OR WITHOUT PROXIMAL ARCH, TOTAL ARCH

Minimally invasive surgical techniques have been described to treat ascending and proximal arch pathology. The access for such repairs is via a right mini-thoracotomy approach or an upper mini-sternotomy.

∞ **Right mini-thoracotomy**

Key points in the literature:

1. The incision is made over the second or third intercostal space with dislocation of the third to fourth costochondral cartilage or entry into the fourth intercostal space.

FIGURE 14.1.3 Transfemoral intraluminal graft implantation.

FIGURE 14.1.5 Gore Tag Thoracic Endoprosthesis.

FIGURE 14.1.4 Transluminal placement of endovascular stent grafts.

FIGURE 14.1.6 Gore receives first FDA approval.

OR

A 5-cm mini-thoracotomy is performed in the right second intercostal space.

2. CPB is achieved via femoral or axillary artery cannulation and femoral vein cannulation.
3. If proximal arch repair is needed, cooling down to 20°C has been described. Once circulatory arrest is initiated, then the long femoral venous cannula is withdrawn into the right atrium to snare the 24 F venous cannula in the superior vena cava for retrograde cerebral perfusion. No antegrade cerebral perfusion is administered.
4. A retractable shaft cross-clamp can be used (Cygnet, Péters Surgical, Bobigny, France).
5. Cardioplegia is delivered antegrade into the root or directly into the coronary ostia.
6. In a 2018 series, mini-thoracotomy was considered to be contraindicated in patients who required coronary revascularization, required a valve-sparing procedure or had pathology that extended into the aortic arch, necessitating total arch replacement [6]. A sternotomy approach was used in such cases (Figure 14.1.7 and Figure 14.1.8).

∞ **Upper mini-sternotomy**

It has been described as

∞ A J-shaped partial upper sternotomy with a 6- to 7-cm skin incision from the sternal notch to the third right intercostal space (Figure 14.1.9).
∞ Or as an L-shaped partial upper sternotomy with an 8-cm midline skin incision starting 1–2 fingers below the sternal notch. The sternum is incised to the left fourth intercostal space.

The sternum can be also incised in an L manner to the right fourth intercostal space (our own preference).

Key points in the literature and based on our own experience:

FIGURE 14.1.7 Right mini-thoracotomy Bentall with traditional and automated suturing devices.

1. Pericardial traction sutures are important to bring the ascending aorta higher into the surgical field.
2. CPB can be achieved via axillary cannulation with an 8- or 10-mm graft or via innominate artery cannulation [7], so the aortic cannula does not occupy space in the small field of the upper mini-sternotomy and femoral vein (our own preference). Others have advocated dual-stage cannula placement in the right atrium.
3. Direct aortic cannulation opposite the origin of the brachiocephalic artery also has been advocated.
4. The left ventricle can be vented via a cannula in the right superior pulmonary vein.
5. Cardioplegia can be administered via the aortic root or directly into the coronary ostia.
6. For brain protection, antegrade cerebral perfusion can be administered unilaterally or bilaterally (it is our own preference to administer it bilaterally via a 9F Pruitt cannula into the left common carotid artery).
7. Pacing wires are placed before the aortic clamp is removed.

ENDOVASCULAR REPAIR OF THE ASCENDING AORTA

Endovascular repair of the ascending aorta has been performed off-label in the United States in patients at high risk from conventional repair. No devices yet have been approved in the US for the endovascular repair of pathologies of the ascending aorta [8,9].

In Europe, a multicenter experience in ten patients has been reported with the Zenith Ascend TAA Endovascular Graft, which is a short (6.5-cm) graft (William Cook Europe, Bjaeverskov, Denmark). All of the patients were considered to be at high risk from open surgery. The indications for

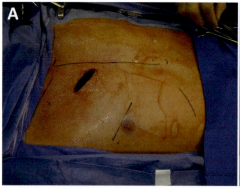
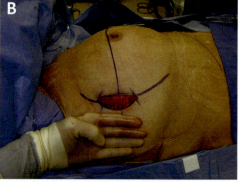

FIGURE 14.1.8 (A, B) Images showing a sternal-sparing minimally invasive mini right thoracotomy incision in two patients. (Reprinted from *Ann Thorac Surg*, 106 (3), Lamelas J, Chen PC, Loor G, LaPietra A, Successful Use of Sternal-Sparing Minimally Invasive Surgery for Proximal Ascending Aortic Pathology, 742-748, © 2018 by The Society of Thoracic Surgeons, with permission from Elsevier.)

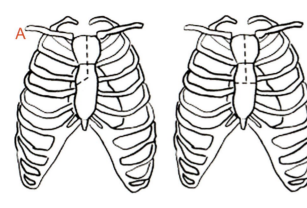
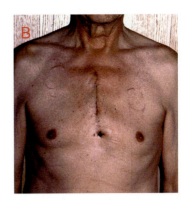

FIGURE 14.1.9 (A) Schematic for "upper J" and "T inverted" mini-sternotomy [Reprinted from Perrotta S, Lentini S. Ministernotomy approach for surgery of the aortic root and ascending aorta. *Interact Cardiovasc Thorac Surg*. 2009;9(5):849-858, with permission from Oxford University Press]. (B) Skin incision for upper hemi-sternotomy [Reprinted from Deschka H, Erler S, Machner M, El-Ayoubi L, Alken A, Wimmer-Greinecker G. Surgery of the ascending aorta, root remodelling and aortic arch surgery with circulatory arrest through partial upper sternotomy: results of 50 consecutive cases. *Eur J Cardiothorac Surg*. 2013;43(3):580-584, with permission from Oxford University Press].

treatment were dissection in five patients, aneurysm in four and fixation of a dislocated aortic valve in one. All endografts were deployed successfully; the 30-day survival rate was 90% (Figure 14.1.9).

Key points for the procedure:

1. In some cases, an existing mechanical aortic valve can be a limitation because the nose cone of the endograft needs to be short so that the device will not cross the valve. The nose cone is shorter on the newer endografts than on the older ones.
2. The stiff wire with which the endograft is delivered occasionally needs to be placed inside the left ventricle, much as it is in percutaneous aortic valve procedures.
3. Temporary pacing can be useful during the deployment of the endovascular stent graft to avoid the windsock effect and permit accurate deployment.
4. Access for endograft delivery can be obtained via the femoral artery, transapical delivery, carotid artery or axillary artery.
5. The ideal length of the endograft for the ascending aorta is approximately 7–8 cm.

ENDOVASCULAR REPAIR OF AORTIC ARCH

Understanding the Ishimaru landing zones 0–4 is important when we plan endovascular procedures (Figure 14.1.12, Figure 14.1.13 and Figure 14.1.14).

- Zone 0 is the ascending thoracic aorta and requires landing the endograft in the ascending aorta.
- Zone 1 is the area between the innominate artery and the left common carotid artery.
- Zone 2 is the area between left common carotid artery and left subclavian artery, and the endograft is covering the left subclavian artery.
- Zone 3 is the proximal descending thoracic aorta distal to left subclavian artery.
- Zone 4 is the remaining descending thoracic aorta (Figure 14.1.15).

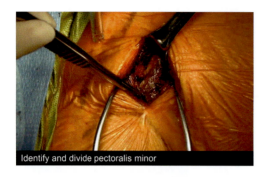

FIGURE 14.1.10 Identification and division of pectoralis minor. (Reprinted from *J Thorac Cardiovasc Surg*, 155(5), Preventza O, Price MD, Spiliotopoulos K, et al. In elective arch surgery with circulatory arrest, does the arterial cannulation site really matter? A propensity score analysis of right axillary and innominate artery cannulation, 1953-1960.e4. © 2017 The American Association for Thoracic Surgery, with permission from Elsevier.)

Hybrid procedures have been developed in an effort to avoid CPB (Figure 14.1.16). Cervical extra-anatomic revascularization is required in the form of left subclavian–to-carotid bypass or left carotid–to–right carotid bypass [10].

Total debranching aortic arch repair can be achieved with cervical debranching and with inflow from the descending thoracic aorta or the iliac artery, or from the ascending aorta via a Y or double Y graft and revascularization of the head vessels. No CPB is required [11–13].

FIGURE 14.1.12 Mini-aortic arch surgery.

Custom-made multibranched grafts have also been used for total arch reconstruction, as have parallel stent grafts in the snorkel or chimney configuration. No arch branched grafts have been approved in the US yet.

Key points for the procedure:

1. In cervical revascularization with left-to-right carotid bypass, the body habitus of the patient is crucial and plays a role in decision-making with regard to the positioning of the graft, that is, whether to tunnel the graft behind or in front of the trachea. Tunneling behind the trachea is preferable.

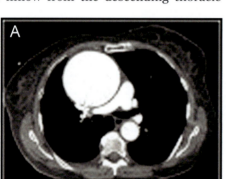
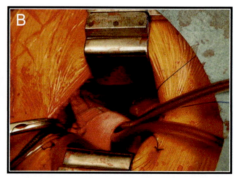

FIGURE 14.1.11 (A) CT scan of giant ascending and aortic arch aneurysm. (B) Subtotal aortic arch replacement with brachiocephalic trunk clamped and bilateral selective antegrade cerebral perfusion. (After Goebel N, Bonte D, Salehi-Gilani S, Nagib R, Ursulescu A, Franke UFW, Minimally Invasive Access Aortic Arch Surgery, *Innovations (Phila)*,12(5), 351-355, © 2017 by the International Society for Minimally Invasive Cardiothoracic Surgery. Reprinted by Permission of SAGE Publications, Inc.)

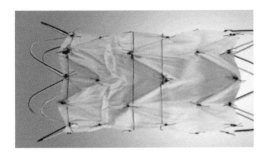

FIGURE 14.1.13 The Zenith Ascend TAA Endovascular Graft is constructed of woven polyester fabric sewn to self-expanding nitinol stents with braided polyester and monofilament polypropylene suture. (Reprinted from *J Vasc Surg*, 63(6), Tsilimparis N, Debus ES, Oderich GS, et al. International experience with endovascular therapy of the ascending aorta with a dedicated endograft, 1476-1482, © 2016 Society for Vascular Surgery, with permission from Elsevier.)

2. In cases of total arch debranching with the Y or double Y graft from the ascending aorta: If the ascending aorta is more than 4–4.3 cm long, then to avoid the risk of aortic dissection, it is advisable to replace the ascending aorta so the ascending graft can be used as a landing zone.
3. The sequence of the total arch debranching with the Y graft is as follows: The proximal anastomosis is performed first with a partial occluding clamp on the ascending aorta. While the clamp is in place, we keep the systolic blood pressure at 80–90 mmHg to prevent ascending aortic dissection. Then we perform the aorta-to–left subclavian artery bypass, aorta-to–left common carotid bypass and aorta-to–innominate artery bypass.
4. During reconstruction of the head vessels, we keep the mean perfusion pressure at 90–100 mmHg.

Operator experience is important to the success of these procedures. Total endovascular ascending repair and arch repair currently are performed in patients deemed high-risk by the cardiovascular surgeons.

DESCENDING THORACIC AORTA

Pathologies of the descending thoracic aorta are currently treated with the various endovascular grafts. Key points for the procedure:

1. Access is achieved via either open exposure or percutaneous access of the femoral artery.
2. The femoral artery needs to be large enough to accommodate the sheath of the endograft for the TEVAR. The newer endografts have a lower profile than grafts of previous generations.
3. Wire and catheter exchanges are performed under direct fluoroscopic vision and not blindly.
4. Endografts and large-bore sheaths are advanced over a stiff wire.
5. Careful and minimal manipulation of the aortic arch, wires and catheters is imperative to avoid retrograde ascending aortic dissection.
6. Intravascular ultrasonography can be a useful tool during TEVAR procedures, especially in cases of aortic dissection. Its use can also reduce the amount of dye contrast material used during the procedure.
7. Proximal and distal Type I and Type III endoleaks should be fixed in the operating room, whereas Type II endoleak can be followed [14].

THORACOABDOMINAL AORTA

Traditionally, thoracoabdominal aortic pathology is treated with open repair via a left thoracoabdominal incision with or without left heart bypass or hypothermic circulatory arrest, which is used in

FIGURE 14.1.14 Endovascular aortic arch repair.

cases in which the transverse aortic arch is large enough and a cross-clamp cannot be applied. This procedure is highly specialized; it is performed at aortic centers of excellence, and it can carry significant morbidity and mortality risk.

Hybrid procedures with snorkels, chimneys and a combination of open and endovascular approaches have been devised to address the morbidity and mortality associated with open repair. No FDA-approved endovascular devices exist today for treating extensive thoracoabdominal pathology. Physician-modified endografts, fenestrated and branched endografts, patient-specific manufactured devices and off-the-shelf devices have been used in purely endovascular approaches, hybrid approaches or both to treat patients with thoracoabdominal aortic aneurysm pathology. No standardized approach exists, and expertise in using catheters and wires is extremely important in performing these procedures [15–17].

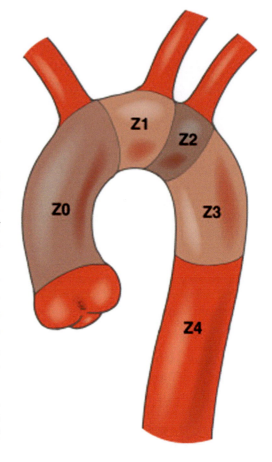

FIGURE 14.1.15 Aortic landing zones for thoracic endovascular aortic repair. The thoracic aorta is divided into five anatomic zones that relate to the landing zone for thoracic endovascular aortic repair. (Reprinted from Perioperative Transesophageal Echocardiography, 1st Ed, John G. Augoustides, Albert T. Cheung, Aneurysms and dissections, 195, © 2013, with permission from Elsevier.)

TOOLS/ INSTRUMENTS AND DEVICES

FDA-APPROVED STENT GRAFTS

Currently, there are seven FDA-approved stent grafts on the market for TEVAR in the descending thoracic aorta: Bolton Medical's (Vascutek, Terumo) RelayPlus and Relay NBS plus, Cook Medical's TX2 with Pro-Form and the Zenith Alpha Thoracic Endovascular Graft, W. L. Gore and Associates' Conformable Gore TAG Thoracic Endoprosthesis, and Medtronic's Valiant Thoracic Stent Graft With Captivia Delivery System and the Medtronic Valiant. Another device, the Navion TEVAR device from Medtronic, very recently received FDA approval.

All of these devices have undergone multiple rounds of design revisions with the goal of better conformability and navigation in the aortic arch and lower profile to allow easy access. More devices are being developed to treat complex lesions of the ascending thoracic aorta, aortic arch and descending thoracic and thoracoabdominal aorta.

PERIOPERATIVE CONSIDERATION

INDICATIONS FOR MINIMALLY INVASIVE AORTIC SURGERY

ASCENDING AORTA AND AORTIC ARCH

No specific guidelines exist for the use of minimally invasive aortic surgery for pathologies of the ascending aorta and aortic arch (aneurysms and dissections), and the expertise of the operator plays a pivotal role. In addition, no endovascular devices are currently approved in the US to treat the ascending aorta and the arch totally endovascularly, so this application is off-label.

DESCENDING THORACIC AORTA

Thoracic endovascular repair (TEVAR) via a percutaneous femoral approach or via a small incision and exposure of the femoral artery has been used to treat various pathologies (acute and chronic dissection, aneurysm, penetrating ulcer, intramural hematoma, coarctation) involving the descending thoracic aorta. The following are indications to treat ascending aortic, aortic arch and descending thoracic pathology with surgery, TEVAR or both according to current practice recommendations as described in the 2014 ESC Guidelines on the diagnosis and treatment of aortic diseases (The Task Force for the Diagnosis and Treatment of Aortic Diseases of the European Society of Cardiology [ESC]) (Figure 14.1.17).

(Note: Each recommendation below is followed by the class of recommendation [I, IIa or IIb] and the level of supporting evidence [A, B or C].)

1. Recommendation for (thoracic) endovascular aortic repair ([T]EVAR)
2. Recommendations for treating acute aortic dissection
3. Recommendations for the management of intramural hematoma
4. Recommendations for the management of penetrating aortic ulcer

FIGURE 14.1.16 Hybrid techniques for complex aortic arch surgery.

FIGURE 14.1.17 2014 ESC Guidelines on the diagnosis and treatment of aortic diseases.

FIGURE 14.1.18 2010 ACCF/AHA Practice Guidelines.

5. Recommendations for treating (contained) rupture of a thoracic aortic aneurysm
6. Recommendations for treating traumatic aortic injury
7. Recommendations for intervention on
   1. Ascending aortic aneurysm
   2. Aortic arch aneurysm
   3. Descending aortic aneurysm
8. Recommendations for follow-up and management of chronic aortic diseases

FIGURE 14.1.19 Endovascular stent graft for the ascending aorta: Gore

4. Chronic aortic dissection
5. Follow-up after endovascular treatment for aortic diseases

2010 ACCF/AHA/AATS/ACR/ASA/SCA/SCAI/SIR/STS/SVM Practice Guidelines for the Diagnosis and Management of Patients with Thoracic Aortic Disease can be found in Figure 14.1.18.

ALTERNATIVE APPROACHES

Alternative approaches to ascending aortic pathology are limited. Many patients need open surgical repair. For patients with high surgical risk, individualized treatment plans are needed. Surgeons' experience and expertise are important in treating this group of patients.

CAVEATS AND CONTROVERSIES

Currently, endovascular repair for treating ascending aortic pathology is limited to off-label use. Surgeons' experience is important for patient selection and intraoperative planning. An ongoing trial, Feasibility of Endovascular Repair of Ascending Aortic Pathologies (PS-IDE) [18], is aiming to determine the feasibility of endovascular repair for ascending aortic pathology. Regarding approaches via incisions other than traditional median sternotomy, to date, published research about mini-sternotomies or right thoracotomies for surgical repairs of ascending aortic pathology is limited to retrospective studies. Retrospective comparative studies have not shown any substantial differences, but these studies are limited by the bias inherent to their retrospective design. Prospective studies and, possibly,

FIGURE 14.1.20 Aortic Surgery Fellowship.

robust meta-analyses comparing minimally invasive and conventional procedures are needed to establish the potential benefits and outcomes of minimally invasive approaches.

RESEARCH, TRENDS AND INNOVATION

CURRENT RESULTS

Mini-sternotomy or right mini-thoracotomy for ascending, proximal arch and aortic arch repair produces acceptable results that are comparable to those of traditional repairs, as reported by experienced groups [6,19,20].

ASCENDING AORTA: ENDOVASCULAR REPAIR

Only isolated reports and case series are currently available regarding endovascular treatment of ascending aortic disease. The technique is limited to patients deemed high-risk by the surgical team. Results in these high-risk patients are respectable, but there is still risk of morbidity and mortality.

A 2018 meta-analysis reported results from a total of 118 patients treated with primary endovascular repair of the ascending aorta. The devices most commonly used were thoracic stents (in 84 patients), abdominal cuffs (13 patients) and custom-made grafts (12 patients). Femoral, transapical, carotid and axillary access routes were used. All-cause mortality was 15.2%, and aorta-related mortality was 5%. Conversion to open surgery occurred in 3.4% of cases [21].

Currently ongoing trials of endovascular stent grafts to treat pathologies of the ascending aorta:

- ∞ Trial for Feasibility of Endovascular Repair of Ascending Aortic Pathologies (PS-IDE) [18].
- ∞ Feasibility of Endovascular Repair of Ascending Aortic Pathologies [22].
- ∞ The Gore ARISE Study for the Gore Ascending Stent Graft (ARISE TBE 14-02) trial: the first multicenter, early feasibility study approved by the FDA to investigate the use of a minimally invasive device to treat type A dissection [23] (Figure 14.1.19).

ARCH AND DESCENDING THORACIC AORTA

HYBRID RESULTS

Acceptable results have been reported, but it is challenging to compare traditional and hybrid repairs because they are used in different patient populations. An individualized approach offers the best results [24–26].

ENDOVASCULAR REPAIR

Currently, there are few ongoing trials of a branched thoracic endograft for treating lesions of the aortic arch:

- ∞ Feasibility trial with GORE TAG Thoracic Branch Endoprosthesis to treat lesions of the aortic arch and descending thoracic aorta [27].
- ∞ Mona LSA (left subclavian artery) trial 00167 [28].

DESCENDING THORACIC AORTA

Excellent results have been reported with the endovascular treatment of aneurysms and other pathologies of the descending thoracic aorta [29–32].

WHERE AND HOW TO LEARN

They are different cardiothoracic surgery programs in the United States, with a high volume of aortic pathology cases, which offer fellowships in aortic surgery (Figure 14.1.20).

The Baylor College of Medicine in Houston, Texas, USA, offers a 1- or 2-year Aortic Surgery Fellowship in which trainees are exposed to complex open and endovascular aortic procedures involving all the segments of the ascending arch and thoracoabdominal aorta. In addition, the trainees are exposed to various percutaneous heart valve interventions.

REFERENCES

1. Nikolay L. Volodos. The First Steps in Endovascular Aortic Repair: How It All Began. 2013, 20(1): I-3-I-23 https://doi.org/10.1583/1545-1550-20.sp1.I-3
2. Nikolay L. Volodos. The 30th Anniversary of the First Clinical Application of Endovascular Stentgrafting. *Eur J Vasc Endovasc Surg.* 2015, 49, 495e497 https://doi.org/10.1016/j.ejvs.2015.02.012
3. Nikolay L. Volodos, Karpovich IP, Troyan VI, et al. Clinical experience of the use of self-fixing synthetic prostheses for remote endoprosthetics of the thoracic and the abdominal aorta and iliac arteries through the femoral artery and as intraoperative endoprosthesis for aorta reconstruction. *Vasa Suppl.* 1991, 33:93–95.
4. Parodi JC, Palmaz JC, Barone HD. Transfemoral intraluminal graft implantation for abdominal aortic aneurysms. *Ann Vasc Surg.* 1991, 5(6):491–499. https://doi.org/10.1007/BF02015271
5. Dake MD, Miller DC, Semba CP, Mitchell RS, Walker PJ, Liddell RP. Transluminal placement of endovascular stent-grafts for the treatment of descending thoracic aortic aneurysms. *N Engl J Med.* 1994, 331(26):1729–1734. https://www.nejm.org/doi/full/10.1056/NEJM199412293312601
6. Lamelas J, Chen PC, Loor G, LaPietra A. Successful Use of Sternal-Sparing Minimally Invasive Surgery for Proximal Ascending Aortic Pathology. *Ann Thorac Surg.* 2018;106(3):742–748. https://doi.org/10.1016/j.athoracsur.2018.03.081
7. Deschka H, Erler S, Machner M, El-Ayoubi L, Alken A, Wimmer-Greinecker G. Surgery of the ascending aorta, root remodelling and aortic arch surgery with circulatory arrest through partial upper sternotomy: results of 50 consecutive cases. *Eur J Cardiothorac Surg.* 2013;43(3):580–584. doi:10.1093/ejcts/ezs341
8. Preventza O, Henry MJ, Cheong BY, Coselli JS. Endovascular repair of the ascending aorta: when and how to implement the current technology. *Ann Thorac Surg.* 2014;97(5):1555–1560. doi:10.1016/j.athoracsur.2013.11.066
9. Roselli EE, Idrees J, Greenberg RK, Johnston DR, Lytle BW. Endovascular stent grafting for ascending aorta repair in high-risk patients [published correction appears in J Thorac Cardiovasc Surg. 2016 Jul;152(1):292. Idrees, Jahanzaib J [corrected to Idrees, Jay J]]. *J Thorac Cardiovasc Surg.* 2015;149(1):144-151. doi:10.1016/j.jtcvs.2014.07.109
10. Faulds J, Sandhu HK, Estrera AL, Safi HJ. Minimally Invasive Techniques for Total Aortic Arch Reconstruction. *Methodist Debakey Cardiovasc J.* 2016;12(1):41–44. doi:10.14797/mdcj-12-1-41
11. Iida Y, Ito T, Misumi T, Shimizu H. Total debranching thoracic endovascular aortic arch repair with inflow from the descending thoracic aorta. *J Vasc Surg.* 2016;63(2):527–528. doi:10.1016/j.jvs.2014.10.095
12. Preventza O, Bakaeen FG, Cervera RD, Coselli JS. Deployment of proximal thoracic endograft in zone 0 of the ascending aorta: treatment options and early outcomes for aortic arch aneurysms in a high-risk population. *Eur J Cardiothorac Surg.* 2013;44(3):446–453. doi:10.1093/ejcts/ezt068

13. Sultan I, Bavaria JE, Szeto W. Hybrid Techniques for Aortic Arch Aneurysm Repair. *Semin Cardiothorac Vasc Anesth.* 2016;20(4):327–332. doi:10.1177/1089253216659701
14. Preventza O, Wheatley GH 3rd, Ramaiah VG, et al. Management of endoleaks associated with endovascular treatment of descending thoracic aortic diseases. *J Vasc Surg.* 2008;48(1):69–73. doi:10.1016/j.jvs.2008.02.032
15. Oderich GS, Ribeiro M, Reis de Souza L, Hofer J, Wigham J, Cha S. Endovascular repair of thoracoabdominal aortic aneurysms using fenestrated and branched endografts. *J Thorac Cardiovasc Surg.* 2017;153(2):S32-S41.e7. doi:10.1016/j.jtcvs.2016.10.008
16. Heidemann F, Tsilimparis N, Rohlffs F, et al. Staged procedures for prevention of spinal cord ischemia in endovascular aortic surgery. *Gefasschirurgie.* 2018;23(Suppl 2):39–45. doi:10.1007/s00772-018-0410-z
17. Banga PV, Oderich GS, Reis de Souza L, et al. Neuromonitoring, Cerebrospinal Fluid Drainage, and Selective Use of Iliofemoral Conduits to Minimize Risk of Spinal Cord Injury During Complex Endovascular Aortic Repair. *J Endovasc Ther.* 2016;23(1):139–149. doi:10.1177/1526602815620898
18. Feasibility of Endovascular Repair of Ascending Aortic Pathologies. ClinicalTrials.gov Identifier: NCT03322033. Retrieved from https://clinicaltrials.gov/ct2/show/NCT03322033.
19. Risteski P, El-Sayed Ahmad A, Monsefi N, et al. Minimally invasive aortic arch surgery: Early and late outcomes. *Int J Surg.* 2017;45:113–117. doi:10.1016/j.ijsu.2017.07.105
20. El-Sayed Ahmad A, Risteski P, Papadopoulos N, Radwan M, Moritz A, Zierer A. Minimally invasive approach for aortic arch surgery employing the frozen elephant trunk technique. *Eur J Cardiothorac Surg.* 2016;50(1):140–144. doi:10.1093/ejcts/ezv484
21. Muetterties CE, Menon R, Wheatley GH 3rd. A systematic review of primary endovascular repair of the ascending aorta. *J Vasc Surg.* 2018;67(1):332–342. doi:10.1016/j.jvs.2017.06.099
22. Feasibility of Endovascular Repair Of Ascending Aortic Pathologies. ClinicalTrials.gov Identifier: NCT02201589. Retrieved from https://clinicaltrials.gov/ct2/show/NCT02201589
23. Aortic Replacement Using Individualised Regenerative Allografts: Bridging the Therapeutic Gap - ARISE (the "Surveillance"). ClinicalTrials.gov Identifier: NCT02527629. Retrieved from https://clinicaltrials.gov/ct2/show/NCT02527629
24. Preventza O, Garcia A, Cooley DA, et al. Total aortic arch replacement: A comparative study of zone 0 hybrid arch exclusion versus traditional open repair. *J Thorac Cardiovasc Surg.* 2015;150(6):1591–1600. doi:10.1016/j.jtcvs.2015.08.117
25. Preventza O, Tan CW, Orozco-Sevilla V, Euhus CJ, Coselli JS. Zone zero hybrid arch exclusion versus open total arch replacement. *Ann Cardiothorac Surg.* 2018;7(3):372–379. doi:10.21037/acs.2018.04.03
26. Andersen ND, Williams JB, Hanna JM, Shah AA, McCann RL, Hughes GC. Results with an algorithmic approach to hybrid repair of the aortic arch. *J Vasc Surg.* 2013;57(3):655–667. doi:10.1016/j.jvs.2012.09.039
27. Evaluation of the GORE® TAG® Thoracic Branch Endoprosthesis in the Treatment of Proximal Descending Thoracic Aortic Aneurysms. ClinicalTrials.gov Identifier: NCT02021812. Retrieved from https://clinicaltrials.gov/ct2/show/NCT02021812.
28. Roselli EE, Arko FR 3rd, Thompson MM; Valiant Mona LSA Trial Investigators. Results of the Valiant Mona LSA early feasibility study for descending thoracic aneurysms. *J Vasc Surg.* 2015;62(6):1465-71.e3. doi:10.1016/j.jvs.2015.07.078
29. Biancari F, Mariscalco G, Mariani S, Saari P, Satta J, Juvonen T. Endovascular Treatment of Degenerative Aneurysms Involving Only the Descending Thoracic Aorta: Systematic Review and Meta-analysis. *J Endovasc Ther.* 2016;23(2):387–392. doi:10.1177/1526602815626560
30. D'Annoville T, Ozdemir BA, Alric P, Marty-Ané CH, Canaud L. Thoracic Endovascular Aortic Repair for Penetrating Aortic Ulcer: Literature Review. *Ann Thorac Surg.* 2016;101(6):2272–2278. doi:10.1016/j.athoracsur.2015.12.036

31. Nienaber CA, Rousseau H, Eggebrecht H, et al. Randomized comparison of strategies for type B aortic dissection: the INvestigation of STEnt Grafts in Aortic Dissection (INSTEAD) trial. *Circulation.* 2009;120(25):2519–2528. doi:10.1161/CIRCULATIONAHA.109.886408

32. Nienaber CA, Kische S, Rousseau H, et al. Endovascular repair of type B aortic dissection: long-term results of the randomized investigation of stent grafts in aortic dissection trial. *Circ Cardiovasc Interv.* 2013;6(4):407–416. doi:10.1161/CIRCINTERVENTIONS.113.000463

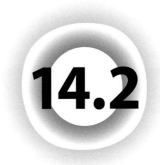

AORTIC SURGERY
Endovascular and Hybrid Approaches for Distal Arch and Descending Thoracic Aorta

CEM ALHAN, SAHIN SENAY, JULIAN WONG AND ANDREW MTL CHOONG

HISTORY OR INTRODUCTION

In 1991, Parodi et al. described the deployment of the first endovascular stent-graft (EVSG) in an infra-renal abdominal aortic aneurysm [1]. By 1994, as a direct evolutionary step, Dake et al. then used an EVSG for isolated descending thoracic aortic aneurysms [2]. This use of EVSG for aortic aneurysms limited to the thoracic segment showed significant early promise. However, their use for extensive distal arch and descending thoracic aortic disease was necessarily limited by the presence of the arch vessels proximally and the visceral and renal vessels distally. Significant advances in endovascular technology have since allowed for total endovascular repairs of both the aortic arch and the visceral segment of the aorta in selected patients. However, hybrid repairs (combining open surgical technologies with endovascular technologies) remain popular, as robust methods and generally applicable methods of dealing with these important aortic branches.

Aortic pathologies involving the distal arch and descending aorta include aneurysm, rupture, traumatic transection, penetrating ulcers, intramural hematoma, coarctation of aorta and type B dissections. The classical management of these pathologies is challenging and may require cardiopulmonary bypass and circulatory arrest. Endovascular and hybrid approaches have been proposed as a less invasive method for the treatment for these pathologies [1–3]. This chapter reviews the endovascular and hybrid treatment strategies for distal arch and descending aortic pathologies.

DISTAL ARCH ANEURYSMS

Aneurysm formation is the second most common disease of the aorta after atherosclerotic lesions. Thoracic aortic aneurysms (TAA) in general are detected with an incidence of 10.4 per 100,000 patient-years [4]. The hospital admission rate due to TAA has been reported as of 9.0 per 100,000 [4]. The rate of major aneurysm-related complications has been reported to occur 10% at the maximum diameter of 60 mm and 43% at 70 mm [4–6]. The most common site for TAA is known to be the ascending aorta. However, the arch aneurysms may accompany both ascending and/or descending aorta aneurysms (Figure 14.2.1).

TAAs grow slowly. Although the mean growth rates for TAAs in general ranged between 0.2 and 4.2 mm/year, the growth rate for aortic arch is reported to be similar to the ascending aorta and ranges between 0.2 and 2.8 mm/years. However, a large presenting diameter, distal aneurysm and history of bicuspid aortic valve or Marfan syndrome increase the risk for accelerated aneurysm growth [4]. TAAs related with elastic tissue diseases may grow faster; the growth rate in patients with Marfan syndrome ranges between 0.5 and 1 mm/year, and in patients with Loeys–Dietz syndrome (LDS) the growth rate is reported to be more than 10 mm/year. Eventually the risk for dissection or rupture rapidly increases when the aortic diameter is 60 mm for the ascending aorta and 70 mm for the descending aorta [2]. Due to the high risk of complication, aneurysm repair is recommended in patients with isolated aortic arch aneurysm with maximal diameter ≥55 mm. The repair of aortic arch aneurysm may also be considered in patients during the repair of adjacent ascending or descending aortic aneurysm [2].

DESCENDING AORTIC ANEURYSMS

The growth rate of the aneurysms at the descending aorta is generally faster (1.9–3.4 mm/year) than those in the ascending aorta. Dissection, urgent procedure and hypertension were associated with an increased growth rate of descending TAAs in patients with Marfan syndrome after aortic valve and proximal aorta surgery for aortic dissection [2–4]. The decision on the timing of repair of descending aortic aneurysms depends on the type of technique to be used. Thoracic endovascular aneurysm repair (TEVAR) is recommended as the first choice of treatment when compared to open surgery in cases with suitable anatomy. TEVAR should be considered, rather than surgery, when anatomy is suitable. In such cases the intervention should be considered in patients with descending aortic aneurysm with maximal diameter ≥55 mm. If TEVAR is not possible, surgical repair should be considered in patients with descending aortic aneurysm with maximal diameter ≥60 mm. In patients with elastic tissue disorders like Marfan syndrome the choice for repair should be surgery [2,3].

TRAUMATIC AORTIC INJURY

Blunt trauma to the thorax may lead to traumatic aortic injury (TAI). Patient history usually reveals a deceleration trauma like a car accident or a fall accident. A widened mediastinum, hypotension (<90 mmHg),

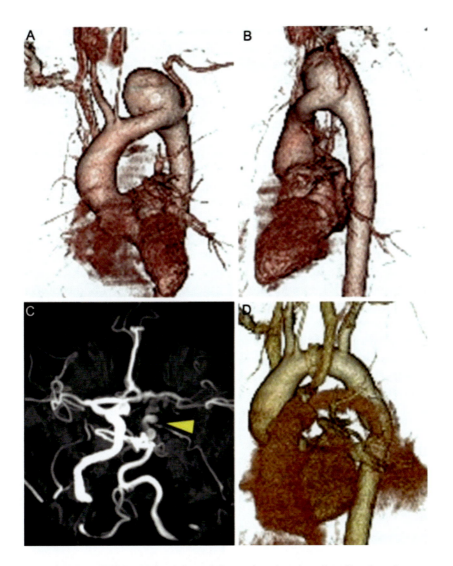

FIGURE 14.2.1 (A) Computed tomography angiography showing the distal arch aneurysm. (B) Sagittal view. (C) Magnetic resonance imaging showing the cerebrovascular aneurysm (delta). (D) Postoperative image. (Reprinted from Tanaka C, Shimura S, Cho Y, Ueda T. Distal aortic arch aneurysm in an adult case of PHACE syndrome. *Interact Cardiovasc Thorac Surg.* 2018;27(4):619-621, with permission from Oxford University Press.)

long bone fracture, pulmonary contusion, left scapula fracture or hemothorax are defined to be risk factors for TAI in such a polytrauma patient. The injured site is usually (up to 90%) the isthmus of aorta. The aortic root and the diaphragmatic portion may also be affected. The aortic lesion can be an intimal tear (Type I TAI), intramural hematoma (Type II TAI), pseudoaneurysm (Type III TAI) or rupture (Type IV TAI) [2,7,8]. Patients with free aortic rupture or large periaortic hematoma need emergency treatment; other cases may be treated within a 24-hour period, performing patient stabilization first and treating any other co-existing emergency pathology. Type 1 lesions may be conservatively managed with serial imaging in stable patients. TEVAR should be the first choice of treatment in patients with suitable anatomy. Hybrid solutions or conventional surgery may be an option for the rest of the patients requiring intervention.

PENETRATING AORTIC ULCERS

Penetrating aortic ulcers (PAU) are usually located at the descending aorta (type B). However, progressive aortic enlargement and the development of saccular or fusiform aneurysms are more common in PAUs located at the ascending aorta (type A). PAUs represent 2–7% of acute aortic syndromes in general and may lead to intramural hematoma (IMH), pseudoaneurysm, aortic rupture or dissection. Urgent surgical therapy is recommended in type A PAU. In cases with pericardial effusion, peri-aortic hematoma or large aneurysms emergency surgery is required. TEVAR over surgical treatment may be considered in complicated type B PAU (Figure 14.2.2).

INTRAMURAL HEMATOMA

Aortic intramural hematoma (IMH) develops in the media of the aortic wall as a circular or crescent-shaped thickening of >5 mm of the wall in the absence of any intimal tear, false lumen or detectable blood flow. About 30% of these are located in the ascending aorta and aortic arch (type A) and 70% of them at the descending thoracic aorta (Type B). Approximately 30–40% of type A IMH may complicate into aortic dissection. Risk factors for developing complications for IMH include persistent and recurrent pain, resistant hypertension, type A PAU, aortic diameter ≥50 mm, aortic wall thickness >11 mm, enlarging aortic diameter, recurrent pleural effusion, associated dissection and organ ischemia. In cases of type A IMH and complicated type B IMH, urgent surgery is indicated. TEVAR over surgical therapy may be considered for type B lesions.

COARCTATION OF AORTA

Coarctation of the aorta (CA) is usually located at the insertion area of the ductus arteriosus. Usually >20 mmHg gradient between the proximal and distal parts of the lesion indicates significant coarctation. Pre- and post-stenotic aneurysm of aorta

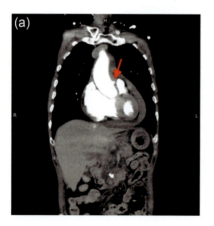
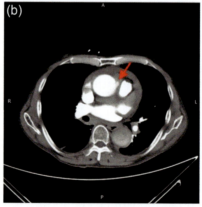

FIGURE 14.2.2 A protruding spot (PAU) in the ascending aorta (red arrow). (A) Coronal view. (B) Axial view. (With kind permission from Springer Science+Business Media, Springer Nature, *J Cardiothorac Surg*, A penetrating atherosclerotic ulcer rupture in the ascending aorta with hemopericardium: a case report, 11, 103, Liu, Y., Ke, H., Lin, Y. et al. © 2016.)

may also be detected. Treatment should be considered in hypertensive patients with >50% aortic narrowing compared to the aortic diameter at the diaphragm level.

TYPE B AORTIC DISSECTIONS

Type B aortic dissection results from a disruption of the medial layer of the aortic wall leading to formation of a true and false lumen at the descending aorta. The lesion may extend distally. In general aortic dissections occur with a rate of 6/100,000 per year, and the risk factors for developing aortic dissections include hypertension, pre-existing aortic diseases or aortic valve disease, family history of aortic diseases, previous cardiac surgery, smoking, chest trauma and use of intravenous drugs. Clinical signs of type B aortic dissections may include chest pain (severe and abrupt chest or back pain), myocardial ischemia, heart failure, pulmonary complications (pleural effusion, aortobronchial fistula and rupture), neurological complications (paraplegia), mesenteric or renal ischemia and leg malperfusion. Specific diagnostic tools include the d-dimer test, echocardiography and magnetic resonance or computed tomographic (CT) angiography. However the gold standard tool for both the diagnostic and preoperative planning processes is CT angiography. In patients with an uncomplicated clinical course and absence of malperfusion, TEVAR should be considered alongside medical treatment as the choice for management. In complicated type B aortic dissections, TEVAR is recommended as the first-line therapy.

OTHER PATHOLOGIES

Other rare pathologies that may affect the distal arch and descending aorta include pseudoaneurysms, aortobronchial fistulas, aortoesophageal fistulas and atherosclerotic or inflammatory lesions. Basically the strategy for treatment of these pathologies depends on the site of the aorta affected. Treatment strategies depending on the aortic zones can be applied for these pathologies.

HOW TO DO IT/STEP BY STEP

ARCH DEBRANCHING

Rerouting of the aortic arch branches is well described and can be performed in an intra- or extra-thoracic manner depending on the debranching required. Here, we discuss the various approaches possible based on the proximal landing zone of the TEVAR.

EVOLUTION OF THE "VISCERAL HYBRID" REPAIR FOR THORACOABDOMINAL AORTIC PATHOLOGY

Thoracoabdominal aortic aneurysms (TAAA) are defined by the involvement of the origins of the coeliac, superior mesenteric and renal arteries. Crawford's classification is universally accepted [1] (Figure 14.2.3), although Safi subsequently added a fifth class of TAAA in his version of the classification system [2] (Figure 14.2.4).

The repair of TAAA has high mortality and morbidity when treated by open techniques [3,4]. These risks have persisted despite advances in operative technique (including cardiopulmonary or left heart bypass, hypothermic cardiopulmonary arrest, selective visceral perfusion, spinal cord protection) and higher standards of perioperative care.

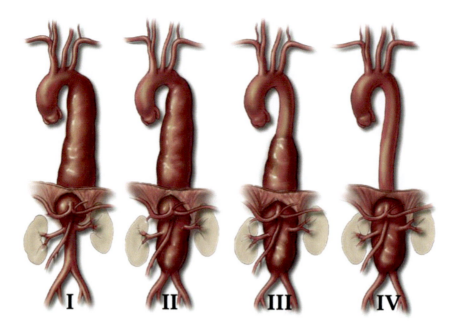

FIGURE 14.2.3 Crawford classification of the extent of thoracoabdominal aortic aneurysms. (Reprinted from *J Thorac Cardiovasc Surg* S0022-5223(20)30200-2, Chatterjee S, Casar JG, LeMaire SA, Preventza O, Coselli JS, Perioperative care after thoracoabdominal aortic aneurysm repair: The Baylor College of Medicine experience. Part 1: Preoperative considerations, © 2020 by The American Association for Thoracic Surgery, with permission from Elsevier.)

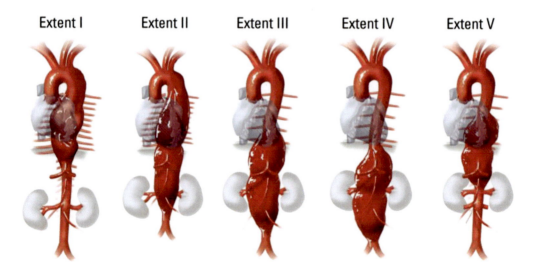

FIGURE 14.2.4 Schematic representation of the modified Crawford classification scheme for thoracoabdominal aortic aneurysm extents. (After Frederick JR, Woo YJ. Thoracoabdominal aortic aneurysm. *Ann Cardiothorac Surg.* 2012;1(3): 277-285. © 2020, with permission from AME Publishing Company.)

In 1999, Quinones-Baldrich et al. were the first to report a combined endovascular and open surgical approach for a type IV TAAA [7]. Previous abdominal aortic surgery and concomitant visceral artery aneurysms precluded an open repair. Retrograde visceral bypasses from a limb of a pre-existing bifurcated aortic tube graft were performed, followed by TAAA stent-grafting. By re-vascularizing the visceral and renal branches first, total endovascular aneurysm exclusion was achieved by completion endo-grafting.

Rimmer et al. in 2003, at St Mary's, used a similar technique of retrograde visceral/renal re-vascularization with completion endo-grafting for a 49-year-old gentleman with a 9-cm aneurysm of native aorta occurring between a previous infra-renal abdominal and an upper descending thoracic aortic aneurysm repair [8]. Three years later, Black et al., from St Mary's, reported the largest published series of these repairs describing a total of 29 attempted *visceral hybrid* procedures [9]. Their unit performs this technique in preference to an open repair for Crawford Type I, II and III TAAA, while an open approach with medial visceral rotation is used for Crawford Type IV aneurysms. These repairs are particularly attractive and deemed less invasive as they avoid the need for a thoracotomy, single-lung ventilation, aortic cross clamp, left or full heart bypass as well as the extensive tissue dissection all associated with an open repair.

GENERAL PRINCIPLES

Preoperative CT angiographic assessment of the lesion is crucial for planning of the intervention. The length of the lesion, the diameter and the length of healthy aortic segments proximal and distal to the lesion (proximal and distal landing zones), the relationship to the side branches and the quality and diameter of the access route for endovascular repair should be evaluated. For a safe stent graft implantation, a landing zone with diameter of <40 mm and a length of ≥20 mm both at the distal and proximal sites is necessary. In some circumstances a safe landing zone may not always be available due to the extension of the aortic lesion through specific side branches. In such cases a hybrid approach including debranching or extra-anatomic bypass for side branches first and stent implantation later can be planned. Debranching of the side branches facilitates the obtaining of a safe landing zone. This part of the operation is usually performed in a minimally invasive fashion. Alternatives for this technique can be branched grafts or the chimney technique [1,2,7,8].

Deciding on the size of the stent graft is a crucial step in planning an endovascular or hybrid procedure. For aneurysm repairs, usually an oversizing of 10–15% is considered when deciding on the stent graft size; however almost no oversizing is recommended for a dissected aorta to prevent further erosion of the aortic wall (Figure 14.2.5). Moreover the stent graft to be used should be flexible and self-expandable without need for any ballooning [7].

In some cases there may be discrepancy between the diameters of the proximal and distal landing zones. Tapered stent grafts (aorto-uni-iliac grafts) may be used in selected cases.

The usual site for access is the femoral artery for stent implantation. The catheter for angiography and sizing can be advanced through the contralateral femoral artery, brachial artery or radial artery. It is very crucial to exactly position the catheter in the true lumen during the repair of a dissection. Echocardiographic guidance can be helpful for this.

When the exact position is obtained, the stent graft is deployed during a reduced

FIGURE 14.2.5 Thoracic endovascular aortic repair – animation

FIGURE 14.2.7 Zone 1, hybrid TEVAR (subclavian-to-subclavian bypass) by Cem Alhan.

FIGURE 14.2.6 Zone 1, hybrid TEVAR (caroticocarotid bypass).

systemic blood pressure (<80 mmHg) period. This can be achieved medically or by a short period of rapid ventricular pacing.

TREATMENT TECHNIQUES

In general, hybrid treatments for aortic arch pathologies are classified into three types according to the extension of the disease. Type 1 operations include debranching of the brachiocephalic truncus and endovascular repair of the aortic arch. Type 2 operations include an open ascending aorta reconstruction, bypass of supraaortic branches and endovascular repair of the arch. Type 3 operations include an elephant trunk procedure with a complete endovascular repair of the thoracoabdominal aorta [1,2]. The proximal extent of arch disease has been found to be a major determinant of outcome [9].

Currently the operative techniques are detailed according to the classification of Ishimaru and Mitchell [10].

ZONE 1 PATHOLOGIES

Zone 1 pathologies involve the diseases of the aortic arch between the innominate and left common carotid arteries. This group of patients accounts for approximately 30% of patients treated with hybrid aortic debranching and endovascular arcus aorta repair. The hybrid approach for this group of patients requires debranching of the left common carotid artery and left subclavian artery. A carotid-carotid bypass via the retropharyngeal or ante-trachea tunnel can be performed with left subclavian artery revascularization (Figure 14.2.6). Transposition or bypass for the left subclavian artery may be an option for operative technique. A second operative option is a subclavian-to-subclavian cross-bypass and ipsilateral subclavian carotid bypass (Figure 14.2.7). Subclavian-to-subclavian bypass necessitates a longer graft; however this technique avoids left common carotid artery clamping and may help prevent cerebral ischemia. In the meantime, if clamping of the internal carotid arteries is found to be risky, then bypass directly to external carotid arteries may be an alternative technique.

In a selected group of patients, debranching of the brachiocephalic truncus may also be needed due to inadequate landing zone distance. A 6- or 8-mm Dacron prostheses can be used for debranching. The left vertebral artery should be preserved to protect collateral function. Supraaortic

FIGURE 14.2.8 Carotid-carotid subclavian bypass, by Maham Rahimi.

FIGURE 14.2.11 Hybrid thoracoabdominal aneurysm repair – CTS.net.

FIGURE 14.2.9 Extra-anatomic bypass: Left carotid to subclavian artery bypass – CTS.net.

FIGURE 14.2.12 Hybrid thoracoabdominal aneurysm repair by Selim Isbir.

FIGURE 14.2.10 Extra-anatomic bypass: Left carotid to subclavian artery bypass by Daniel GN.

FIGURE 14.2.13 Hybrid technique: Reoperative thoracoabdominal aneurysm repair – CTS.net.

reconstructions should always be controlled with intraoperative angiography. Afterwards, zone 0 or partially zone 1 can be used as a landing zone for endovascular stent graft implantation. A transfemoral approach can be used for endovascular stent implantation. In selected patients (patients with >20 cm length of aortic coverage or a prior aortic procedure with a synthetic graft), spinal drainage can be used. Early postoperative computed tomographic angiography should be performed to demonstrate the patency of the supra-aortic reconstruction and the exclusion of aortic disease. Retrograde dissection, stroke and type 1a endoleak may complicate the perioperative period and should be monitored carefully. Postoperative type 1a endoleaks have been shown to be an independent risk factor for mortality. The rate of type 1 endoleaks tends to decrease from zone 0 to distal zone repairs (zone 0 > zone 1 > zone 2) [1,9,11,12]. However some reports demonstrate an increased stability of the stent graft when proximal zones are used for landing [13]. The prominent aortic angle may have an impact on this finding. Nevertheless, it is crucial to establish a healthy zone with a sufficient length before implantation of the stent.

FIGURE 14.2.14 Hybrid technique: Reoperative thoracoabdominal aneurysm repair by Derek RB.

FIGURE 14.2.16 Insertion ProGlides: Preclose technique by Alan BL.

FIGURE 14.2.15 Total percutaneous thoracic endovascular aortic repair.

FIGURE 14.2.17 Retroperitoneal exposure: Iliac artery and conduit case by Alan BL.

ZONE 2 PATHOLOGIES

Zone 2 pathologies involve the diseases of the aortic arch between the left common carotid artery and left subclavian artery. This group of patients also accounts for approximately 30% of patients treated with hybrid aortic repair. Hybrid approaches for this group of patients require debranching of the left subclavian artery. Carotid subclavian bypass or transposition the subclavian artery can be performed (Figure 14.2.8). The left subclavian artery can be proximally ligated or occluded with endovascular devices (coiling or plugs). In some selected group of patients, debranching for the left carotid artery may be needed. Zone 1 or partially zone 2 is used as a landing zone for stent graft implantation [1,9].

ZONE 3 PATHOLOGIES

Zone 3 pathologies involve the diseases of the proximal portion of descending aorta. A hybrid approach for this group of patients may require debranching of the left subclavian artery, and zone 2 (or partially zone 3) is used as a landing zone for stent graft implantation (Figure 14.2.9 and Figure 14.2.10). One of the most common pathologies at this region is type B dissection. The entry tear of the dissection is usually located in the immediate vicinity of the orifice of the left subclavian artery. Treatment in selected cases may require debranching of the left subclavian artery. In some patients the dissected segments may extend proximally to the arch. In such cases zone 1 or 2 repair may be needed to secure a safe proximal landing zone according to the extent of the dissected segment [14,15].

ST MARY'S VISCERAL HYBRID REPAIR TECHNIQUE

The patient is placed in a supine position under general and epidural anesthesia. Cerebrospinal fluid drainage is always used. We routinely use cell salvage techniques with rapid infusers available. Arterial and central venous lines, urethral catheterization and transesophageal echocardiography are all mandatory in perioperative invasive monitoring (Figure 14.2.11, Figure 14.2.12 and Figure 14.2.13).

FIGURE 14.2.18 Zenith thoracic product portfolio.

FIGURE 14.2.20 Terumo RELAY® endovascular devices

FIGURE 14.2.19 Medtronic Valiant Navion™ thoracic stent graft system.

FIGURE 14.2.21 JOTEC: E-Vita THORACIC 3G.

A midline laparotomy allows for adequate exposure of the abdominal aorta, the origins of the renal arteries, the coeliac axis and the superior mesenteric artery (SMA). The in-flow site for retrograde visceral bypass grafting is determined by the distal extent of aneurysmal disease and previous abdominal surgery. If a previous infrarenal repair has been undertaken, the bypass grafts are anastomosed in an end-to-side fashion to the existing graft. If an infrarenal repair is possible, this is completed first, and bypass grafts are subsequently sutured as before. If the infrarenal aorta is normal, an arteriotomy is performed, and the bypass grafts anastomosed in an end-to-side fashion to the native aorta. If the aneurysmal disease extends to the bifurcation, one external iliac artery can provide the in-flow to the bypass grafts.

Two inverted (14 by 7 mm or 16 by 8 mm) Dacron® trouser-grafts can function as the conduits. Otherwise, a single trouser-graft is used with additional side-limbs sutured in an end-to-side manner. This four-limbed "spaghetti graft" is fashioned in a bespoke fashion during the procedure. The renal arteries are sequentially anastomosed in an end-to-side fashion. The two remaining graft limbs are routed along the base of the small bowel mesentery to the coeliac axis and SMA in an end-to-side fashion. If Doppler signals are satisfactory in the bypass grafts (with the origins of the native vessel clamped), they are subsequently suture-ligated to prevent retrograde flow into the aneurysm sac (type II endoleak) (Figure 14.2.14).

Following successful visceral and renal bypass, a suitable access site is chosen for endovascular stent deployment. A dedicated conduit attached to the common iliac artery or the abdominal aorta is common, but native vessels are also used provided they are of suitable caliber. An angiogram catheter is introduced on the contralateral side, and the stents are deployed in a sequential fashion from the left subclavian artery through the thoracic aorta to the landing zone. Completion angiography after adjunctive procedures (extension cuff, giant Palmaz stent, balloon molding) then confirms exclusion of the aneurysm.

ALTERNATIVE APPROACHES

STANDARD APPROACH (TRANSFEMORAL)

Most modern TEVAR stent grafts are small enough to be delivered transfemorally. The two standard approaches are either a traditional open femoral artery exposure (horizontal or longitudinal incision) or a totally percutaneous one (Figure 14.2.15).

CONDUITS

Conduits usually take the form of an 8-mm Dacron graft to facilitate the insertion of larger-bore TEVAR devices (an 8-mm graft will allow the passage of a device up to 24 F in size). They are usually anastomosed onto a suitable target vessel in an end-to-side fashion (Figure 14.2.16).

ILIAC/INFRA-RENAL ABDOMINAL AORTIC APPROACH

In situations where the femoral or external iliac is occluded, a common iliac artery or infra-renal abdominal aortic exposure ± a conduit can be used to facilitate access. If only an iliac exposure is required, then the retroperitoneal exposure provides good access (14.2.17).

THORACIC AORTIC APPROACH

In the presence of total abdominal aortic occlusion, a conduit can be put on the ascending aorta and the stent graft inserted retrograde via the conduit. This can be done via a left lateral thoracotomy or median sternotomy depending on the situation.

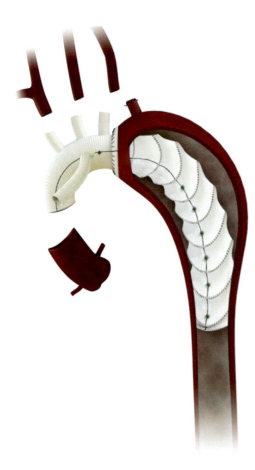

FIGURE 14.2.22 Scheme showing proximalization of the descending anastomosis by leaving the left subclavian artery origin intact by using Thoraflex™ Hybrid graft system. Reprinted from Czerny M, Rylski B, Kari FA, et al. Technical details making aortic arch replacement a safe procedure using the Thoraflex™ Hybrid prosthesis. *Eur J Cardiothorac Surg.* 2017;51(suppl 1):i15-i19, with permission from Oxford University Press

FIGURE 14.2.23 JOTEC: E-Vita Open Plus.

FIGURE 14.2.24   NEXUS™ Aortic Arch Stent Graft System.

FIGURE 14.2.26   Relay™ deployment technique.

FIGURE 14.2.25   Nexus deployment technique.

FIGURE 14.2.27   Cydar Medical – AI-powered image fusion platform.

TOOLS/INSTRUMENTS AND DEVICES

TOOLS/INSTRUMENTS

A standard endovascular toolkit is all that is required for the TEVAR procedures, including the following:

- ∞ Access sheath (5 F or 6 F)
- ∞ 035 hydrophilic floppy wire (Terumo)
- ∞ Straight flush exchange catheter
- ∞ Pigtail angiographic catheter
- ∞ Extra-stiff long wire (Lunderquist/Amplatz/Meier)

DEVICES

With regards to TEVAR devices however, there are many available globally. The ones listed here are all FDA approved. The choice of device depends on a number of different factors including, but not limited to, graft availability, patient anatomy and individual surgeon practice.

Both Cook Medical and Bolton Medical offer custom-made devices for total endovascular solutions at the arch as well as "off-the-shelf" TEVAR solutions. However, Vascutek and JOTEC offer hybrid open arch devices for treating more complex aortic pathology. There is a further recent advancement in which a new hybrid total arch graft offers extra-thoracic debranching and does not require a sternotomy. This is the new Nexus graft (Endospan) which has just been granted FDA approval.

STANDARD TEVAR DEVICES

Cook Medical: Zenith Alpha Thoracic™ Endovascular Graft (Figure 14.2.18)
Medtronic: Valiant Navion™ thoracic stent graft system (Figure 14.2.19)
Terumo (Bolton Medical): RELAY® endovascular devices (Figure 14.2.20)
JOTEC: E-Vita THORACIC 3G (Figure 14.2.21)

CUSTOM-MADE TEVAR DEVICES

Cook
Bolton Medical

HYBRID OPEN TEVAR DEVICES

JOTEC: E-Vita Open Plus
Terumo: Thoraflex™ Hybrid graft system

Endospan, Israel: NEXUS™ Aortic Arch Stent Graft System (Figure 14.2.22 to Figure 14.2.26)

PERIOPERATIVE CONSIDERATIONS

DEVICE AND STOCK CONSIDERATIONS

The most important thing about starting a TEVAR program is to make sure you are familiar with one single device and all its characteristics. When setting up a TEVAR program, keeping enough stock at your unit is particularly important, especially for emergency situations of rupture and transection.

RADIATION PROTECTION

Recent studies have demonstrated that the radiation doses used in TEVAR can affect the endovascular operator at a genetic level. This has caused understandable concern in the endovascular world. Apart from the normal lead gown protection on the operator, there are disposable lead-lined drapes available, which can be used to protect the patient as well as operator from scatter radiation.

In recent years, modern hybrid operating theaters have gained the ability to overlay CT images to reduce the use of both fluoroscopy and DSA and hence further reduce radiation. Other navigation systems like Cydar can be used on existing X-ray systems to also reduce radiation (Figure 14.2.27).

LUMBAR SPINAL DRAINAGE

One of the most important techniques in doing TEVAR is prevention of spinal ischemia using spinal drainage. If coverage of TEVAR is very long and the case is elective, this should be done routinely. However it is not recommended in the emergency setting. Drainage should be no more than 240 ml per day and the pressure should be monitored closely (Figure 13.28).

CAVEATS AND CONTROVERSIES

SUBCLAVIAN ARTERY COVERAGE

Intentional subclavian artery coverage remains controversial. We recommend that in routine cases, the subclavian artery should always be revascularized (except for emergency cases). In the emergency settings like aortic rupture, revascularization of the left subclavian artery may not be performed and stent graft implantation should be performed urgently. However collateral circulation from subclavian arteries to the spine has been defined to be crucial for preventing spinal cord ischemia. Thus, whenever possible, the left subclavian artery should be revascularized [16].

CHIMNEY TECHNIQUES

Endovascular and hybrid therapies for arcus aorta pathologies involving the distal arch segments and descending aorta are currently performed with a low rate of late aorta-related death and reinterventions, and acceptable midterm survival, even when compared to open repair techniques [17,18]. The early results of the endovascular chimney technique are even more encouraging when compared to the hybrid technique [19,20]. Moreover extra-thoracic debranching techniques using the iliac arteries as inflow source have also been described for high-risk patients with previous sternotomies or in the presence of large aneurysms next to the sternum [21].

A 5-year survival report of around 70% has been reported [17]. However retrograde type A dissection and stroke still remain concerns. Retrograde dissection and stroke following TEVAR occur in 1–10% of cases [22–25]. Ischemic cerebral events have been reported in the range of 0.8–25% [15,17]. Alternative methods for cerebral protection including temporary external carotid artery bypass or axillary bypass during debranching of the supraaortic vessels have been described to prevent this complication [26,27].

Fenestrated devices and the chimney graft techniques may be alternatives for

FIGURE 14.2.28 Becker External Drainage and Monitoring System

hybrid techniques requiring debranching of the supraaortic vessels. However the risk of endoleaks from fenestrations and missing outcome data are concerns regarding these techniques [28,29].

Hybrid or endovascular repair for distal arch and descending aorta pathologies is still a target for technological improvement. Current studies focus on branched devices and improved delivery systems, and supplement devices like gels for fixation, which will enable surgeon more and more to perform these kinds of procedures with high-quality standards and safety [14].

REFERENCES

1. Parodi JC, Palmaz JC, Barone HD. Transfemoral intraluminal graft implantation for abdominal aortic aneurysms. *Ann Vasc Surg* 1991;5(6):491–9.
2. Dake MD, Miller DC, Semba CP, Mitchell RS, Walker PJ, Liddell RP. Transluminal placement of endovascular stent-grafts for the treatment of descending thoracic aortic aneurysms. *N Engl J Med* 1994;331(26):1729–34.
3. Boodhwani M, Andelfinger G, Leipsic J, et al. Canadian Cardiovascular Society position statement on the management of thoracic aortic disease. *Can J Cardiol* 2014;30(6):577–89.
4. Oladokun D, Patterson BO, Sobocinski J, Karthikesalingam A, Loftus I, Thompson MM, Holt PJ. Systematic review of the growth rates and influencing factors in thoracic aortic aneurysms. *Eur J Vasc Endovasc Surg* 2016;51(5):674–81.
5. Elefteriades JA, Farkas EA. Thoracic aortic aneurysm clinically pertinent controversies and uncertainties. *J Am Coll Cardiol* 2010;55:841e57.
6. Davies RR, Goldstein LJ, Coady MA, et al. Yearly rupture or dissection rates for thoracic aortic an- eurysms: simple prediction based on size. *Ann Thorac Surg* 2002;73:17e27.
7. Sun L, Qi R, Zhu J, et al. Total arch replacement 20. Combined with stented elephant trunk implantation: a new "standard" therapy for type a dissection involving repair of the aortic arch? *Circulation* 2011;123:971–8.

8. Benedetto U, Melina G, Angeloni E, et al. Current results of open total arch replacement versus hybrid thoracic endovascular aortic repair for aortic arch aneurysm: a meta-analysis of comparative studies. *J Thorac Cardiovasc Surg* 2013;145:305–6.
9. De Rango P, Cao P, Ferrer C, et al. Aortic arch debranching and thoracic endovascular repair. *J Vasc Surg* 2014;59(1):107–14.
10. Mitchell RS, Ishimaru S, Ehrlich MP, et al. First international summit on thoracic aortic endografting: round table on thoracic aortic dissection as an indication for endografting. *J Endovasc Ther* 2002;9(Suppl 2):II98–105.
11. Ockert S, Eckstein G, Lutz B, Reeps C, Eckstein HH. Aortic hemiarch hybrid repair. *J Vasc Surg* 2015;62(4):907–13.
12. Bünger CM, Kische S, Liebold A, et al. Hybrid aortic arch repair for complicated type B aortic dissection. *J Vasc Surg* 2013;58:1490–6.
13. De Rango P, Ferrer C, Coscarella C, et al. Contemporary comparison of aortic arch repair by endovascular and open surgical reconstructions. *J Vasc Surg* 2015;61(2):339–46.
14. Kuratani T. Best surgical option for arch extension of type B dissection: the endovascular approach. *Ann Cardiothorac Surg* 2014;3(3):292–9.
15. Cao P, De Rango P, Czerny M, et al. Systematic review of clinical outcomes in hybrid procedures for aortic arch dissections and other arch diseases. *J Thorac Cardiovasc Surg* 2012;144:1286–300, 1300.e1–2.
16. Eagleton MJ, Shah S, Petkosevek D, et al. Hypegastric and subclavian artery patency affects onset and recovery of spinal cord ishemia associated with aortic endografting. *J Vasc Surg* 2014;59:89–94.
17. Zerwes S, Leissner G, Gosslau Y, et al. Clinical outcomes in hybrid repair procedures for pathologies involving the aortic arch. *Vascular* 2015;23(1):9–16.
18. Chiesa R, Bertoglio L, Rinaldi E, Tshomba Y. Hybrid repair of aortic arch pathology. *Multimed Man Cardiothorac Surg* 2014;2014. pii: mmu003.
19. Yang J, Xiong J, Liu X, Jia X, Zhu Y, Guo W. Endovascular chimney technique of aortic arch pathologies: a systematic review. *Ann Vasc Surg* 2012;26(7):1014–21.
20. Cires G, Noll RE Jr, Albuquerque FC Jr, Tonnessen BH, Sternbergh WC 3rd. Endovascular debranching of the aortic arch during thoracic endograft repair. *J Vasc Surg* 2011;53(6):1485–91.
21. Morishita K, Kuroda Y, Uehara M, Mawatari T. Endovascular repair of a proximal aortic arch aneurysm with extrathoracic debranching. *J Vasc Surg* 2012;56(2):508.
22. White RA, Miller DC, Criado FJ, et al. Report on the results of thoracic endovascular aortic repair for acute, complicated, type B aortic dissection at 30 days and 1 year from a multidisciplinary subcommittee of the Society for Vascular Surgery Outcomes Committee. *J Vasc Surg* 2011;53:1082–90.
23. Thrumurthy SG, Karthikesalingam A, Patterson BO, et al. A systematic review of mid-term outcomes of thoracic 33. endovascular repair (TEVAR) of chronic type B aortic dissection. *Eur J Vasc Endovasc Surg* 2011;42:632–47.
24. Eggebrecht H, Thompson M, Rousseau H, et al. Retrograde ascending aortic dissection during or after 34. thoracic aortic stent graft placement: insight from the European registry on endovascular aortic repair complications. *Circulation* 2009;120 Supplement:S276–81.
25. Madenci AL, Ozaki CK, Belkin M, McPhee JT. Carotid-subclavian bypass and subclavian-carotid transposition in the thoracic endovascular aortic repair era. *J Vasc Surg* 2013;57(5):1275-1282.e2.
26. Ugurlucan M, Sayin OA, Onalan MA, et al. Cerebral protection with a crossover external carotid artery bypass during arch debranching. *Ann Thorac Surg* 2015;99(2):725–7.
27. Mizuno T, Hachimaru T, Oi K, et al. Easy and safe total debranching of arch aneurysms using axilloaxillary arterial bypass. *Ann Thorac Surg* 2015;100(4):1476–8.
28. Kitagawa A, Greenberg RK, Eagleton MJ, et al. Fenestrated and branched endovascular aortic repair for chronic type B aortic dissection with thoracoabdominal aneurysms. *J Vasc Surg* 2013;58:625–34.
29. Moulakakis KG, Mylonas SN, Dalainas I, et al. The chimney-graft technique for preserving supra-aortic branches: a review. *Ann Cardiothorac Surg* 2013;2:339–46.

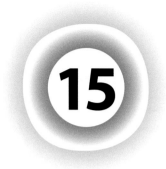

MINIMALLY INVASIVE HEART FAILURE SURGERY

FAIZUS SAZZAD AND THEO KOFIDIS

INTRODUCTION

The 2005 American College of Cardiology/American Heart Association (ACC/AHA) guideline update for the diagnosis and management of chronic heart failure in the adult defines heart failure as a "complex clinical syndrome that can result from any structural or functional cardiac disorder that impairs the ability of the ventricle to fill with or eject blood".

Heart failure is a huge health care problem that becomes more prevalent with age [1]. The main aim of the heart failure treatment strategy is to improve the cardiac output through various means. As far as surgery for heart failure is concerned, the approach for the improvement of cardiac output can be achieved either by removing the primary ventricular insult (i.e. revascularization surgery or valve repair/replacement) or by reforming the damaged ventricle (ventricular restoration surgery).

The main surgical goal should be to either achieve reverse remodeling or restore the ventricle to its normal shape and size [2]. If this is not completely achievable, then the compromise is to aim for reducing the size of the heart toward normal as much as possible.

OPERATIONS FOR HEART FAILURE

A. Surgical strategies to reduce left ventricular size (LA PLACE surgery):
   1. The myosplint (not available now)
   2. The Acorn CorCap device
   3. Partial left ventricular resection
   4. Left ventricular aneurysmectomy

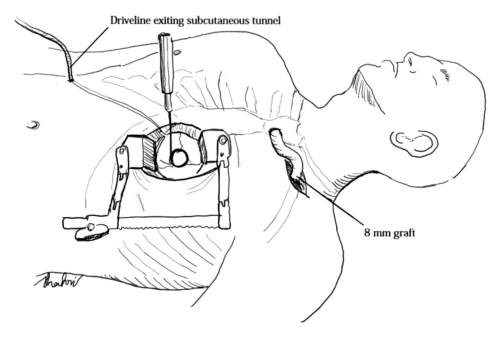

FIGURE 15.1 Schematic of minimally invasive LVAD implantation. Left mini-thoracotomy for device placement and small left subclavian incision for insertion of inflow anastomosis. [Courtesy: Shaghayegh Shahrigharahkoshan, 2019].

  5. Mitral repair for secondary mitral regurgitation
B. Mechanical support to re-power the failing heart:
  1. Ventricular assist devices (VAD)
C. Surgical strategies (biological) to re-power the failing heart:
  1. Dynamic cardiac myoplasty
  2. Heart transplantation
  3. Cellular transplantation
  4. Others: Gene therapy or upregulation of natural pathways

HOW TO DO IT/STEP BY STEP

MINIMALLY INVASIVE LVAD IMPLANTATION

The LVAD devices that were first used in a clinical setting were far too bulky, with designs that were too large and complex for minimally invasive implantation (Figure 15.1). The current generation of LVAD devices is less heavy, which not only made implantation in a minimally invasive fashion possible, but also increased the prospects of its future development [3].

There are different techniques for minimally invasive LVAD implantation that have been reported. These different approaches to the left ventricular apex can be combined with different techniques and locations for the outflow anastomosis [4,5].

Minimally invasive LVAD implantation techniques are associated with several benefits, namely lower rates of transfusion, smaller incisions, less intraoperative blood loss and less need for blood transfusion [6].

FIGURE 15.2 LVAD implantation animation.

Reported mortality rates during the first 30 days postoperatively were also observed to be lower after minimally invasive LVAD implantation [4] (Figure 15.2).

TECHNIQUE

SURGICAL ACCESS

Bilateral mini-thoracotomy or left thoracotomy + left A. subclavian or subcostal incision + right thoracotomy or right A. subclavian. Access to LV apex: Left subcostal incision, left anterior thoracotomy for insertion of the inflow device and LVAD pump (Figure 15.3). Access to ascending aorta: Upper hemisternotomy, right mini-thoracotomy. If the outflow graft is attached to the descending aorta or the aortic arch, both the in- and the outflow devices can be implanted via a left anterior thoracotomy.

CIRCULATORY SUPPORT

ECMO, off pump or CPB.

OPERATION

General anesthesia and single-lumen endotracheal intubation, TEE. Upper mini J-sternotomy with extension into the right third intercostal space for aortic access. The left anterior thoracotomy at the fifth or the sixth intercostal space. Pericardiotomy over the apex as well as the aorta and an umbilical tape is passed through the pericardium, which is subsequently used to pull the outflow graft through the pericardium.

The insertion site of LVAD: Determined by echocardiography on the left ventricle (LV). The apical swing ring is placed by using interrupted pledgeted sutures, usually done off-pump. After this stage heparin can be given; it will reduce the apex-associated bleeding. CO_2 insufflation and establishment of CPB. Subsequently, the LVAD is inserted into the LV via the apical sewing ring and secured with its connecting tubing. The outflow graft is brought out to the

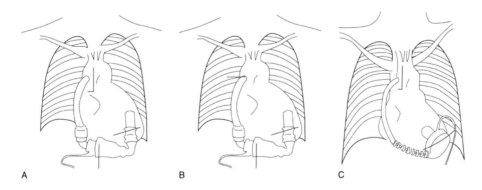

FIGURE 15.3 Three sets of incisions expose structures for cardiopulmonary bypass as well as placement of left ventricular assist device inflow cannula and outflow graft. Mini-laparotomy facilitates HeartMate II pump pocket dissection (A&B). The outflow graft lies intrapericardial except in patients with previous cardiac surgery. Incision for HeartWare HVAD insertion (C). (After Cheung A, Soon JL, Bashir J, Kaan A, Ignaszewski A. Minimal-access left ventricular assist device implantation. *Innovations (Phila)*, 9(4):281-285. © 2014 by the International Society for Minimally Invasive Cardiothoracic Surgery. Reprinted by Permission of SAGE Publications, Inc.)

FIGURE 15.4 Minimally invasive LVAD implantation.

SPECIAL CONCERNS

1. Apical sewing ring: Place the apical sewing ring of the LVAD on the insertion site of the LV, which is determined beforehand, and mark all around the ring with a surgical pen. Subsequently, remove the ring from the LV apex and put the sutures on the marked apex like in a valve replacement procedure.
2. For a smaller thoracotomy: Do not cut the threads of the sutures, and stabilize the LV apex position with uncut sutures instead of using your fingers during insertion of the device.
3. Closure of the pericardium: After placement of the device, let the perfusion technician fill the LV to make it easier to check for bleeding from the LV apex. Afterward, let the perfusion technician empty the LV and finally, the heart can be placed back into the pericardial space.

upper incision using the umbilical tape; then an end-to-side fashion anastomoses to the ascending aorta can be done through the upper hemisternotomy. The outflow graft is commonly placed lateral to the right atrium and within the pericardium (Figure 15.4 and Figure 15.5). The adequacy of the length of the tubing should be assessed carefully. The pericardium should be closed over the LVAD whenever possible. Sometimes the LVAD may need to be covered with a polytetrafluoroethylene membrane in order to facilitate dissection at the time of transplant and to avoid adhesion (Figure 15.6).

TOOLS/INSTRUMENTS AND DEVICES

ACORN CORECAP

The Acorn CoreCap is a device that achieves ventricular remodeling through reducing the wall shear stress of the heart. A randomized clinical trial (the Acorn trial) has evaluated the safety and efficacy of the device in patients [7]. The study concluded that the Acorn CoreCap was able to achieve sustained ventricular remodeling of the left ventricle with few adverse post-implantation outcomes (Figure 15.7).

HEARTWARE VAD (HVAD)

The HVAD is currently the smallest CE-marked and FDA-approved pump on the market (Figure 15.8 and Figure 15.9).

HEARTMATE III

The HeartMate III is an LVAD that was recently approved by the FDA for use in patients with advanced heart failure (Figure 15.10 and Figure 15.11).

ALTERNATIVES

CONVENTIONAL FULL STERNOTOMY APPROACH

Should the minimally invasive approach be unachievable, a full sternotomy procedure can be carried out, and an LVAD designed for median sternotomy implantation can be implanted instead.

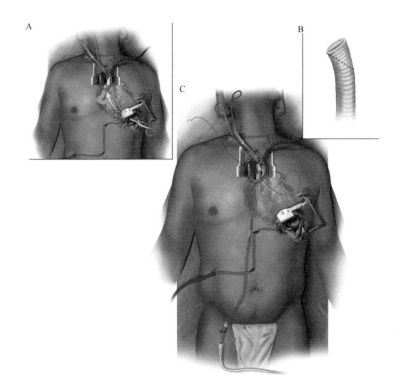

FIGURE 15.5 The outflow vascular graft is distally tied and tunneled extrapericardially and retrosternally toward the ascending aorta (A). A partial cross clamp is placed on the ascending aorta. The graft is measured, cut obliquely, and the anastomosis with the ascending aorta is performed using a continuous 4-0 prolene suture through the upper hemisternotomy (B). The driveline is tunneled within the sheath of the rectus muscle in umbilical direction and then subcutaneously to the right or left upper quadrant (C) to decrease infection rates. (Reprinted from *Operative Techniques in Thoracic and Cardiovascular Surgery*, 21(1), Schmitto JD, Deniz E, Rojas SV, Maltais S et al. Minimally Invasive Implantation: The Procedure of Choice! 65-78, © 2016, with permission from Elsevier.)

CAVEATS AND CONTROVERSIES

ABANDONED SURGICAL OPTIONS

Dynamic cardiomyoplasty used to performed by wrapping the heart with the latissimus dorsi muscle and stimulating the muscle to assist contraction. It appears that those who can survive the operation do not need it, and those who need it, cannot survive it [8].

Passive cardiomyoplasty was aimed to reduce ventricular enlargement due to ventricular remodeling with the help of an elastic net, called a cardiac support device, slipped over the myocardium, like an elastic girdle around the heart, to help reverse chamber remodeling. ACORN CorCap do not allow a definitive assessment of the technique of passive cardiomyoplasty. So, it is not a proven therapeutic alternative for patients with end-stage heart failure [7,8].

Partial left ventriculectomy, which was an acute removal of a portion of the lateral wall, has been introduced by Batista but the results are controversial if not intriguing, thus, it almost disappeared because of high operative mortality and frequent recurrence of heart failure [8].

FIGURE 15.6 Less invasive implantation of HeartWare – MMCTS.

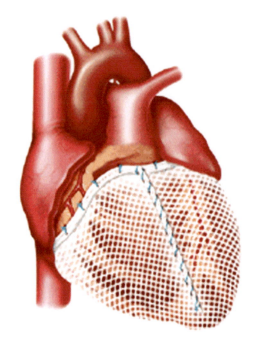

FIGURE 15.7 Implantation of the cardiac support device (CSD) as the sole surgical procedure. (Reprinted from *Ann Thorac Surg*, 75(6 Suppl), Sabbah HN. The cardiac support device and the myosplint: treating heart failure by targeting left ventricular size and shape, S13-S19, © 2003 The Society of Thoracic Surgeons with permission from Elsevier.)

FIGURE 15.8 HeartWare ventricular assist system video.

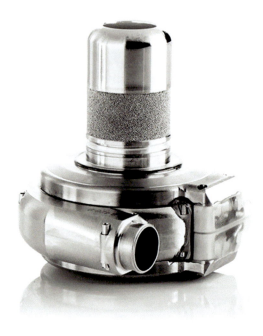

FIGURE 15.9 HeartWare ventricular assist system. Reproduced with permission of Medtronic, Inc.

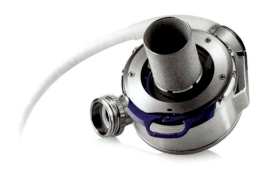

FIGURE 15.10 HeartMate 3™ LVAD, Abbott. Reproduced with permission of Abbott, © 2020.

FIGURE 15.11 HeartMate 3 animation.

FIGURE 15.12 Managing arrhythmias in LVAD patients.

FIGURE 15.14 Bilateral mini-thoracotomy vs separate incisions.

FIGURE 15.13 Park's plication stitch for AI at the time of LVAD.

FIGURE 15.15 Sternal-sparing LVAD.

MANAGING ARRHYTHMIAS IN LVAD PATIENTS

Figure 15.12 provides a lecture on the methods of managing arrythmias in LVAD patients and the outcomes and evidence for each. Some studies have reported with safe and reproducible good clinical outcomes with less invasive approach [9,10].

PARK'S PLICATION STITCH FOR AI AT THE TIME OF LVAD

A lecture explaining the method of utilizing the Park's plication stitch for aortic insufficiency at the time of implantation of LVAD can be found in Figure 15.13.

BILATERAL MINI-THORACOTOMY VS SEPARATE INCISIONS

An article with a detailed description of the bilateral mini-thoracotomy technique for LVAD implantation of the HeartMate 3 can be found in Figure 15.14.

STERNAL-SPARING APPROACH

The sternal-sparing approach described in a paper (Figure 15.15) details a case series of ten consecutive patients who underwent the complete sternal-sparing (CSS) HeartMate 3 (Abbott Laboratories, Abbott Park, IL) LVAD implantation method using bilateral mini-thoracotomies. The authors concluded that the CSS approach produced favorable results, with shorter intubation times, lengths of stay in the intensive care unit and less incidence of right ventricular failure and bleeding. Mohite et al. described in a report additional benefit of sternal sparing avoids dilatation of right ventricle and reduces chances of right ventricular failure requiring temporary right ventricular assist [11].

OFF-PUMP VS ON-PUMP LVAD IMPLANTATION

Figure 15.16 is linked to a case study performed on a method of minimally invasive HeartMate 3 LVAD implantation that does

FIGURE 15.16 Off-pump vs on-pump LVAD implantation.

FIGURE 15.18 What's new in heart failure therapy?

FIGURE 15.17 Minimally invasive vs conventional LVAD.

not require a sternotomy to be performed or cardiopulmonary bypass to be established.

MINIMALLY INVASIVE VS CONVENTIONAL LVAD IMPLANTATION

A systematic review comparing literature on the minimally invasive and conventional LVAD implantation methods can be found in Figure 15.17.

RESEARCH, TRENDS AND INNOVATION

HEART FAILURE THERAPY UPDATE

A review that summarizes the current evidence for the various treatments of heart failure can be found in the link embedded in Figure 15.18 based on the most up-to-date recommendations for medical therapy and interventional strategies.

WHERE AND HOW TO LEARN

ISHLT

A link to the ISHLT academy core competencies course on heart failure and cardiac transplant medicine is available for access in Figure 15.19.

FIGURE 15.19 ISHLT Academy core competencies course.

FIGURE 15.20 Postgraduate course in Heart Failure London.

POSTGRADUATE COURSE IN HEART FAILURE LONDON

For more information on postgraduate courses on heart failure in London, please visit the link in Figure 15.20.

REFERENCES

1. George Makdisi, I-Wen Wang. Minimally invasive is the future of left ventricular assist device implantation. *Journal of Thoracic Disease* 2015;7(9): E283–E288. doi: 10.3978/j.issn.2072-1439.2015.08.30.
2. Stephen Large. Surgery for heart failure. *Heart* 2007;93:392–402. doi: 10.1136/hrt.2005.078543.
3. Dominik Wiedemann, Thomas Haberl, Philipp Angleitner, Kamen Dimitrov, Günther Laufer, Daniel Zimpfer. Minimally invasive approaches for implantation of left ventricular assist devices. *Indian Journal of Thoracic and Cardiovascular Surgery* 2018;34(Suppl 2):S177–S182 doi: 10.1007/s12055-017-0639-2.
4. J Schmitto, G Dogan, SJ Hanke, J Riebandt, M Ozbaran, C Engin, U Kervan, M Paç, V Orvath, S Klotz, F Wagner, CJ Roussel, M Shrestha, C Feldmann, A Chatterjee, A Martens, D Zimpfer. A multicenter analysis of implantation via a thoracotomy approach of a left ventricular assist system for the treatment of advanced heart failure. *Journal of Thoracic and Cardiovascular Surgery* 2019;67(S 01): S1–S100. doi: 10.1055/s-0039-1678824
5. Antonio Loforte, Jacopo Alfonsi, Gregorio Gliozzi, Gianluca Folesani, Mariafrancesca Fiorentino, Mauro Biffi, Giuseppe Marinelli, Roberto Di Bartolomeo, Davide Pacini. Less invasive ventricular enhancement (LIVE) as potential therapy for ischaemic cardiomyopathy end-stage heart failure. *Journal of Thoracic Disease* 2019 Apr; 11(Suppl 6): S921–S928. doi: 10.21037/jtd.2019.02.86.
6. Haitham Mutlak, Birgit Assmus, Aron-Frederik Popov. Minimally invasive embolectomy of HeartWare left ventricular assist device outflow graft. *Journal of Thoracic Disease* 2019; 11(Suppl 6):S957-S959. doi: 10.21037/jtd.2019.03.82.
7. Michael A Acker, Steven Bolling, Richard Shemin, James Kirklin, Jae K Oh, Douglas L Mann, Mariell Jessup, Hani N Sabbah, Randall C Starling, Spencer H Kubo& Acorn Trial Principal Investigators and Study Coordinators. Mitral valve surgery in heart failure: insights from the Acorn Clinical Trial. *The Journal of thoracic and cardiovascular surgery*, 2006;132(3): 568–577.e5774. https://doi.org/10.1016/j.jtcvs.2006.02.062
8. EM Delmo Walter, R Hetzer. Surgical treatment concepts for heart failure. *HSR Proceedings in Intensive Care & Cardiovascular Anesthesia* 2013;5(2):69–75.
9. Sinan Sabit Kocabeyoglu, Umit Kervan, Dogan Emre Sert, Ertekin Utku Unal, Burcu Demirkan, Yesim Guray, Emre Aygun, Osman Fehmi Beyazal, Mehmet Karahan, Mustafa Pac. Is it possible to implant heart mate 3 less invasively? New pump, new approach. *Artificial Organs* 2018;42(12):1132–1138. doi: 10.1111/aor.13289.
10. K Wachter UFW Franke, J Christian. Rustenbach1 hardy Baumbach1, minimally invasive versus conventional LVADImplantation—an analysis of the literature. *Journal of Thoracic and Cardiovascular Surgery* 2019;67:156–163. doi: 10.1055/s-0038-1627455.
11. PN Mohite, A Sabashnikov, B Raj, R Hards, G Edwards, D García-Sáez, B Zych, M Husain, A Jothidasan, J Fatullayev, M Zeriouh, A Weymann, AF Popov, F De Robertis, AR Simon. Minimally invasive left ventricular assist device implantation: a comparative study. *Artificial Organs* 2018;42(12):1125–1131. doi: 10.1111/aor.13269.

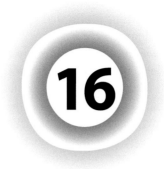

EPILOGUE

THEO KOFIDIS

EPILOGUE

It is with pleasure that we see a global wave towards the employment of less invasive techniques, as well as a surge in the invention and manufacture of minimally invasive tools. Even though we find the adoption to be slower than initially anticipated, we established that this is not because of lack of interest or technology, but rather entropy, habit and the comfort zone, or fear of the unknown. On a positive note, thousands and thousands of patients around the world have increasingly come to harvest the results of this – not anymore so novel – platform.

In contrast, it is with concern that we also witness controversial behaviors by many colleagues, who have not made an effort to learn MICS or hybrid cardiac surgery, and dismiss it injudiciously. In some cases, they have participated in conferences and lectures, or even took courses and proctorships, but for obscure and potentially unethical reasons, do not disclose to the enquiring patient that this method is available in the vicinity or available altogether, to avoid "losing" the patient. Patients have changed, as have technology and skill in the last decade: they do not depend on the divine opinion of the old surgeon-guru; they Google, read, take multiple insights and go to their surgeon prepared, with specific queries. It is our duty to reveal that there are surgeons around who may be performing MICS surgery safely and efficiently, though it is a newer method compared to the so-called "golden standard", the median sternotomy. No colleague should be accused for not adopting MICS or hybrid; however, it is in the sense of the most primary Hippocratic principles to disclose all information to the patient, when he comes asking for an MICS alternative. We have seen this issue occurring over and over again, and it is so pressing, as it impedes self-improvement and progress in the field, that it afforded the main bulk of the epilogue.

If we do not take charge of the future of the field, it will take charge of us and our craft. No heart surgeon professional will be able to resist this trend, wherever it validly qualifies. The train of MICS and hybrid heart surgery is bound north. The present effort utilizes new link and multimedia tools to provide an easier, more vibrant learning experience, without claiming perfection or completeness. We view it as "work in progress", constantly renewing, as do knowledge and skill in the field.

It remains to thank the contributors to this endeavor, for their time and effort, as well as their faith and pursuit of progress, for the benefit of our patients; the latter are the true "authors" of the ever-evolving opus of MICS and hybrid cardiac surgery.

For the authors,

Theo Kofidis

ANNEX

MINIMALLY INVASIVE INSTRUMENTS AND DEVICES

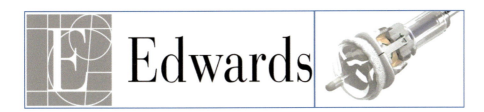

Rapid Deployment Valve Prosthesis:
EDWARDS INTUITY valve system
EDWARDS INTUITY Elite valve system

Transcatheter Heart Valve Prosthesis:
Edwards SAPIEN 3 transcatheter heart valve system
Edwards SAPIEN XT transcatheter heart valve system

FIGURE 17.1   Edwards cardiovascular products.

Transcatheter Heart Valve Repair:
Edwards Cardioband Mitral valve reconstruction system
Edwards Cardioband Tricuspid valve reconstruction system

FIGURE 17.2   Edwards contacts.

Atraumatic Occlusion:
Fogarty-Hydragrip clamps
Fogarty-Hydragrip surgical clamp insert sets
Cosgrove Flex clamps
Cosgrove QuickBend clamp
Cosgrove SlimFit clamp

FIGURE 17.3   Edwards education and training.

Edwards ThruPort Systems:
IntraClude intra-aortic occlusion device
ProPlege peripheral retrograde cardioplegia device
EndoVent pulmonary catheter kit
EndoReturn arterial cannula
QuickDraw venous cannula
ThruPort Soft tissue retractor
ThruPort Knot pusher

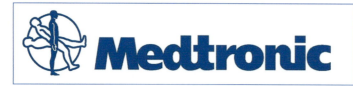 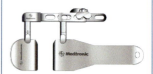

Ablation:
CARDIOBLATE™ 68000 SURGICAL ablation system generator
CARDIOBLATE™ IRRIGATED surgical ablation pens
CARDIOBLATE™ BP2 irrigated RF surgical ablation system

Aortic Stent Graft:
ENDURANT™ II AAA stent graft system
VALIANT NAVION™ thoracic stent graft system
VALIANT™ THORACIC stent graft system with Captivia™ delivery system
RELIANT™ stent graft balloon catheter

Cannula:
EXTRACORPOREAL CIRCUIT
CARDIOPLEGIA CIRCUIT
SUCTION AND SUPPORT PRODUCTS

Heart valve systems
CONTOUR 3D™ annuloplasty ring
CG FUTURE™ annuloplasty system
DURAN ANCORE™ annuloplasty system
PROFILE 3D™ annuloplasty system
AVALUS™ bioprostheses
CONTEGRA™ PULMONARY VALVED CONDUIT — HDE
FREESTYLE™ Aortic root bioprosthesis
HANCOCK™ II AND HANCOCK™ II ULTRA bioprostheses
MOSAIC™ AND MOSAIC™ ULTRA bioprostheses
MEDTRONIC OPEN PIVOT™ mechanical heart valves
MEDTRONIC OPEN PIVOT™ aortic valved graft (AVG)

Tissue Stabilizer:
OCTOPUS™ tissue stabilizers
OCTOPUS™ NUVO tissue stabilizer
STARFISH™ HEART positioners
STARFISH™ NS heart positioner
URCHIN™ heart positioners

Retractors:
OCTOBASE™ sternal retractor
THORATRAK™ MICS retractor system

FIGURE 17.4 Medtronic cardiovascular products.

FIGURE 17.5 Medtronic contacts.

FIGURE 17.6 Medtronic education and training.

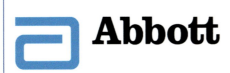

Cardiac Rhythm Management
MR conditional Entrant™ HF CRT-D
MR conditional Gallant™ HF CRT-D
Quadra Allure MP™ CRT-P
Quadra Assura MP™ CRT-D
Conform Rx™ Insertable patient monitor
Merlin.net™ Patient Care Network (PCN)

FIGURE 17.7   Abbott cardiovascular products.

Electrophysioylogical
Advisor™ HD Grid Mapping Catheter Sensor Enabled™
Agilis™ NxT steerable introducers
EnSite Precision™ cardiac mapping system
FlexAbility™ irrigated ablation catheter
FlexAbility™ irrigated ablation catheter, SE™
Perclose ProGlide™ Suture-Mediated Closure System

FIGURE 17.8   Abbott contacts.

Heart Failure:
CentriMag™ Acute Circulatory Support System
CardioMEMS™ HF System
HeartMate II™ Left Ventricular Assist Device
HeartMate 3™ Left Ventricular Assist Device

FIGURE 17.9   Abbott education and training.

Structural Heart
Amplatzer™ PFO Occluder
Epic™ Mitral Valve
MitraClip Transcatheter Mitral Valve Repair
Trifecta™ GT Aortic Valve

Peripheral Intervention
Emboshield NAV6™ Embolic Protection System
RX Acculink™ Carotid Stent System
Perclose ProGlide™ SMC System

ANNEX   **403**

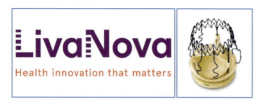

Advanced Circulatory Support

EXTRACORPOREAL LIFE SUPPORT (ECLS)
- TandemLife®
- LifeSPARC®
- TandemLung®
- SCPC®

MECHANICAL CIRCULATORY SUPPORT
- ProtekDuo®
- TandemHeart®

Cardiopulmonary

Autotransfusion
- XTRA®

Cannula
- Bio-Flow® Ecmo
- Bi-Flow® Arterial Cannulae
- PureFlex™ Arterial Cannulae
- Conventional adult cannula
- Conventional paediatric cannula

MICS Cannula
- Dual stage venous femoral RAP® cannulae
- Optiflow® direct venous cannula
- EasyFlow® cannulae
- EasyFlow DUO® cannulae

Other cannula
- Aortic Root Cannulae
- Coronary Ostia Perfusion Cannulae with Balloon Tip
- Coronary Ostia Perfusion Cannulae with 3D Tip
- Vents
- ATRA® Sump vent

Endoscopic Vessel Harvesting
- VascuClear®

Heart Valves

Aortic
- Perceval®
- Solo Smart®
- Carbomedics®

Mitral
- Memo 4D® Mitral annuloplasty ring
- Memo 3D ReChord®
- Memo 3D®
- AnnuloFlex®
- AnnuloFlo®

FIGURE 17.10 LivaNova cardiovascular products.

FIGURE 17.11 LivaNova contacts.

FIGURE 17.12 LivaNova education and training.

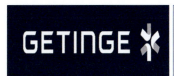 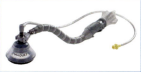

Beating Heart Surgery
Acrobat SUV Vacuum Stabilizer
Acrobat V Vacuum Stabilizer
Acrobat-i Stabilizer
Ultima OPCAB Stabilizer System
Acrobat-i Positioner
Xpose 3 Positioner
Axius Blower Mister
Axius Coronary Shunts
Heartstring III Proximal Seal System
Endoscopic Vessel Harvesting:
Vasoview 7xB Endoscopic Vessel Harvesting System
Vasoview Hemopro 2 Endoscopic Vessel Harvesting System
IABP:
CARDIOSAVE® IABP Hybrid
CARDIOSAVE® IABP Rescue
CS300® IABP
Extracorporeal Life Support
Cardiohelp System
HLS Set Advanced
HLS Cannulae
Avalon Elite Bi-Caval Dual Lumen Catheter
Rotaflow Console
PLS System
Cardiac Intervention Set (CiSet)
Knitted Vascular Grafts
Intergard Knitted
Hemagard Knitted
Intergard Knitted Ultrathin
Intergard Knitted Trifurcated/Quadrifurcated
Hemashield Gold Knitted Microvel Double Velour
Woven Vascular Grafts
Hemashield Platinum Woven Double Velour
Hemashield Platinum Woven Double Velour Aortic Branch
Cardioroot
Intergard Woven
Intergard Woven Aortic Arch and Hemabridge
Intergard Woven Thoracic Aortic Graft
Antimicrobial Vascular Graft
Intergard Synergy
Intergard Silver
Heparin Coated Vascular Grafts
Fusion Bioline
Intergard Heparin Knitted
ePTFE Geafts
Flixene Vascular Grafts
Advanta VXT Vascular Graft
Advance monitoring
PiCCO Technology

FIGURE 17.13 GETTINGE cardiovascular products.

FIGURE 17.14 GETTINGE contacts.

FIGURE 17.15 GETTINGE education and training.

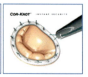

Cardiovascular Products:
The RAM® DEVICE is an automated dual curved needle annular suturing device
Ti-KNOT® DEVICE
The RD180® line of suturing devices
The SEW-EASY® DEVICE is a dual needle device
COR-KNOT® DEVICE
The miniARM® SYSTEM

FIGURE 17.16   LSI Solutions.

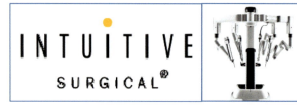

Robotic System
Da Vinci Xi; Da Vinci X;
Da Vinci SP
Instruments:
Force Bipolar with DualGrip
First entry accessories
Da Vinci Single-Site
EndoWrist technology
Clip Appliers
Bipolar Instruments
Monopolar Instruments
Suction and Irrigation
Needle Drivers
Stapling:
SureForm 45 and 60
EndoWrist Staplers 30 and 45
Energy:
SynchroSeal
Vessel Sealer Extend
Vision:
Procedure planning with Iris
Firefly fluorescence imaging
Da Vinci endoscope

FIGURE 17.17   INTUITIVE robotic system.

FIGURE 17.18   INTUITIVE contacts.

FIGURE 17.19   INTUITIVE education and training.

OPERATIVE CARDEX

PREFERENCE CARD FOR MINIMALLY INVASIVE CABG SURGERY

Surgeon:	Prof Theo Kofidis	
Procedure:	MIS CABG	
Position:	Supine with one gel-roll under the left chest. Ensure patient's hand can be flexed. For female patient - to lift up left side of breast during draping The rest of positioning as per conventional CABG	
Glove Size/Gown:	Biogel #8 / XL Non-reinforced Gown	
Equipment:	• Camera System for EVH • CO_2 machine (for EVH) • Wall Mounted Suction Device x 2 for Octopus Nuvo Stabilizer and Starfish (pressure at 400mmHg)	
Supplies:	• Cardiovascular Drape (Customized) • Single Bowl • Suction Tubing x2 • Suture Counter • Cautery Tip Cleaner • Disposable Yankuer Tip • Hypodermic Needle 19G x2, 27G x1 • Diathermy Tip (Long, non-insulated) • Nylon Tape 6mm x2 • Vessel Loop Maxi x2 • Purple Skin Marker (Devon, Covidien) • Tonsil Square, Lahey Swab • Titanium Hemostatic Clip Blue x3 (MIS) • Titanium Hemostatic Clip Yellow x3 (MIS) • Titanium Hemostatic Clip Blue x2 • Titanium Hemostatic Clip Yellow x2	• Major Cleansing Set • Diathermy Cables x2 • Irrigation Bulb Syringe • Raytex Sponge x3, • Penny Towel x1 • Surgiboots • Syringes 20ml x7 • Chest Tube #28 • Jackson Pratt Drain
Instrumentation:	• Cardio Basic Set • Open Heart Set • CTVS MIS CABG Set • CTVS MIS Supplementary Set • Rultrak Retractor • ThoraTrak Retractor • AVF set	• Cardio Receptacles Set • Dietrich Set • Sternal Saw with Battery • Single Bowl • Defibrillation Paddle • Micro-Instrument Set
If needed camera system on standby to record the procedure: prepare 5mm 30^0 Telescope, 5.5mm Thoracoport, light cable, camera sleeve, TV system, anti-fog kit, need static arm and clamp knot from HV Heart Retractor to hold telescope		
Blades & Sutures:	Blades: #10x2, #11x3	
	BD Beaver 376400 x 1, BD Green Micro Sharp 5.0mmx1	
	Ties: Silk 1, 4/0	

	Pericardial Stay:	Silk 0 (W334 x3)
	Femoral Cannulation (Arterial & Venous)	Prolene 5/0 W8556 x2 (FH/SL)
	Cardioplegia Purse string:	Prolene 4/0 W8761 x1 (FH/DL) with MIS-NH
	Anastomosis: Distal	Prolene 7/0 W8704 (BH/ SL)
	Anastomosis: Proximal	Prolene 6/0 W8706 (BH/SL)
	Decannulation: Cardioplegia	Prolene 4/0 W8761 (FH/DL)
	Decannulation: Femoral Site (Arterial & Venous)	Prolene 5/0 W8556
	Closure (Chest):	• Ethibond 5 (FH) • Vicryl 1 x 1 • Vicryl 2/0 x 1 • Monocryl 4/0 x 1
	Closure (Leg):	• Vicryl 2/0 x 1 • Vicryl 3/0 (Cutting) x 1
	Pacing Wire:	Osypka
	Chest Tube:	Prolene 2/0 W295 x2 and Silk 0 W782 x2
Special Consumables:	• Octopus NUVO TSMICS1 • Blower Mister (Medtronic Clearview) 22150 • StarFish NS HP 102 (200) Heart Positioner • Evicel Fibrin Sealant	
Medications:	• Papaverine 60mg in 55ml of 0.9 NaCl • Gentamycin 80mg in 20ml of 0.9 NaCl • Heparin 5000 units in 500ml of 0.9 NaCl	
Skin Prep:	Hexodane 2% followed by Providone Iodine with Alcohol	
Dressings:	Opsite (Small) x7	

Procedural Considerations:
1. Bulldog and Parsonet retractor to be tied with Silk 1, keep long length
2. Cardio drape for the chest, keep slightly to the left side
3. Surgeon will stand on the left side of patient
4. Tonsil square to be folded all the corner & clip on the Roberts x2
5. Lahey swab to clip on the Roberts x2
6. Rultrack Retractor to be fixed immediately after draping
7. ThoraTrak Pole (long) usually on the right side at mid-thigh of the patient
8. ThoraTrak Pole (short) usually on the left side at the hip region of the patient
9. Octopus Nuvo's bullet tie with Silk-1 tie
10. For on-pump beating heart or off-pump use Prolene 4/0 W8761 1 site Pledget with snare or Prolene 4/0 without Pledget catch with suture boots x 2 sets for proximal occluder; use new Prolene 4/0 for every anastomosis
11. Aortic Sling: Nylon Tape 6mm x1 (spencer well to clip) (if more than one vessel)
12. Blade #11 for incision of Octopus and Starfish follow by Kelly to dilate

Legend: NH - Needle Holder, SL - Single Load, BH – Backhand, DL - Double Load, FH - Forehand

PREFERENCE CARD FOR MINIMALLY INVASIVE MITRAL VALVE SURGERY

Surgeon:	Prof Theo Kofidis
Procedure:	Minimally Invasive Mitral Valve Repair/Replacement
Position:	Supine with right side elevated. Place gel roll on right side laterally. Right arm slightly hangs down. Left arm wraps with gel pad and tuck at the side. Shoulder roll under both shoulders
Glove Size/ Gown:	Biogel #8 / XL Non-reinforced Gown
Equipment:	• Camera System (Standby) • CO_2 Machine
If needed camera system on standby to record the procedure - prepare 5mm 30⁰ Telescope, 5.5mm Thoracoport, light cable, camera sleeve, TV system, anti-fog kit. Static arm and clamp knot from HV Heart Retractor to hold telescope may also need.	
Supplies:	• Cardiovascular Drape (Customized) • Ioban 6650 x1 • Major Cleansing Set • CO_2 Tubing • Adult Pledget (9.6mm x4.8mm) • Lahey Swab • Irrigation Bulb Syringe x2 • Foley catheter F14 x1 (cut 1-inch x6) • Raytex Sponge x3, • Saw Blade Diathermy Cables x2 • Cautery Tip Cleaner • Suction Tubing x2 • Disposable Yankuer Tip • Suture Counter x2 • Hypodermic Needle 19G x2 • Penny Towel x1 • Long Diathermy Tip (non-insulated) • Surgiboots • Chest Tube #28 curve x1 • Syringes 20ml x2 • Vessel Loop Maxi (Red & Blue) • Teflon Felt • Purple Skin Marker • Jackson Pratt Drain • Clips: Blue Vita clip x1, Yellow vita clip x1 • Nelaton Catheter F14 x1
Instrumentation:	• Cardio Basic Set • Cardio Receptacle Set • Open Heart Set • Valve Set • AVF Set • MIS Supplementary Set • HV Heart Valve Retractor • Intercostal Retractor • MIS Fehling Instruments • Valve Sizers • Defibrillator Cable (Paeds) • Sarns Sternal Saw with Battery
Blades & Sutures:	Blades: #10 x2, #11 x3
	Ties: Silk 1
	Diaphragmatic Stitch: Ethibond 2/0 x1 pledgetted (Teflon TAVI pledget)
	Pericardial Stay Suture: Silk O W334 x5
	Femoral Cannulation: Prolene 5/0 W8556 x2
	Cardioplegia Purse String: Prolene 4/0 W8761 x2 pledgetted

	Valve Sutures:	• Ethibond 2/0 (Standby both big and small needle) • Non pledgetted for repair, pledgetted for replacement
	Closure of Atrium:	• Prolene 3/0 W8522 x1 • Prolene 3/0 W8558 x1
	Cardioplegia Decannulation:	Prolene 4/0 W8761
	Femoral Decannulation:	Prolene 5/0 W8556 x2
	Pacing Wire:	Osypka Pacing Wire
	Chest Drain Sutures:	• Prolene 2/0 W295 x2 • Silk O W782 x2
	Chest Closure:	• Ethibond 5/0 x2 • Vicryl 1 x2 • Monocryl 4-0 x2
	Femoral Closure:	• Vicryl 2-0 9136 x1 • Vicryl 3-0 9571 x1
Special Consumables:	• Cor-knot-5mm • Alexis Wound Protector (Small) • Evicel Fibrin Sealant, On-Q Pump Pain Buster (Standby)	
Medications:	• Gentamycin 80mg/2ml in 20ml of 0.9 NaCl • Heparin 5000 units in 500ml of 0.9 NaCl • For On-Q Pump Pain Buster • Naropin 0.2% 2mg/ml 200ml x 2 packs (Standby)	
Skin Prep:	Hexodane 2% followed by Providone Iodine with Alcohol	
Dressings:	Opsite (Small) x7	
Procedural Considerations		
Femoral Cannulation:	**Venous:** Prolene 5/0 W8556 purse string • Puncture needle • Long guide wire • Dilators - give smallest to biggest • Venous cannula in, guide wire out • Snare down • Tubing clamp and connect to venous line • Secure the cannula with big sharp towel clip	
	Arterial: • Prolene 5/0 W8556 purse string • Puncture needle • Short guide wire • Dilators – give smallest to biggest • Aortic cannula in, guide wire out • Snare down and tie • Tubing clamp and connect to arterial line • Secure the cannula with big sharp towel clip	
Chest:	• Skin incision at the right chest • Small Alexis and Intercostal Retractor (Fehling) • Diaphragmatic stitch using Ethibond 2/0 with TAVI pledget, cut the needles, Blade #11 to the skin, MICS suture hook to bring out the Ethibond stitch and tie it in the Foley's catheter rubber.	

• Open the pericardium, use Silk O W334 as pericardial stay suture. Cut the needle, blade #11, MICS suture hook to bring out the silk stitch and tie it in the Foley's catheter rubber. • CARDIOPLEGIA: Prolene 4/0 W8761 x2 pledgetted for purse string, long snares x2, long cardioplegia needle. Give 1 sternal wire without needle to anchor CP line. • Blade #11, Kelly artery forceps to dilate, Chitwood clamp. • Blade #11, Kelly artery forceps y to dilate, CSS needle from perfusionist connected to the CO2 tubing • Blade #11, Kelly artery to dilate, HV Retractor • Opening of Left Atrium: Blade #11, Curve Scissors (from Fehling set), Potts Scissors (from Fehling set), Prof will choose the appropriate size of HV retractor blade to use. • Valve or Ring sutures - single load for repair, double load for replacement, backhand first until surgeon ask for forehand or hook • Uses 5mm Cor-knot • Uses bulb syringe with F14 Nelaton Catheter as valve tester • Gentamycin wash to the valve	
• Closure of Left Atrium	Prolene 3/0 8522 Backhand; Prolene 3/0 W8558 Forehand
• Cardioplegia Decannulation	Will sometimes reinforce with Prolene 4/0 W8761
• Osypka pacing wire	Mostly ventricular pacing wire only
• Chest Drain	JP drain x1 and Portex Curve #28 x1
• Femoral Decannulation	noindent Standby small Derra clamp and Vascular clamp; Prolene 5/0 W8556

PREFERENCE CARD FOR MINI J-STERNOTOMY FOR AORTIC VALVE REPLACEMENT

Surgeon:	Prof Theo Kofidis
Procedure:	Aortic Valve Replacement-Mini (J) Sternotomy
Position:	Supine, both arms wrap with gel pad and tuck at the side. Shoulder roll under both shoulders.
Glove Size/Gown:	Biogel #8 / XL Non-reinforced Gown
Equipment:	• CO_2 machine
Supplies:	• Cardiovascular Drape (Customized) • Diathermy Cable x1 • Suction Tubing x2 • Suture Counter x2 • Cautery Tip Cleaner • Disposable Yankuer Tip • Hypodermic Needle 19G x2 • Chest Tube #28 • Nelaton Catheter F14 x1 • Clips • CO_2 tubing • Major Cleansing Set • Adult Pledget (9.5mm x 4.8mm) • Irrigation Bulb Syringe x2 • Raytex Sponge x3 • Penny Towel x1 • Surgiboots • Syringes 20ml x2 • Long Diathermy Tip (non-insulated) • Straight x1, curve x1 • Saw Blade x1 • Lahey swab • Blue Vita clip x1 • Yellow vita clip x1 • Tubing x1

Instrumentation:	• Cardio Basic Set • Open Heart Set • Cygnet FlexibleClamp (Standby) • Valve Sizers • Defibrillator cable (Paeds) • Malleable • Valve Leaflet Retractor • Cardio Towel • Castrovejo x2	• Cardio Receptacle Set • Valve Set • Oscillating Saw • Sarn Sternal Saw • Bone hook x2 • Long Ronguer x1 • Sharp Towel clip x1 • Ball Tip Diathermy • Valve Needle Holder x2 • Knot pusher (Standby)

Blades & Sutures:	Blades: #10 x2, #11x2	
	Ties: Silk 1	
	Pericardial stay suture:	Silk O W334 x2
	Aortic Cannulation:	Prolene 3-0 8332 x2 (Forehand, Single load)
	Venous Cannulation:	Prolene 4-0 7581 x1 (Forehand, Single Load)
	Vent Cannulation:	Prolene 4-0 8761 x1 (Backhand, Double Load)
	Cardioplegia Cannulation:	Prolene 4-0 7581 x1 (Forehand, Single Load) or Direct Ostial Cardioplegia Delivery
	Aortic Stay Suture:	Prolene 5-0 8556 x2
	Valve Sutures:	Ethibond 2-0 W10B55
	Closure of Aorta:	Prolene 4-0 8761 Pledgetted x2 (1st-Backhand, 2nd Forehand)
	Pacing Wire:	Osypka Pacing Wire
	Vent Decannulation:	Prolene 4-0 8761 x1
	Venous Decannulation:	Prolene 4-0 7581 x1
	Aortic Decannulation:	Prolene 3-0 8332 x1
	Drain Stitch:	Prolene 2-0 295 x2
		Silk O W782 x2
	Sternum:	Steel wire (4 pcs)
	Subcutaneous & Muscle:	Vicryl 1 x2
	Skin Closure:	Monocryl 4-0

Special Consumables:	• Cor-knot-4mm
Medications:	• Gentamycin 80mg/2ml in 20ml of 0.9 NaCl • Heparin 5000 units in 500ml of 0.9 NaCl • Evicel glue
Skin Prep:	Hexodane 2% followed by Providone Iodine with Alcohol
Dressings:	Opsite Long x1
	Opsite Small x3

PREFERENCE CARD FOR AORTIC VALVE REPLACEMENT VIA RIGHT ANTERIOR THORACOTOMY

Surgeon:	Prof Theo Kofidis
Procedure:	Right Anterior Thoracotomy Aortic Valve Replacement
Position:	Supine with right side elevated. Place gel roll on right side laterally. Both arms wrap with gel pad and tuck at the side. Shoulder roll under both shoulders
Glove Size/Gown:	Biogel #8 / XL Non-reinforced Gown
Equipment:	• Camera System (Standby) • CO_2 machine
Supplies:	• Cardiovascular Drape (Customized) • Diathermy Cables x2 • Adult Pledget (9.5mm x 4.8mm) • Suction Tubing x2 • Irrigation Bulb Syringe x2 • Suture Counter x2 • Raytex Sponge x3, • Penny Towel x1 • Cautery Tip Cleaner • Disposable Yankuer Tip • Hypodermic Needle 19G x2 • Foley's catheter F14 x1 (cut 1inch x6) • Major Cleansing Set • Surgiboots • Syringes 20ml x2 • Long Diathermy Tip (non-insulated) • Chest Tube #28 straight x1 • Saw Blade x1 • Vessel Loop Maxi (Red & Blue) • Jackson Pratt Drain • Green Hemoclip x1 • Nelaton Catheter F14 x1 • Blue Vita clip x1, Yellow vita clip x1 • Ioban 6650 x1 • CO_2 tubing • Lahey swab
Instrumentation:	• Cardio Basic Set • Open Heart Set • AVF Set • Cygnet Flexible Cross Clamp • MIS Fehling Instruments • Defibrillator cable (Paeds) • Thoracotomy Set • Cardio Receptacle Set • Valve Set • MIS Supplementary Set • Intercostal Retractor • Valve Sizers • Sarns Sternal saw (Standby) • Green hemoclip applicator (Standby orange clip applicator)
Blades & Sutures:	Blades: #10x2, #11x3
	Ties: Silk 1
	Pericardial stay suture: Silk O W334 x5
	Femoral Cannulation suture: Prolene 5-0 8556 x2
	Vent purse string: Prolene 4-0 8761 x1 pledgetted
	Aorta Stay Suture: Prolene 5-0 8556 x2
	Valve Sutures: Ethibond 2-0 W10B55
	Closure of Aorta: • Prolene 4-0 8761 x1 (Backhand) • Prolene 4-0 8761 x1 (Forehand)
	Vent Decannulation: Prolene 4-0 8761
	Pacing Wire: Osypka Pacing Wire

	Femoral Decannulation:	Prolene 5-0 8556 x2
	Chest Drain Sutures:	• Prolene 2-0 295 x2 • Silk O W782 x2
	Chest Closure:	• Ethibond 5-0 • Vicryl 1 x1 • Monocryl 4-0 x1
	Femoral Closure:	• Vicryl 2-0 9136 x1 • Vicryl 3-0 9571
Special Consumables:	• Cor-knot- 4mm • Alexis Wound Protector Small (Standby XS) • Pain Buster On-Q Pump	
Medications:	• Gentamycin 80mg/2ml in 20ml of 0.9 NaCl • Heparin 5000 units in 500 ml of 0.9 NaCl • On-Q Pump (pain buster) with Naropin 0.2% 2mg/ml 200ml x2 packs • Evicel glue	
Skin Prep:	Hexodane 2% followed by Providone Iodine with Alcohol	
Dressings:	Opsite (Small) x5	
Procedural Considerations		
Femoral Cannulation:	**Venous** • Prolene 5-0 8556 purse string • Puncture needle • Long guide wire • Dilators-smallest to biggest • Venous cannula in, guide wire out • Snare down • Tubing clamp and connect to venous line • Secure the cannula with big sharp towel clip **Aortic** • Prolene 5-0 8556 purse string • Puncture needle • Short guide wire • Dilators-smallest to biggest • Aortic cannula in, guide wire out • Snare down and tie • Tubing clamp and connect to arterial line • Secure the cannula with big sharp towel clip	
Chest:	• Right anterior mini thoracotomy incision • Small Alexis and intercostal retractor • Open the pericardium, use silk O W 334 as pericardial stay suture • Vent stitch: Prolene 4-0, Pledgetted x1 • Flexible Cygnet Clamp (Standby Chitwood clamp) • Blade 11, Kelly artery to dilate, CSS needle from perfusionist connected to the CO_2 tubing • Direct ostial cardioplegia delivery • Opening of Aorta: Blade 11, Curve scissors (Fehling), Potts scissors (Fehling), Standby metzenbaum scissors	

• Aorta stay suture: Prolene 5-8556 x2 • Ethibond 2-0 Valve sutures- backhand first (forehand or hook) • Uses 4mm Cor-knot • Gentamycin wash to the valve	
• Closure of Aorta	• Prolene 4-0 8761 Pledgetted Backhand • Prolene 4-0 8761 Pledgetted Forehand
• Vent Decannulation	Reinforce with Prolene 4-0 8761
• Osypka pacing wire	Mostly ventricular pacing wire only
• Chest drains	Jackson Pratt x 1 and Portex Straight size 28 x1
• Femoral decannulation	Standby Derra clamp x1 and vascular clamps; Prolene 5-0 8556
• Chest closure	• Ethibond 5-0 • Vicryl 1 • Monocryl 4-0

INDEX

A

ACC, *see* American College of Cardiology
ACCESS-EU phase I, 250–251
ACCESS-EU phase II, 250–251
ACCESS-Europe, 249–250
Accufit
    TMVR prosthesis, 206
    valve, 204–205
AccuMist® blower/mister device, 44
Acorn CoreCap, 392
Acrobat-i stabilizer, 311
ACS, *see* Annals of cardiothoracic surgery
Activated clotting time (ACT), 146
ACURATE neo valve system, 178
Acute kidney injury (AKI), 151, 154
Aesculap FLEXHeart, 45
AF, *see* Atrial fibrillation
Aggressive cardiology, 2
AHA, *see* American Heart Association
Airway management, 62
AKI, *see* Acute kidney injury
Alexis O wound protector, 261
Alexis® soft tissue retractor, 261
Alexis wound atraumatic protectors, 225
Alternative caval isolation technique, 84
American Association for Thoracic Surgery (AATS) cardiac surgery robotic program, 305, 306
American College of Cardiology (ACC), 139, 144, 389
American Heart Association (AHA), 113, 324, 389
Anaortic/no-touch OPCAB (anOPCAB), 311
Anaortic OPCAB surgical technique, 314–316
Anesthesia, 282–283
    alternative approaches, 63
    caveats and controversies, 63–65
    challenges, 51, 53
    history, 51–53
    implication of MICS, 51, 53
    importance, 51, 52
    monitoring, 53–54
    perioperative considerations, 61–63
    positioning, 62
    postoperative management, 62–63
    pre-anesthetic evaluation, 61
    preparation, 53–55
    principles, 59
    research, trends and innovation, 65–66
    surgical techniques
        deairing of heart, 64
        long-acting cardioplegia, 65
        mitral valve and right mini-thoracotomy, 64–65
    tools/instruments and devices, 60–61
Annals of cardiothoracic surgery (ACS), 232
Antiarrhythmic drug therapy, 341
Anticoagulation strategy, 349
Aortic annulus, 157
Aortic clamping, 258
Aortic cross clamping, 127
Aortic landing zones, 366
Aortic non-touch proximal anastomosis, 81
Aortic regurgitation (AR), 148, 158, 160
Aortic root angiogram, 145, 146
Aortic stenosis (AS), 143, 155
Aortic surgery
    alternative approaches, 368
    cardiovascular surgeons, 359
    caveats and controversies, 368
    endovascular aortic repair, 360
    endovascular stent graft, 360
    fellowship, 368
    history, 359–360
    hybrid techniques, 367
    indications, 367
    infrarenal aortic pathologies, 359
    perioperative consideration, 367–368
    research, trends and innovation, 369
    surgical approach, 360–362
    tools/instruments and devices, 366–367
Aortic valve area (AVA), 151
Aortic valve crossing, 146–147
Aortic valve replacement (AVR)
    alternative approaches, 94
    aortotomy, aortic valve exposure and replacement, 90–93
    catheter-based techniques, 87
    caveats and controversies, 94–96
    challenging patient characteristics, RAT approach, 93
    endoscopic (*see* Endoscopic AVR)
    J-shaped upper mini-sternotomy (*see* Upper "J" mini sternotomy)
    life expectancy, 107
    meta-analysis, 95
    outcomes, 107
    patient preparation and exposure, 88–89
    perioperative considerations, 92–94
    prosthesis implantation, 91, 92
    removal and annular decalcification, 91, 92
    research, trends and innovation, 96
    right infra-axillary mini-thoracotomy, 75–76
    right parasternal approach, 77
    sternotomy and cannulation, 88, 89
    supra-sternal approach, 76–77
    sutureless (*see* Sutureless valves)
    tools/instruments and devices, 92
    total sternum-sparing technique, 88
Aorto-ilio-femoral atherosclerotic disease, 227
AR, *see* Aortic regurgitation
AS, *see* Aortic stenosis
Atheromatous plaque, 310
Atherosclerotic disease, 62
Atrial fibrillation (AF), 10
    alternative approaches, 340–345
    caveats and controversies, 345–349
    history, 331–333
    hybrid maze ablation, 345
    hybrid surgery, 352–355
    perioperative considerations, 337–340
    pulmonary vein isolation, 333–336
    recurrent, 350, 353
    research, trends and innovation, 349–355

tools/instruments and devices, 336–337
Atrial lift system, 272
AtriClip®, 83
AtriClip Pro-V device, 83
AtriCure education and training, 355, 356
AVA, *see* Aortic valve area
AVR, *see* Aortic valve replacement
AVR *vs.* TAVI, 107
Awake cardiac bypass/valve surgery, 18
Axillary artery cannulation, 45, 46

B

Balloon aortic valvuloplasty (BAV), 137, 146, 147, 157
Balloon-expandable valve, 149
Balloon valvuloplasty catheter, 164
BAV, *see* Balloon aortic valvuloplasty
Beating heart (BH), 297
Bentall procedure, 103
Bilateral internal thoracic arteries (BITA) harvesting, 80, 81
Bilateral mini-thoracotomy *vs.* separate incisions, 395
Biomedicus™ next-gen demo, 54
Bio-Medicus™ NextGen femoral venous cannula, 42, 43
Bioprosthetic valve, 102
Bipolar RF maze, 12
Bipolar unidirectional ablation device, 340
BIS™ monitor, 61
Bispectral Index (BIS), 53
Blower mister, 42
"Box principle," 88, 90

C

CABG, *see* Coronary artery bypass graft
CAD, *see* Coronary artery disease
Cannulation technique
 axillary artery, 45
 conventional, 46
 peripheral, 46
 SVC, 45
Cardiac atrioventricular conduction abnormalities, 160
Cardiac catheterization, 151–155
Cardiac electrophysiology epicardial GP ablation, 336
Cardiac support device (CSD), 394
Cardiac surgeon's training, 2
Cardiac surgery
 Cleveland Clinic, Cleveland, Ohio, USA, 97

University of Miami, FL, USA, 97
University of Ottawa, Canada, 97
Cardiac Surgery Bible, 1
CardiAQ™ transcatheter mitral valve implantation (TMVI) system, 208
Cardiaq valve, 206
Cardioband procedure, 210, 211
Cardiology-cardiac surgery spectrum, 28
Cardioplegia, 46, 51, 90, 127, 188, 230, 258, 297
Cardiopulmonary bypass (CPB), 7, 51, 90, 91, 126–127, 135, 144, 220–223, 277, 291, 333, 359
Cardiovalvulotome, 202
Cardiovascular outcomes assessment of the mitraclip percutaneous therapy (COAPT), 251
Cardiovascular valve repair system (CVRS), 247
Carillon mitral contour system, 206–207, 210
Carotid-carotid subclavian bypass, 381
Carpentier–Loulmet classification, 70
Catheter ablation techniques, 348
Cath lab procedure, 186
Caval
 isolation, 269–270, 273, 274
 occlusion, 270
Centers for Medicare and Medicaid Services (CMS), 251
Central cannulation, 74, 75, 103
Chagas disease, 14
Chest wall deformity, 104, 105
Chimney techniques, 386–387
Chitwood
 aortic cross-clamp, 14
 clamp, 9, 40–41, 258
 Debakey aortic cross-clamp, 226
 transthoracic aortic cross clamp, 41
Chronic obstructive pulmonary disease (COPD), 227
Cineangiography, 158
Circumflex artery, 55, 56
Cleveland clinic training program, 197, 198
Clinically significant functional mitral regurgitation, 249
CME, *see* Continuing medical education
CMS, *see* Centers for Medicare and Medicaid Services

COAPT, *see* Cardiovascular outcomes assessment of the mitraclip percutaneous therapy
COBRA fusion 150 ablation system, 14, 15, 341
Combined heart valve surgery
 concomitant cardiac procedures, 267
 conventional full sternotomy approach, 272
 double valve repair/replacement, 268–269
 minimally invasive *vs.* conventional approaches, 273
 research, trends and innovation, 273–275
 tools/instruments and devices, 272
 upper J sternotomy approach, 268–269
 upper T mini sternotomy, 269
Comorbidities, 339–340
Complete sternal-sparing (CSS), 395
Concomitant minimally invasive AF ablation, 345, 348
Concomitant procedures, 271–272
Confounding variables, 28
Continuing medical education (CME), 5
Conventional cannulation, 46
Conventional prostheses *vs.* TAVI, 112
Conversion to sternotomy, 273
COPD, *see* Chronic obstructive pulmonary disease
CoreVista, 106
Corknot®, 102, 104, 105, 224
Coronary
 anastomosis, 300–301
 angiogram, 155
 grafting options, 298
 revascularization, 310
 sinus-based percutaneous mitral annuloplasty, 206–207
 sinus catheter, 54
Coronary artery bypass graft (CABG), 7, 8, 111, 118, 323
Coronary artery disease (CAD), 8, 17, 151
Corridor procedure, 331
Cosgrove clamp, 41
Cosgrove™ flexible aortic clamp, 42
Cosgrove malleable aortic cross-clamp, 90
Cosgrove Quick BendT Flex Clamp, 92, 94

Cox Maze IV demonstration, 10, 12
Cox Maze procedure, 10, 12, 331–333, 349
CPB, *see* Cardiopulmonary bypass
CPB cannulation, 46
Cross-clamp, 230
Cryoablation, 12
CryoLife boot camps, 109
CSD, *see* Cardiac support device
CSS, *see* Complete sternal-sparing
CTSNet, 1
Cumulative survival, 301
Custom-made multibranched grafts, 364
Cut-and-sew technique, 331, 333
CVRS, *see* Cardiovascular valve repair system
Cygnet™ aortic cross clamp, 104, 105
Cygnet flexible aortic clamp, 41–43

D

Dallas lesion set, 335, 337, 338, 341, 351
DA-TAVI, *see* Direct aortic transcatheter aortic valve replacement
David procedure, 103
Da Vinci robotic system, 9, 11
Da Vinci Xi surgical system, 46–47, 216, 225, 297
DBP, *see* Diastolic blood pressure
Delivery sheath
　design, 164
　insertion, 146
Descending aortic aneurysms, 374
Descending thoracic aorta, 365, 367–369
Dexamethasone, 64
Diastolic blood pressure (DBP), 158
Digital subtraction angiography (DSA), 149, 156
Direct aortic transcatheter aortic valve replacement (DA-TAVI), 174–175
Double lumen
　endotracheal tube insertion, 186
　ET tube training, 73
DSA, *see* Digital subtraction angiography
Dual antiplatelet therapy, 328
Dynamic cardiomyoplasty, 393

E

EACTS, *see* European Association for Cardio-Thoracic Surgery
E-AVR, *see* Endoscopic AVR

EBAC, *see* European Board for Accreditation in Cardiology
ECC, *see* Extracorporeal circulation
Echocardiography, 136–138
Echo-guided endoclamp placement, 189
EchoNavigator software, 204
EGFR, *see* Estimated glomerular filtration rate
ELI, *see* Energy loss index
Endoballoon, 36, 299–300
　vs. transthoracic clamp, 48, 49
Endocardial catheter ablation, 333, 345–348
Endoclamping, 187, 188
Endo Close™ traction device, 220, 221, 223, 225
Endoscopic AVR (E-AVR)
　caveats and controversies, 128–129
　clamping, cardioplegia and ventricular venting, 127
　concomitant procedures, 130
　CPB, 126–127
　history, 125
　operative setting, 127
　OT setup and instrumentation, 126
　prosthetic choice, 128
　simulation-based training methods, 129
　soft tissue retractor, 126
　summarized experience, 128
　surgical technique, 127
　video-guided approach, 127
Endoscopic mitral valve surgery, 196
Endoscopic radial artery harvesting (ERH), 9, 11, 80, 81
Endoscopic vein harvesting (EVH), 80
Endovascular aortic arch repair, 363–366
Endovascular repair of ascending aorta, 362–363, 369
Endovascular stent-graft (EVSG)
　aortic aneurysms, 373
　aortic pathologies, 373–374
　arch debranching, 377
　caveats and controversies, 386–387
　coarctation of aorta, 376–377
　conduits, 384
　descending aortic aneurysms, 375–376
　device and stock considerations, 386
　distal arch aneurysms, 374–375

endovascular technology, 373
ILIAC/infra-renal abdominal aortic approach, 384
IMH, 376
lumbar spinal drainage, 386
pathologies, 377
PAU, 376
perioperative considerations, 386
principles, 379–380
radiation protection, 386
standard approach (transfemoral), 384
ST Mary's visceral hybrid repair technique, 382–383
TAI, 376
thoracic aortic approach, 384–385
tools/instruments and devices, 385–386
treatment techniques, 380
type B aortic dissection, 377
visceral hybrid repair, 377–379
zone 1 pathologies, 380–381
zone 2 pathologies, 382
zone 3 pathologies, 382
EndoWrist stabilizer, 297
Energy loss index (ELI), 151
Energy modalities, 11
Enhanced recovery after surgery (ERAS), 302
EOPA™ aortic cannula, 104
Epicor cardiac ablation system, 12
ERAS, *see* Enhanced recovery after surgery
ERH, *see* Endoscopic radial artery harvesting
ESC, *see* European Society of Cardiology
Esmolol administration, 301
Estimated glomerular filtration rate (eGFR), 154
European Association for Cardio-Thoracic Surgery (EACTS), 18, 108, 305, 306
European Association of Cardiothoracic Anesthesiology, 66
European Board for Accreditation in Cardiology (EBAC), 140
European Heart Survey on valvular heart study, 111
European Society of Cardiology (ESC), 113, 144, 166, 324
EuroSCORE, 144
EVEREST II REALISM study, 248
EVH, *see* Endoscopic vein harvesting

INDEX   **419**

Evolut™ R valve, 148, 150, 179
EVSG, *see* Endovascular stent-graft
External defibrillator pads, 218, 272
Extra-anatomic bypass, 381
Extracorporeal cannula, 195
Extracorporeal circulation (ECC), 184–186, 300
Extra-thoracic debranching techniques, 387

F

FDA-approved stent grafts, 366–367
Felhing cardiovascular instruments, 38
Fem-fem bypass, 35
Femoral arterial cannula, 262
Femoral cannulation technique, 42, 102, 187
   advantage, 34
   cardiopulmonary bypass, 34
   endoballoon (thruport), 36
   insertion technique, 36
   mini incision, 34
   percutaneous, 36–38
   positioning, 36
   securing, 36
   selection, 35
   sizing, 34
   ultrasound-guided insertion, 34
   without distal perfusion, 36
Flail P2 leaflet, 55
FLEXHeart tissue stabilizer, 45
Fluoroscopy, 135
FMR, *see* Functional mitral regurgitation
Focus valve workshops, 197
FORE-SIGHT, 61
Functional mitral regurgitation (FMR), 206

G

Ganglionated plexi (GP), 335
GDS Accucinch, 208
GE healthcare cardiovascular ultrasound, 60
Glauber aortic cross clamp, 41
Glauber clamp, 41
Gore Tag thoracic endoprosthesis, 361
Gore-Tex NeoChord, 224
Gore-Tex sutures, 186, 194–195
GP, *see* Ganglionated plexi
Gynecological equipment, 25

H

Haptic/tactile feedback system, 231
HCR, *see* Hybrid coronary revascularization

Heart failure
   abandoned surgical options, 393–395
   cardiac output, 389
   caveats and controversies, 393–396
   complex clinical syndrome, 389
   concerns, 392
   conventional full sternotomy approach, 392
   managing arrhythmias in LVAD patients, 395
   minimally invasive LVAD implantation, 390–392
   operations, 389–390
   Park's plication stitch, 395
   research, trends and innovation, 396
   sternal-sparing approach, 395
   technique
      circulatory support, 391
      operation, 391–392
      surgical access, 391
   tools/instruments and devices, 392
HeartMate III, 392, 394
Heart surgeons, 1
Heart valve surgery
   MICS-CABG, 48–49
   MINI MVR *vs.* robotic-assisted, 48
   MIS AVR, upper J sternotomy *vs.* RATS, 47
   TAVI *vs.* SAVR, 47–48
Heartware VAD (HVAD), 392
HeartWare ventricular assist system, 394
Hemisternotomy, 74, 75
Hemodynamic instability, 298
Hepatic vein, 186
High risk registry (HRR), 248–249
Histidine-tryptophan-ketoglutarate (HTK), 127
History of MICS
   alternative approaches, 17
   caveats and controversies, 17–18
   complementary circulation, 7
   CPB, 7
   EACTS course calendar, 19
   establishment, 19
   experimental period, 7
   heart-lung machine (IBM II), 8
   multimedia platform, 19
   perioperative consideration, 15–16
   procedures, 9, 10
   research, trends and innovation, 18

   saphenous vein grafts, 7
   STS course 2019, 19
   tools/instruments and devices, 12–15
HRR, *see* High risk registry
HTK, *see* Histidine-tryptophan-ketoglutarate
HVAD, *see* Heartware VAD
Hybrid ablation
   catheter ablation techniques, 348
   epicardial and endocardial ablation, 340, 348
   postoperative arrhythmia, 349
   subxiphoid pericardioscopic approach, 344–345
   thoracoscopic approach, 341–344
   transdiaphragmatic combined subxiphoid and laparoscopic approach, 345
Hybrid atrial ablation, 14
Hybrid convergent procedure, 344
Hybrid coronary procedure, 298
Hybrid coronary revascularization (HCR), 17, 48
   alternative approaches, 327
   caveats and controversies, 327
   clinical benefits and technologies, 324
   high-risk coronary patients, 328
   minimally invasive staged CABG, 325
   perioperative consideration, 326
   perioperative mortality, 326
   research, trends and innovation, 328
   robot-assisted heart bypass, 326
   summary, 324
   thoracic aorta and heart, 324
   tools/instruments and devices, 326
   vein grafting, 323
Hybrid electrophysiology laboratory, 350
Hybrid operating room, 145
Hybrid operating theatre setup, 325
Hybrid thoracoabdominal aneurysm repair, 381

I

ICS, *see* Intercostal space
Ideal valve morphology, 243
IE, *see* Infected endocarditis
Iliofemoral disease, 139
IMA, *see* Internal mammary artery

IMA harvesting technique, 290
IMH, see Intramural hematoma
Infected endocarditis (IE), 245
Inferior vena cava (IVC), 53, 186, 269
Innovative technology, 310
Institutional review board (IRB), 249
Instrumentation/operating theater set up
  alternative stabilizers, 45
  cannulation technique, 45–47
  caveats and controversies, 47–49
  cerebral oximetry, 31
  femoral cannulation technique, 34–37
  MICS operating room, 32
  minimally invasive CABG surgery, 33–34
  minimally invasive mitral valve surgery, 38–39
  minimally invasive valve surgery, 32–33
  perioperative consideration, 44–45
  TAVI, 34
  team work, 31, 32
  tools/instruments and devices, 37–38
Intercostal space (ICS), 184, 219
Intermediate-risk TAVR approval, 140
Internal mammary artery (IMA), 145, 289–290
International Society for minimally invasive cardiothoracic surgery (ISMICS), 23, 275, 305, 306, 354, 356
International Valvular Surgery Study Group (IVSSG), 122
IntraClude intra-aortic occlusion device, 36, 37
Intramural hematoma (IMH), 376
INTUITY™ preparation, 115–117, 119
Invasive/perceived-traumatic experience, 17
INVOS™ 5001C, cerebral/somatic oximetry, 61
IRB, see Institutional review board
ISHLT academy, 396
ISMICS 2014 annual meeting presentation, 328
ISMICS webpage, 3
IVC, see Inferior vena cava
IVSSG, see International Valvular Surgery Study Group

J
Joseph Lamelas Intercostal Retractor System, 261
Journal of innovations in cardiac rhythm management (JICRM), 355, 356
Judkins right (JR), 145

K
Key opinion leaders (KOL), 5
Kofidis technique, 269–270

L
LAA, see Left atrial appendage
Lateral endoscopic approach using robotics (LEAR), 228–230
LDS, see Loeys-Dietz syndrome
Leadership principles, 22
LEAR, see Lateral endoscopic approach using robotics
Left atrial appendage (LAA), 334, 345
Left internal mammary artery to the left anterior descending artery (LIMA-LAD), 48, 65
Left internal thoracic artery (LITA), 8, 278–279
Left ventricular end-diastolic pressure (LVEDP), 158
Left ventricular outflow tract (LVOT), 151
LIMA-LAD, see Left internal mammary artery to the left anterior descending artery
LITA, see Left internal thoracic artery
LivaNova venous return cannula, 225
Loeys–Dietz syndrome (LDS), 374
Long-acting cardioplegia, 65
Long saphenous veins (LSV), 80
Lotus Edge aortic valve system, 148, 150, 177
Lower partial sternotomy, 107
LSV, see Long saphenous veins
Lumbar spinal drainage, 386
LVEDP, see Left ventricular end-diastolic pressure
LVOT, see Left ventricular outflow tract

M
Major adverse cardiac or cerebral events (MACCE), 302–303
Manubrium limited MiAVR, 106
McGinn technique, 16
Mean transvalvular pressure gradient, 118
Median sternotomy (MS), 51, 253
Medtronic extracorporeal cannula, 195
Medtronic TAVI course, 166
Medtronic TAVI workshop, 140
Medtronic ThoraTrak MICS retractor system, 92, 93, 197
Medtronic tissue stabilizer, 282
MI, see Myocardial infarction
Miami method, 75, 76, 270–271
MiAR™ cardioplegia cannula, 226
MiAVR, see Minimally invasive aortic valve replacement
Micropuncture® Access Set, 150
MICS, see Minimally invasive cardiac surgery
MICS AVR, see Minimally invasive aortic valve replacement
MICS-CABG, see Minimally invasive multivessel coronary surgery-coronary artery bypass grafting
MICS IMA retractor, 40
MICS retractor system, 38
MIDCAB, see Minimally invasive direct coronary artery bypass
MIDCAB/hybrid vs. multivessel CABG, 48
Migrated TAVR valve, 140
MIMVS, see Minimally invasive mitral valve surgery
Mini-aortic arch surgery, 364
Minimal-access right chest approach, 227
Minimal-access techniques, 215
Minimal incision valve surgery (MIVS), 195
Minimalist TF-TAVI Workshop, 140, 141
Minimally invasive aortic valve replacement (MiAVR), 9, 44, 75, 87, 88
Minimally invasive aortic valve replacement myth vs. fact, 73, 74
Minimally invasive aortic valve surgery, 9, 32, 74–78
Minimally invasive ASD closure, 82, 83
Minimally invasive atrial ablation, 81
Minimally invasive CABG surgery, 16
  aortic surgery, pros and cons, 34
  considerations, 33

coronary artery bypass
grafting, 33
  instruments and
    consumables, 34
  positioning draping of
    patient, 33
  preoperation to incision, 34
Minimally invasive cardiac
  surgery (MICS)
  aortic clamps, 40
  CABG anastomoses, 2
  heart teams, 2
  history (*see* History of
    MICS)
  hybrid theatre and/or trans-
    catheter arena, 3
  patient demand, 3
  primary Hippocratic
    principles, 2
  QR codes, 3–6
  surgeon and trainee, 5
  updated educational tool, 4
Minimally invasive combined
  open heart procedure,
  82, 83
Minimally invasive coronary
  artery bypass grafting
  surgery (MICS CABG),
  78–81
  alternative approaches, 283
  caveats and controversies, 284
  chest closure, 281
  chest marking and
    incision, 278
  considerations, 283
  distal anastomoses, 280–281
  LITA, 278–279
  patient positioning, 277–278
  perioperative consideration,
    282–283
  post-operative care, 281
  proximal anastomosis,
    279–280
  research, trends and
    innovation, 284
  robotic/thoracoscopic
    equipment, 277
  tools/instruments and
    devices, 282
Minimally invasive direct
  coronary artery bypass
  (MIDCAB), 15, 16, 18,
  48, 78, 80, 327
Minimally invasive endoscopic
  mitral valve surgery, 125
Minimally invasive heart valve
  surgery, 69, 70
Minimally invasive LAA exclusion
  with LARIAT, 15
Minimally invasive LVAD
  implantation, 81–82,
  390–392

Minimally invasive mitral valve
  surgery (MIMVS), 9,
  32–34, 38–39
  caveats and controversies,
    196–197
  exposure, 188–193
  installing ECC, 184–186
  invasive procedures, 183
  left atrioventricular valve, 201
  mini-thoracotomy, 184
  mitral valve repair technique,
    193–195
  myocardial preservation,
    187–188
  patient positioning, 184, 185
  percutaneous
    interventions, 183
  perioperative considerations,
    196, 209–210
  research, trends and
    innovation, 197
  three Cs, 184
  tools/instruments and
    devices, 195
  totally endoscopic, 184
Minimally invasive multivessel
  coronary surgery–
  coronary artery bypass
  grafting (MICS-CABG),
  39, 48–49, 65, 78–80
Minimally invasive program setup
  alternative approaches, 28
  caveats and controversies,
    28–29
  considerations, 23, 25
  entropy, 23
  harmonious and dedicated
    team, 26
  history, 21–22
  instruments, 25
  left atrial retractor, 26
  operation theater, 24
  perioperative consideration,
    26–27
  practical tips, good and safe
    start, 27
  sample armamentarium, 26
  simulation/hands-on
    training, 22
  technicalities and tools, 29
  tools/instruments and devices,
    23–26
Minimally invasive robotic mitral
  valve repair, 47
Minimally invasive surgical
  vs. catheter ablation,
  338–339
Minimally invasive techniques in
  adult cardiac surgery
  (MITACS), 275
Minimally invasive tricuspid valve
  repair technique, 258

Minimally invasive valve surgery
  aortic valve surgery, 33
  mitral valve surgery, 32–33
Minimally invasive *vs.*
  conventional LVAD
  implantation, 396
Mini maze procedure, 81, 82
Mini mitral MICS, 34
Mini-right thoracotomy, 126
Ministernotomy, 113, 115, 121
Mini-Stern trial, 95, 95
Mini-thoracotomy incision, 80
Mini- *vs.* full sternotomy,
  106–107
MiraQ Cardiac transit time flow
  measurement, 319
MITACS, *see* Minimally invasive
  techniques in adult
  cardiac surgery
MitraClip EXPAND study, 251
MitraClip procedure
  animation, 239
MitraClip system, 203–204
  alternative approaches,
    244–245
  anatomy of septum, 238–240
  caveats and controversies,
    245–247
  clinical trials, 247
  contraindications, 243, 246
  development, 237
  echo measurements, 240
  edge-to-edge technique, 241
  first patient implanted, 236
  fluoroscopic and
    transesophageal
    echocardiographic
    guidance, 235
  indication, 242
  late-breaking data, 246
  MICS procedure, 241–242
  morphology, 245
  patient selection, 243
  perioperative consideration,
    241–242
  research, trends and
    innovation, 247–252
  safety and effectiveness
    data, 236
  steps, 236
  surgical approach, 236–237
  TMVr, 236
  tools/instruments and
    devices, 240
  transcatheter mitral valve
    repair, 236, 244
MitraFlex mitral repair
  system, 204
Mitral heart valve surgery, 202
Mitralign percutaneous
  annuloplasty system
  (MPAS), 207–208

Mitralign procedure, 210
Mitral quadrangular repair, 194
Mitral regurgitation (MR), 240, 250
Mitral valve disease, 250
Mitral valve regurgitation, 203
Mitral valve repair techniques, 2, 193–195
Mitral valve surgery, 9, 345, 355
Mitra-Spacer, 209, 212
MIVS, *see* Minimal incision valve surgery
Mixed tricuspid valve disease, 253
Mohr technique, 194
MPAS, *see* Mitralign percutaneous annuloplasty system
MR, *see* Mitral regurgitation
MS, *see* Median sternotomy
Multimedia Manual of Cardiothoracic Surgery, 19
Myocardial infarction (MI), 155, 313
Myocardial preservation, 187–188
Myocardial protection, 220–222

N

National Institutes of Health (NIH), 161
National University Health System (NUHS), 108, 109
National University Hospital of Singapore (NUHS), 97, 263
Near-infrared spectroscopy (NIRS), 60–61, 291
Neurapraxic/traction injury, 219
Neurologic injury, 310
Neutrophil elastase inhibitor, 66
New England Journal of Medicine, 201
Nexus deployment technique, 385
NIH, *see* National Institutes of Health
NIRS, *see* Near-infrared spectroscopy
Nonin Medical, Inc., 61
Non-rib-spreading technique, 197
Non-ventilated lung, 59
Normal sinus rhythm (NSR), 331
NUHCS Singapore minimally invasive mitral valve programme, 197

O

Obesity, 106
Octopus Nuvo tissue stabilizer, 39–42
Ocular tactility, 229
Off-pump coronary artery bypass (OPCAB), 17
alternative approaches, 319
anaortic surgical technique, 314–316, 317
cardiac positions
 anterior wall vessels, 315
 high-lateral wall vessels, 314
 inferior wall vessels, 315
 low-lateral wall vessels, 314
EACTS fellowship, 319
EBM Beat + Youcan simulator, 319, 320
high-risk patients, 311–313
history, 310
intracoronary shunts, 319
research, trends and innovation, 310–313
revascularization and long-term outcomes, 313
stroke and perioperative complications, 310–311
technical innovation, 310
tools/instruments and devices, 317
Off-pump *vs.* on-pump LVAD implantation, 395–396
One-lung ventilation (OLV), 55, 63–64, 72
Online video resources, 19
On-pump *vs.* off-pump coronary artery bypass grafting (CABG), 309
On-Q pump, 63
OPCAB, *see* Off-pump coronary artery bypass
OPCAB with Heartstring device (OPCAB-HS), 310–311
OPCAB with partial-clamp (OPCAB-PC), 310–311
Open anesthesia, 66, 67
Open heart surgery, 201
Open heart *vs.* MICS, 18
Operation theater layout, MICS heart valve surgery, 33
Operating room setup, 186
Operative technique, 135–136
Optisite arterial cannula, 225–226
Oscillating saw, 104
Ozaki technique, 103

P

Papillary muscle repositioning (PMR), 195
Paravalvular leak (PVL), 58, 59, 148
Paravalvular regurgitation (PVR), 134, 158–160
Paroxysmal *vs.* persistent AF, 337–338
Partial left ventriculectomy, 393
Passive cardiomyoplasty, 393
Patent foramen ovale (PFO), 57
Patient positioning
 heart valve surgery, 70–71
 lateral decubitus, 71
 marking thoracotomy, 71
 MIS CABG, 71, 72
 robotic surgery, 71–73
 trans-axillary approach, 71
PAU, *see* Penetrating aortic ulcers
PCI, *see* Percutaneous coronary intervention
PCR online TAVI Atlas, 166
Penetrating aortic ulcers (PAU), 376
Perceval S, 102, 112, 114–117, 119
Perceval *vs.* intuity, 119–120
Percu-Pro Mitra-Spacer, 212
Percutaneous coronary intervention (PCI), 156, 285
Percutaneous coronary sinus catheter, 54
Percutaneous femoral vessel approach, 270
Percutaneous heart valve (PHV), 112, 143
Percutaneous mitral valve repair, 211–213
Perfusion techniques, 31
Pericardial heart strings, 314, 315
Pericardioscopic technique, 344
Perioperative transesophageal echocardiography, 59
Peripheral cannulation technique, 46
Peripheral vascular disease, 186
PERSIST-AVR clinical trial, 121
Persistent left superior vena cava (PLSVC), 54
PFO, *see* Patent foramen ovale
Philips Live 3D TEE course, 66, 67
PHT, *see* Pulmonary hypertension
PHV, *see* Percutaneous heart valve
Pigtail catheter, 145
Placement of aortic transcatheter valve, 144
PLSVC, *see* Persistent left superior vena cava
PMA, *see* Pre-market approval
PMR, *see* Papillary muscle repositioning
Polytetrafluoroethylene (PTFE), 146, 205
Polyvinylidene fluoride (PVDF), 205
Port-access method, 13
Portico valve, 150, 179
Postgraduate course in heart failure, London, 396, 397
Post-radiation therapy, 106

Post-valve implantation assessment, 148
Predicted risk score of mortality (PROM), 137
Pre-market approval (PMA), 251
Premature ventricular ectopics (PVCs), 147
Professional education, 108
ProGlide perclose vascular closure device, 37
PROM, see Predicted risk score of mortality
ProPlege device, 197
Protamine, 136
Proximal pulmonary artery, 280
PTFE, see Polytetrafluoroethylene
Pulmonary
   artery systolic pressure, 55, 57
   edema, 64, 66
   function, 62
   vein isolation
      autonomic denervation, 335–336, 351–352
      five box ablation, 335–336, 352
      Pruitt box lesion, 334, 349
      PVI via right minithoracotomy, 334
      right minithoracotomy, 350
      Wolf mini maze, 334, 335, 349
Pulmonary hypertension (PHT), 253
Pump oxygenators, 201
Puncture-guidewire-dilation-introduction technique, 185
PVCs, see Premature ventricular ectopics
PVDF, see Polyvinylidene fluoride
PVL, see Paravalvular leak
PVR, see Paravalvular regurgitation

Q

QuickDraw venous cannula, 42, 43
Quick response (QR) codes, 3–6

R

RACAB, see Robotic-assisted coronary artery bypass
Radiation protection, 386
Radiofrequency, 11
Rapid-deployment bioprostheses, 128
RAT, see Right anterior thoracotomy
RBBB, see Right bundle branch block
Recurrent ventricular tachycardia, 14
Redo MiAVR, 106
Regional wall motion abnormalities (RWMA), 55, 56, 58
Relay™ deployment technique, 385
Reoperative surgery, 230
Residual regurgitation, 58
Retrograde approach, 144
Revascularization progression, 287
Rheumatic heart disease, 27
Rheumatic mitral stenosis, 201
Right anterior thoracotomy (RAT), 75, 76, 88, 92, 96, 111, 114, 115
Right axillary artery cannulation, 126
Right bundle branch block (RBBB), 160
Right-lung isolation, 218
Right mini-thoracotomy approach
   caval isolation, 269–270
   caval occlusion, 270–271
   incision, 78
   patient positioning, 77–79
   patient preparation, 77
   surgical approach, 360–362
Right paramedian approach, 202–203
Right thoracotomy approach, 203
Right ventricular outflow tract (RVOT), 280
Risk determination, 243
Robot facilitated coronary artery bypass grafting
   anesthetic considerations, 295
   cannulation, 297
   cardioplegia, 297
   cardiopulmonary bypass, 291
   caveats, 301–302
   endoscopic coronary anastomosis, 293–294
   final actions, 294
   history, 285–288
   identification and exposure of target vessels, 291–293
   IMA, 289–290
   intermediate-and long-term outcomes, 302–303
   patient placement and operative start-up, 288
   patient selection, 288
   peripheral vascular cannulation and application of endoclamp (endoballoon occlusion), 291
   port insertion and robot docking, 288–289
   postoperative care, 295
   precordial fat pad resection and pericardial exposure, 290–291
   predictors of success and safety, 303–304
   preoperative assessment and work-up, 294–295
   preparation, 288
   reduced surgical trauma advantages, 302
   research, trends and innovation, 302–306
   TECAB approaches, 297
   time demand, 295–296
   tools/instruments and devices, 294
   utility port placement, 290
Robotic-assisted coronary artery bypass (RACAB), 302
Robotic CABG, 12–13, 48, 49
Robotic cardiac surgery, 46–47
Robotic MiMVR animation, 78, 79
Robotic mitral valve surgery
   alternative approaches, 230
   anti-atrial fibrillation procedure, 215
   cardiopulmonary bypass and myocardial protection, 220–223
   caveats and controversies, 230–231
   clinical outcomes, 227–229
   contraindications, 231
   minimal-access techniques, 215
   operating room, 216, 222–224
   operative efficiency, 217
   patient selection, 216–218
   preoperative assessment, 226–227
   preparation, 218–219
   previous cardiac surgery, 227
   research, trends and innovation, 231
   surgical exposure and access, 219–220
   three-dimensional (3D) stereoscopic visual systems, 216
   tools/instruments and devices, 225–226
   valve repair, 218, 219
Robotic technology, 31
Rultract Skyhook surgical retractor system, 39, 42–44
RVOT, see Right ventricular outflow tract
RWMA, see Regional wall motion abnormalities

S

SAC, *see* Systemic arterial compliance
SAM, *see* Systolic anterior motion
Sapien 3 transcatheter heart valve, 148, 150
SAPIEN valve, 136, 178
SAVR, *see* Surgical aortic valve replacement
SCANLAN Chitwood Debakey clamp, 41
SC-TAVI, *see* Subclavian transcatheter aortic valve replacement
Seldinger technique, 36, 47, 53, 73, 185, 218, 257
Shiley™ endobronchial tube, 60
Silastic intracoronary shunts, 315
Simulation (in-silico) training, 27
Single-lung ventilation, 55, 62
Sinning index, 148
SMA, *see* Superior mesenteric artery
Society of Thoracic Surgeons (STS), 19, 118, 137, 139
Society of Thoracic Surgeons Adult Cardiac Surgery Database, 228
Society of Thoracic Surgeons Workshop on Robotic Cardiac Surgery, 305, 306
Society of Thoracic Surgery Predicted Risk of Mortality (STS-PROM), 144
Soft robotics, 273–275
Soft tissue retractors, 191, 272, 273
Spaghetti graft, 383
Starfish NS heart positioner, 39–42
Sternal-sparing approach, 395
Sternotomy sparing LVAD, 82
ST Mary's visceral hybrid repair technique, 382–383
Stroke, 160–161
Stroke Volume Index (SVI), 151
Structural valve degeneration, 107–108
StrykeFlow II laparoscopic suction/irrigation system, 223, 226
STS, *see* Society of Thoracic Surgeons
STS-PROM, *see* Society of Thoracic Surgery Predicted Risk of Mortality
STS Workshop on robotic cardiac surgery, 232
SU-AVR-IR, *see* Sutureless Aortic Valve Replacement International Registry
Subclavian artery cannulation, 186
Subclavian artery coverage, 386
Subclavian transcatheter aortic valve replacement (SC-TAVI), 172–173
Subcutaneous video-assisted saphenous vein harvest, 8
Subxiphoid/laparoscopic approach, 355
Subxiphoid pericardioscopic approach, 344–345, 355
Superior mesenteric artery (SMA), 383
Superior vena cava (SVC), 45, 53, 186, 269
Suprasternal AVR approach, 106
Surgical ablation (SA) *vs.* catheter ablation (CA), 341
Surgical aortic valve replacement (SAVR), 48, 133
Surgical approaches, MICS
  adopting, 70
  alternative caval isolation for right heart, 84
  Carpentier–Loulmet classification, 70
  patient positioning, 70–72
  patient selection, 72
  perioperative considerations
    aortic valve, incisions and exposure, 73–77
    intraoperative considerations and monitoring, 72–73
    mitral valve, incisions and exposure, 78–79
    potential complications and troubleshooting, 85
    pre-operative considerations, 70
    self-adhesive external defibrillator pads, 72, 73
    tools/instruments and devices, 83
    trans-areolar endoscopic approach, 84, 85
Sutureless aortic bioprostheses, 112
Sutureless Aortic Valve Replacement International Registry (SU-AVR-IR), 122
Sutureless valves
  alternative approaches, 117–118
  caveats and controversies, 118–119
  history, 111–113
  intuity elite valve, 114–115
  patient selection, 113
  perceval, 113–114
  perioperative consideration, 117
  research, trends and innovation, 119–122
  tools/instruments and devices, 115–117
Sutureless *vs.* rapid deployment valves, 120
SVC, *see* Superior vena cava
SVC cannulation, 45, 46
SVI, *see* Stroke Volume Index
Systemic arterial compliance (SAC), 151
Systolic anterior motion (SAM), 55, 56, 58

T

TAA, *see* Thoracic aortic aneurysms
TAAA, *see* Thoracoabdominal aortic aneurysms
TAI, *see* Traumatic aortic injury
TAPSE, *see* Tricuspid annular plane systolic excursion
TA-TAVI, *see* Transapical transcatheter aortic valve implantation
TAVI, *see* Transcatheter aortic valve implantation
TAVR, *see* Transcatheter aortic valve replacement
TAX-TAVI, *see* Transaxillary transcatheter aortic valve replacement
TCA-TAVI, *see* Transcaval transcatheter aortic valve replacement
TCD, *see* Transcranial Doppler
TCRF, *see* Temperature-controlled radiofrequency
TCT, *see* Transcatheter cardiovascular therapeutics
TECAB, *see* Totally endoscopic coronary artery bypass
TEE/TOE, *see* Transesophageal echocardiography
Temperature-controlled radiofrequency (TCRF), 15
Temporary pacemaker placement, 146
Tendyne™ valve, 205
TF-TAVI, *see* Transfemoral transcatheter aortic valve implantation
TF-TAVI Linkoping, Sweden, 149
3D mini-mitral surgery, 229

INDEX 425

Thoracic aortic aneurysms (TAA), 374–375
Thoracic aortic approach, 384–385
Thoracic endovascular repair (TEVAR), 367
Thoracoabdominal aorta, 365–366
Thoracoabdominal aortic aneurysms (TAAA), 377–379
Thoracoscopic approach, 341–344, 353–355
Thoracoscopic LITA harvesting, 13
Thoratec® Heartmate III left ventricular assist device (LVAD), 15, 16
ThoraTrak® MICS retractor system, 12, 13, 39, 40, 80
ThruPort IntraClude, 187, 194, 195
Thruport™ system, 36
TIA, *see* Transient ischemic attacks
Tiara valve, 204, 205, 213
TOE, *see* Transesophageal echocardiography
Totally endoscopic coronary artery bypass (TECAB), 13–14, 285, 298–299
Total percutaneous thoracic endovascular aortic repair, 382
TR, *see* Tricuspid regurgitation
Transapical approach, 134–136
Transapical off-pump neochord implantation, 208–209
Trans-apical Tiara bioprosthesis, 205
Transapical transcatheter aortic valve implantation (TA-TAVI), 108, 171
Trans-areolar endoscopic approach, 84
Transaxillary transcatheter aortic valve replacement (TAX-TAVI), 173–174
Transcarotid approach, 176
Transcatheter aortic valve implantation (TAVI), 10, 12, 34, 35, 47, 48, 66, 87, 112
  alternative approaches, 138
  caveats and controversies, 138–140
  fellowship, 180
  history, 133–134
  low-risk patients, 165, 166
  operative technique, 135–136
  PARTNER 1A study, 134
  peri-procedural considerations, 179
  preoperative assessment and planning, 137–138
  round table, aortic stenosis, 134
  tools/instruments and devices, 137
  transapical approach, 134–136
  transfemoral (*see* Transfemoral transcatheter aortic valve implantation)
  vascular complications, 159
Transcatheter aortic valve replacement (TAVR), 48, 211
Transcatheter aortic valve system, 137
Transcatheter cardiovascular therapeutics (TCT), 210
Transcatheter mitral interventions, 251
Transcatheter mitral valve implantation, 207, 213
Transcatheter mitral valve repair, 236, 244–245, 252
Transcatheter mitral valve replacement (TMVR), 210–211, 213–214
Transcatheter valve therapies (TVT), 139
Transcatheter Valve Therapy Registry (TVT Registry), 251
Transcaval transcatheter aortic valve replacement (TCA-TAVI), 176
Transcranial Doppler (TCD), 160
Transesophageal echocardiography (TEE/TOE), 13, 32, 54–59, 60, 73, 74, 126, 145, 151, 218, 227
Transfemoral intraluminal graft implantation, 361
Transfemoral transcatheter aortic valve implantation (TF-TAVI), 171
  alternative approaches, 157
  aortic root angiogram, 146
  aortic valve crossing, 146–147
  associated co-morbidities, 156
  BAV, 147
  bioprosthetic valves, 152–153
  cardiac catheterization, 151–155
  caveats and controversies, 158–162
  CT angiography, 155–156
  delivery sheath insertion, 146
  echocardiogram, 151
  history, 143–144
  patient selection, 144
  post-valve implantation assessment, 148
  preoperative assessment and screening, 151
  research, trends and innovation, 162–166
  setup and equipment, 144–145
  temporary pacemaker placement, 146
  tools/instruments and devices, 148–150
  valve deployment, 149
  valve implantation, 147–148
  vascular access, 145–146
TRANSFORM trial, 119, 120
Transient ischemic attacks (TIA), 160
Trans-septal catheterization, 143
Transseptal puncture, 236
Trans-thoracic Chitwood® clamp, 127
Transthoracic echocardiography (TTE), 145, 151
Transvalvular regurgitation, 158
Traumatic aortic injury (TAI), 374–375
Tricuspid annular plane systolic excursion (TAPSE), 55, 56
Tricuspid regurgitation (TR), 253–254
Tricuspid stenosis (TS), 253, 254
Tricuspid valve replacement, 256
Tricuspid valve surgery (TVS), 53, 186
  alternative approaches, 260
  cannulation and cardiopulmonary bypass, 257–258
  caveats and controversies, 260–261
  chest, 256
  completion of procedure, 259
  coronary artery bypass surgery, 254
  double mini valve repair, 255
  exposure of heart and right atrium, 256–257
  groin, 256
  left-sided heart surgery, 254
  main operation, 258–259
  perioperative consideration, 260
  peripheral cannulation, 255
  REDO right mini thoracotomy TV surgery, 259
  research, trends and innovation, 261–262
  right mini thoracotomy approach, 255

single-lung ventilation, 255
tools/instruments and devices, 259–260
TR, 253–254
TS, 254
TS, *see* Tricuspid stenosis
TV repair/replacement, 258–259
TVS, *see* Tricuspid valve surgery
TVT, *see* Transcatheter valve therapies
TVT Registry, *see* Transcatheter Valve Therapy Registry
2010 ACCF/AHA Practice Guidelines, 368
Type B aortic dissection, 377

U

UHS, *see* Upper hemisternotomy
Upper hemisternotomy (UHS), 75
Upper "J" mini sternotomy, 74, 75, 268–269, 361–363
   aortic valve and root boot camp, 108
   benefits, 100
   caveats and controversies, 106–108
   chest wall deformity, 104, 105
   considerations, 102
   EACTS Academy, 108
   long-term outcomes, 99
   manubrium limited MiAVR, 106
   MMCTS, 100
   NUHS training hub, 108, 109
   obesity, 106
   post-radiation therapy, 106
   preoperative CT scan patient, 104, 105
   principles, 100–102
   professional education, 108
   reoperations/redo surgery, 105
   research, trends and innovation, 108
   severely calcified ascending aorta, 104–106
   status post-pneumonectomy, 105–106
   suprasternal AVR approach, 106
   technological innovations, 99
   tools/instruments and devices, 104
   trans-apical TAVI, 108
   transfusion requirement, 100
   valve-in-valve, 108
Upper partial hemisternotomy (UPS), 88
Upper partial sternotomy, 101
Upper sternotomy approach, 203
Upper "T" mini sternotomy, 74, 75, 268, 269, 361–363
UPS, *see* Upper partial hemisternotomy
USB HV retractor, 38–39

V

Vacuum-assisted venous drainage, 257
VADs, *see* Ventricular assist devices
Valtech Cardioband system, 207
Valtech V-Chordal, 209
Value-driven outcomes (VDOs), 23–24
Valve Academic Research Consortium-2 (VARC-2), 161
Valve implantation, 147–148
Valve-in-valve (ViV), 107, 108, 164
Valve XS atrium retractor, 45, 46
Valvulo arterial impendence, 151
Vanermen maneuver, 192
VARC-2, *see* Valve Academic Research Consortium-2
Vascular access, 145–146
Vascular complication (VC), 161–162
Vasculography, 174
Vasodilating drugs, 188
VC, *see* Vascular complication
V-18 ControlWire Guidewire, 145, 148, 150
VDOs, *see* Value-driven outcomes
Venous cannulation, 186
Ventilation strategy, 59
Ventricular assist devices (VADs), 15
Ventricular fibrillation, 187
Ventricular venting, 127
Video-laryngoscope, 55, 60
Vinberg procedure, 8
ViV, *see* Valve-in-valve
VuMedi, 1

W

Webinars, 1, 5
Wet lab, 130
Wire to SVC, 56, 57
Wolf mini-maze, 12, 334, 335, 349

Z

Zone 1 pathologies, 380–381
Zone 2 pathologies, 382
Zone 3 pathologies, 382

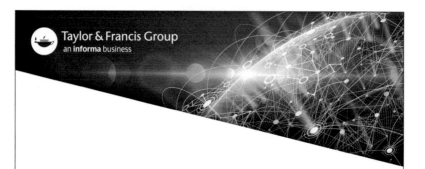